W9-BME-161

American Association of Critical-Care Nurses

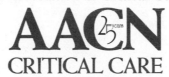

AACN
CRITICAL CARE

THE
Clinical Nurse
Specialist Role
IN
Critical Care

EDITED BY

Anna Gawlinski, RN, DNSc, CS, CCRN
Clinical Nurse Specialist
Cardiac Care Unit/Cardiac Observation Unit
University of California, Los Angeles, Medical Center
Assistant Clinical Professor
University of California, Los Angeles, School of Nursing
Los Angeles, California

Leslie S. Kern, RN, MN
Cardiac Critical Care Clinical Nurse Specialist
Lakewood Regional Medical Center
Lakewood, California
Assistant Clinical Professor
University of California, Los Angeles, School of Nursing
Los Angeles, California

W.B. SAUNDERS COMPANY
A Division of Harcourt Brace & Company
Philadelphia London Toronto Montreal Sydney Tokyo

W.B. SAUNDERS COMPANY

A Division of
Harcourt Brace & Company

The Curtis Center
Independence Square West
Philadelphia, Pennsylvania 19106

Library of Congress Cataloging-in-Publication Data

The clinical nurse specialist role in critical care / American
   Association of Critical-Care Nurses : [edited by] Anna Gawlinski,
   Leslie S. Kern. — 1st ed.
      p.   cm.
   Includes bibliographical references.
   ISBN 0-7216-3715-9
   1.   Intensive care nursing.   2.   Nurse practitioners.
I.   Gawlinski, Anna.   II.   Kern, Leslie S.   III.   American Association
of Critical-Care Nurses.
   [DNLM: 1.   Critical Care.   2.   Nurse Clinicians.   WY 154 C641   1994]
RT 120.I5C564   1994
610.73′61 — dc20
DNLM/DLC
                                93-30391

The Clinical Nurse Specialist Role in Critical Care   ISBN 0-7216-3715-9

Copyright © 1994 by W.B. Saunders Company

All rights reserved. No part of this publication may be reproduced or transmitted in any form or
by any means, electronic or mechanical, including photocopy, recording, or any information
storage and retrieval system, without permission in writing from the publisher.

Printed in United States of America

Last digit is the print number: 9 8 7 6 5 4 3 2

To the critically ill
patients and families
whom we serve
and
to our husbands,
Ronald Philip Ramus
and
Aaron Robert Kern

Contributors

Thomas S. Ahrens, RN, DNS, CCRN

Clinical Specialist, Critical Care, Barnes Hospital, St. Louis, Missouri; Assistant Professor, Adjunct Faculty, Southern Illinois University, Edwardsville, Illinois; Clinical Instructor, Adjunct Faculty, St. Louis University and University of Missouri, St. Louis, St. Louis, Missouri

Working in an Era of Cost Containment

Rochelle L. Boggs, RN, MS, CS, CCRN

Trauma/Critical Care Clinical Nurse Specialist, Surgical Trauma and Critical Care Associates, Parkersburg, West Virginia

Defining the Critical Care Clinical Nurse Specialist: A Collaborative Practice Model

Tess L. Briones, RN, MS, CCRN

Clinical Nurse Specialist, Surgical Intensive Care Unit, University of Michigan Hospital; Clinical Associate Faculty, University of Michigan, Ann Arbor, Michigan

Career Opportunities for the Critical Care Clinical Nurse Specialist

Deborah Caswell, RN, MN, CCRN

Quality Management Coordinator, Division of General Surgery, University of California, Los Angeles, Center for the Health Sciences, Los Angeles, California

The Critical Care Clinical Nurse Specialist Role in Ethical Dilemmas

Diane K. Dressler, RN, MSN, CCRN, CCTC

Senior Transplant Coordinator, St. Luke's Medical Center, Milwaukee, Wisconsin

The Critical Care Clinical Nurse Specialist in Joint Practice with Physicians

Linda Faber, RN, PhD

Director, Nursing Research and Education, University of California, Los Angeles, Medical Center; Assistant Clinical Professor, University of California, Los Angeles, School of Nursing, Los Angeles, California

The Critical Care Clinical Nurse Specialist in Continuous Quality Improvement

Anna Gawlinski, RN, DNSc, CS, CCRN

Clinical Nurse Specialist, Cardiac Care Unit/ Cardiac Observation Unit, University of California, Los Angeles, Medical Center; Assistant Clinical Professor, University of California, Los Angeles, School of Nursing, Los Angeles, California

Research Utilization in the Critical Care Setting

Teresa Halloran, RN, MSN, CCRN

Head Nurse, Neonatal Intensive Care Unit, St. John's Mercy Medical Center, St. Louis, Missouri

The Unit-based Critical Care Clinical Nurse Specialist

J. Keith Hampton, RN, MSN, CS

Nurse Manager, Dialysis Services, University of Minnesota Hospital and Clinic; Adjunct Faculty, School of Nursing, University of Minnesota, Minneapolis, Minnesota

Career Opportunities for the Critical Care Clinical Nurse Specialist

Elizabeth A. Henneman, RN, MS, CCRN

Clinical Nurse Specialist, University of California, Los Angeles, Medical Center; Assistant Clinical Professor, University of California, Los Angeles, School of Nursing, Los Angeles, California

Research Utilization in the Critical Care Setting

Ann N. Hotter, RN, MSN, CS, CCRN

Clinical Nurse Specialist–Critical Care, Mayo Foundation Hospitals; Assistant Professor of Nursing, Mayo Medical School, Rochester, Minnesota

Securing and Implementing the Clinical Nurse Specialist Role in Critical Care

Janet C. Howard, RN, MSN, CEN, CCRN

Trauma Clinical Nurse Specialist, Memorial Hospital, Southbend, Indiana

The Critical Care Clinical Nurse Specialist as Leader

Maureen Keckeisen, RN, MN, CCRN
Clinical Nurse Specialist, Surgical Specialties
Intensive Care Unit, University of California,
Los Angeles, Medical Center; Assistant Clinical
Professor, University of California, Los Angeles,
School of Nursing, Los Angeles, California
**The Critical Care Clinical Nurse Specialist in
Critical Care Staff Education**

Leslie S. Kern, RN, MN
Cardiac Critical Care Clinical Nurse Specialist,
Lakewood Regional Medical Center, Lakewood,
California; Assistant Clinical Professor,
University of California, Los Angeles, School of
Nursing, Los Angeles, California
**The Critical Care Clinical Nurse Specialist in
Continuous Quality Improvement**

Deborah Goldenberg Klein, RN, MSN, CS, CCRN
Clinical Nurse Specialist, Trauma/Critical Care
Nursing, MetroHealth Medical Center; Clinical
Instructor, Acute and Critical Care Nursing,
Frances Payne Bolton School of Nursing, Case
Western Reserve University, Cleveland, Ohio
**Critical Care Clinical Nurse Specialist: Novice to
Expert**

Denise M. Lawrence, RN, MS, CS
Acute Care Practitioner, Critical Care, Hartford
Hospital, Hartford, Connecticut
**The Critical Care Clinical Nurse Specialist and
Delivery Systems and Practice Models in Transition**

Patricia A. O'Malley, RN, MS, CCRN
Primary Nurse Level II, Coronary Intensive Care
Unit, Cardiothoracic Surgical Intensive Care
Unit, Miami Valley Hospital; Adjunct Faculty,
School of Nursing, Wright State University,
Dayton, Ohio
**The Role of the Critical Care Clinical Nurse
Specialist in Critical Care Research**

Anna Omery, RN, DNSc
Clinical Research Manager, Liver Transplant
Program, Dumont Transplant Center, University
of California, Los Angeles, Medical Center;
Assistant Clinical Professor, University of
California, Los Angeles, School of Nursing, Los
Angeles, California
**The Critical Care Clinical Nurse Specialist Role in
Ethical Dilemmas**

Anne Padwojski, RN, MSN, MBA, CCRN
Clinical Nurse Specialist, Critical Care Nurse
Fellowship Program, St. John's Mercy Medical
Center, St. Louis, Missouri
**The Unit-based Critical Care Clinical Nurse
Specialist**

Suzanne S. Prevost, RN, PhD, CCRN
Director of Patient Care Outcomes Evaluation
and Research and Associate Professor, University
of Texas Medical Branch, Galveston, Texas
**The Critical Care Clinical Nurse Specialist Role in
Student Education**

Susan L. Smith, RN, MN, CCRN
Clinical Nurse Specialist, Liver Transplantation,
Emory University Hospital, Atlanta, Georgia
**Defining the Critical Care Clinical Nurse Specialist:
A Collaborative Practice Model**

Patricia S.A. Sparacino, RN, MS, FAAN
Clinical Nurse Specialist, Cardiovascular
Surgery, and Associate Clinical Professor, The
Medical Center at the University of California,
San Francisco, San Francisco, California
**Issues and Future Trends for the Critical Care
Clinical Nurse Specialist**

Karen M. Stenger, RN, MA, CCRN
Clinical Nurse Specialist, Surgical Intensive Care
Unit, University of Iowa Hospitals and Clinics,
Iowa City, Iowa
**Role Evaluation for the Critical Care Clinical
Nurse Specialist**

Sandra L. Tidwell, RN, MN
Clinical Nurse Specialist, Cardiothoracic
Surgery, Virginia Mason Medical Center;
Clinical Instructor, Department of Physiological
Nursing, University of Washington; Graduate
Advisory Board, Seattle Pacific University,
Seattle, Washington
**The Critical Care Clinical Nurse Specialist as Case
Manager**

Marita G. Titler, RN, PhD
Associate Director, Nursing Research, and
Clinical Nurse Specialist, Critical Care,
University of Iowa Hospitals and Clinics, Iowa
City, Iowa
**Role Evaluation for the Critical Care Clinical
Nurse Specialist**

Debbie Tribett, RN, MS, CCRN
Clinical Nurse Specialist, Infectious Disease
Physicians, Inc., Edgewater, Maryland
**The CNS as Change Agent in Today's Political
Health Care Environment**

Joan M. Vitello-Cicciu, RN, MSN, CS, CCRN
Critical Care Clinical Nurse Specialist, Boston
University Medical Center Hospital, Boston,
Massachusetts
**Networking: Making It Successful for the Critical
Care Clinical Nurse Specialist**

Susan M. Walsh, RN, MSN, CS, CCRN
Clinical Nurse Specialist, Quality Resource
Associates, Inc., and Carlisle Hospital,
Harrisburg, Pennsylvania; Instructor Call
Messiah College, Grantham, Pennsylvania
**The Critical Care Clinical Nurse Specialist Role in
Consultation**

Pamela Becker Weilitz, RN, MSN(R)
Pulmonary Clinical Nurse Specialist, Barnes
Hospital at Washington University Medical
Center; Assistant Clinical Professor, St. Louis
University; Adjunct Faculty, Barnes College, St.
Louis, Missouri; Adjunct Clinical Faculty,
University of Missouri, Kansas City, Missouri
**The Critical Care Clinical Nurse Specialist Role in
Patient Education**

Reviewers

CHAPTER REVIEWERS

Barbara Stevens Barnum, RN, PhD, FAAN
Consultant/Editor,
Division of Nursing,
Columbia Presbyterian Hospital,
New York, New York

Randy M. Caine, RN, EdD, CS, CCRN
Professor of Nursing and
Director of Critical Care Clinical Nurse
Specialist Program,
California State University, Long Beach, Long
Beach, California

Suzanne Clark, RN, MSN, MA, CS
Clinical Nurse Specialist,
Department of Psychiatry, Consultation and
Liaison Service,
Kaiser Permanente,
Los Angeles, California

Diane Hawley, RN, MS, CCRN
Critical Care Clinical Nurse Specialist,
Sierra Medical Center,
El Paso, Texas

Elizabeth A. Henneman, RN, MS, CCRN
Clinical Nurse Specialist,
University of California, Los Angeles,
Medical Center,
Los Angeles, California

Patricia Hooper, RN, MSN
Doctoral Candidate,
University of California, San Francisco,
San Francisco, California

Mary Kay Jiricka, RN, MSN, CCRN
Critical Care Clinical Nurse Specialist,
Milwaukee County Medical Complex,
Milwaukee, Wisconsin

Peggy Kalowes, RN, MSN, CCRN
Critical Care Clinical Nurse Specialist,
Government Relations Specialist,
American Association of Critical-Care Nurses,
Aliso Viejo, California

Karin T. Kirchhoff, RN, PhD, FAAN
Professor and Director of Nursing Research,
College of Nursing and University Hospital,
University of Utah,
Salt Lake City, Utah

Debra Lynn-McHale, RN, MSN, CS, CCRN
Clinical Nurse Specialist,
Surgical Cardiac Care Unit,
Thomas Jefferson University Hospital,
Pittsburgh, Pennsylvania

Susan O'Brien Norris, RN, MS, CCRN
Cardiovascular Clinical Nurse Specialist,
Mercy Medical Center,
Oshkosh, Wisconsin

Susan G. Osguthorpe, RN, MS, CNA
Associate Chief, Nursing Services,
Department of Veterans Affairs Medical Center,
Salt Lake City, Utah

Ann Petlin, RN, MSN, CCRN
Clinical Nurse Specialist, Critical Care,
St. Francis Memorial Hospital,
San Francisco, California

Kathy Brown-Saltzman, RN, MN
Clinical Nurse Specialist,
University of California, Los Angeles,
Medical Center,
Los Angeles, California

Ginger Schafer-Wlody, RN, EdD, FCCM
Quality Manager, Medical Staff,
Department of Veteran Affairs Medical Center,
Los Angeles, California

Linda Searle, RN, MN, CNAA
Doctoral Candidate and
Assistant Professor of Clinical Nursing,
University of Southern California,
Los Angeles, California

Marita G. Titler, RN, PhD
Clinical Nurse Specialist,
University of Iowa Hospitals and Clinics,
Iowa City, Iowa

Madeline Wake, RN, PhD
Dean, College of Nursing,
Marquette University,
Milwaukee, Wisconsin

Cathy Rodgers Ward, RN, MS, CNAA
Director of Nursing Systems and
Assistant Clinical Professor,
University of California, Los Angeles,
School of Nursing,
Los Angeles, California

BOOK REVIEWERS

Pauline Beecroft, RN, PhD
Editor, *Clinical Nurse Specialist,*
Roland Heights, California;
Nurse Researcher, Childrens Hospital,
Los Angeles, California

Pamela F. Cipriano, PhD, FAAN
Patient Care Manager,
Hollings Oncology Center,
Hollywood, South Carolina

Constance Engelking, RN, MS
Oncology Clinical Nurse Specialist,
Westchester County Medical Center;
Adjunct Instructor of Medicine,
New York Medical College,
Mt. Kisco, New York

Marguerite R. Kinney, RN, DNSc, FAAN
Professor of Nursing,
University of Alabama School of Nursing,
Birmingham, Alabama

Debra J. Lynn-McHale, RN, MSN, CS, CCRN
Clinical Nurse Specialist,
Surgical Cardiac Care Unit,
Thomas Jefferson University Hospital,
Lower Gwynedd, Pennsylvania

Foreword

During the 1980s, the Clinical Nurse Specialist (CNS) role was under considerable scrutiny. Reimbursement systems based on diagnosis-related groups (DRGs) and other changes in health care financing led to examination and reexamination of CNS roles, particularly since many of those positions were staff, not line, positions. This reassessment occurred at a time when many specialists had been removed from any direct care responsibilities and were tending projects, not patients. Some specialists lost their jobs; some departments reorganized so that the contributions of CNSs would be more visible in the accomplishment of organizational goals related to patient outcome and cost containment.

The naysayers predicted the demise of the CNS role, while believers shepherded key publications to life.[1-4] The decade closed with the American Nurses Association's taking an important step: uniting the Council of CNSs and the Council of Primary Care Practitioners into one Council of Nurses in Advanced Practice.[5] This union was important. It represented a solid commitment to *practice* as the focus of CNSs, nurse practitioners, nurse-midwives, and other nurses in advanced practice. For CNSs, whose organizational and change agent talents often led them away from the bedside (while retaining the practice title), it meant reclaiming areas in nursing that demand expert clinical skills and judgment. These dilemmas did not seem to be such an issue for our colleagues in other advanced practice roles. The intellectual, clinical, research, and political work of the 1980s with respect to advanced practice affirms that advanced practice is here to stay. The challenge to specialties is to take these contributions from the last decade (and before) to articulate existing advanced practice in the specialty and to shape the specialty's future. In developing this textbook, the AACN and the editors, Gawlinski and Kern, are meeting this challenge.

The Clinical Nurse Specialist Role in Critical Care builds on the work done on the role of the CNS over the last 15 years. The book affirms that this advanced practice role continues to be multifaceted. The subroles, skills, and competencies articulated by Hamric and Spross are applied and extended in this text.[1p.39] Of significance is the description of these aspects of CNS practice from the perspective of the CNS in critical care. This perspective includes a summary of literature within the critical care specialty and relevant literature on advanced practice in general and from other specialties. In addition to giving the reader theoretical background, the contributors provide exemplars, advice, and ideas that come from the lived experience of being a critical care CNS. This information is important for students and novice CNSs who want to know "What is it going to be like for me in my specialty?" as well as for the experienced CNS who has grasped the general framework of advanced practice and wishes to develop further in the role.

Each chapter covers theoretical perspectives, literature review, practice implications, and case examples. The chapter on research utilization makes an important contribution to an area often given short shrift in graduate students' education. The case management chapter is an elegant illustration of why we need to keep the *practice* in advanced practice. The author makes a clear case for having CNSs who "take the pulse" of the clinical environment. There "are clients who cannot afford *not* to be taken care of by CNSs,"[6p.39] and this chapter provides clinical and financial data to support that conviction. Chapters on ethics, networking, and career opportunities are important additions to this specialty-based text.

The integration of AACN position statements, standards, and other practice publications together with the diverse practice experience of the contributors make this the authoritative text on advanced practice in critical care. *The Clinical Nurse Specialist Role in Critical Care* will be indispensable to many experienced CC-CNSs as well as to graduate students and novice CNSs in critical care. The documentation in a single text of advanced practice in a particular specialty is essential to developing specialty-based research and practice agendas. *The Clinical Nurse Specialist Role in Critical Care* is such a text and will surely shape the future of advanced practice in critical care.

Judith A. Spross RN, MS, OCN, FAAN
Arlington, Massachusetts

References

1. Hamric A, Spross JA, editors: *The clinical nurse specialist in theory and practice,* ed 2, Philadelphia, 1989, WB Saunders Co.
2. The *Clinical Nurse Specialist* journal was established.
3. Sparacino PSA, Cooper DM, Minarik PA: *The clinical nurse specialist: Implementation and impact,* Norwalk, Conn, 1990, Appleton & Lange.
4. Styles MM: *On specialization in nursing: Toward a new empowerment,* Kansas City, Mo, 1989, American Nurses' Foundation.
5. Hawkins J, Rafson J: Council of nurses in advanced practice established, *Synergy* 1(1):1, 5, 1991 (published by American Nurses' Association Council of Nurses in Advanced Practice).
6. Hamric A: History and overview of the CNS role. In Hamric A, Spross JA, editors: *The clinical nurse specialist in theory and practice,* ed 2, Philadelphia, 1989, WB Saunders Co, pp. 3–18.
7. Spross JA, Baggerly J: Models of advanced nursing practice. In Hamric A, Spross JA editors: *The clinical nurse specialist in theory and practice,* ed 2, Philadelphia, 1989, WB Saunders Co, pp. 19–40.

Preface

The success of any health care facility depends on the quality of nursing care provided. The role of critical care clinical nurse specialist (CC-CNS) is an integral part of nursing. The CC-CNS elevates standards of nursing practice, furthers quality of nursing care, and can move nursing practice from a tradition-based practice to a research-based practice. The ability of the CC-CNS to function is dependent on integration of the role components. In the position statement adopted by the American Association of Critical Care Nurses, "The Critical Care Clinical Nurse Specialist: Role Definition," the AACN delineates the role components as practitioner, educator, consultant, researcher, and manager. The AACN further published "AACN Competence Statements for the Critical Care Clinical Nurse Specialist." These statements provide a framework for advanced practice and delineate the required knowledge, skills, and abilities of the CC-CNS. This book expands on these documents, leading the CC-CNS through the framework in a logical progression. The chapters are organized according to the role components and address the critical issues affecting CNSs in a rapidly changing health care environment. Since effective development of the CC-CNS depends on integration of theory, research, and practice, chapters are written to reflect this integration. Each chapter incorporates theoretical perspectives, related literature and research, practice implications, and critical care case studies. Together they provide an effective method for CC-CNS role development.

Part I introduces a collaborative practice model for the CC-CNS in Chapter 1. In this model the CC-CNS is the link between the critically ill patient and family and other health care professionals. This model sets the stage for the chapters that follow. "The Critical Care Clinical Nurse Specialist: Role Definition" describes the five role components of the CC-CNS. These essential role components are discussed in Chapter 2 along with the historical

context from which the role evolved. The "AACN Competence Statements for the Critical Care CNS" are then presented and provide practicing CC-CNSs with essential descriptors that are amenable to assessment and evaluation of role performance. Chapter 3 further elaborates on strategies for role implementation and development. These strategies address the needs of the novice and expert CNS. Suggestions follow for marketing the role of the CC-CNS within the institution, community, and nation.

Part II presents the practitioner role of the CC-CNS. Strategies are presented that demonstrate how CC-CNSs can follow a patient caseload. Techniques for integrating both the nursing process and the AACN's standards of nursing practice (structure, process, and outcome) with a patient caseload are provided. The practitioner unit-based (Chapter 4), population (Chapter 5), and case manager (Chapter 6) roles in critical care are described. Direct and nondirect patient care activities of the CC-CNS are delineated. Chapter 7 further discusses the role of the CC-CNS in continuous quality improvement. Examples of multidisciplinary monitors and reporting methods are provided. Emphasis is placed on how the CC-CNS develops staff in the continuous quality improvement process.

Part III presents the educator role of the CC-CNS. Practical ideas for staff education, orientation, and internship programs are provided in Chapter 8. Theory and practice implications for patient and family education, discussed in Chapter 9, broaden the scope of the educator role of the CC-CNS. Chapter 10 deals with the roles of the CC-CNS in working with graduate nursing students as their mentor and in joint appointments.

Part IV discusses the CC-CNS as consultant. Types of consultation activities are provided with emphasis on actual examples of critical care consultation activities. In Chapter 11, methods of documenting consultation activities are described as well as techniques for obtaining fees for consultation services. Chapter 12 is dedicated to the discussion of the consultative role of the CC-CNS in ethical decision making. Specifically, Chapter 12 addresses the role of the CC-CNS while consulting on ethical issues such as maintaining life-sustaining equipment and withholding and withdrawing treatment in the critical care setting.

Part V presents the CC-CNS role as researcher. Research journal clubs and research critique sessions, examples of how CC-CNSs can get started in the researcher role, are discussed in Chapter 13, as well as the "how to's" in conducting research. The unique needs of the novice and the advanced CC-CNS researcher are addressed. Practical steps for grant writing and examples of grants obtained by CC-CNSs are given along with a list of available AACN research grants. Chapter 14 focuses on the role of the CC-CNS in research utilization (RU). RU is an important vehicle the CC-CNS can use to move nursing from tradition-based to research-based practice. How a CC-CNS applied the research results of AACN's Thunder project to change clinical practice is given as an example of RU.

Part VI describes the leader/manager role of the CC-CNS. Key management concepts are presented in Chapter 15. Emphasis is placed on the CC-CNS role in empowering and developing staff. A technique to achieve this is via the mentorship activities of the CC-CNS. Chapter 16 provides content on the art of negotation and techniques to manage conflict. The CC-CNS role as change agent in a political environment is addressed. Practical examples of changes implemented by CNSs in the critical care setting give practicing CNSs the con-fidence and skill to be effective change agents. Techniques to reduce cost and generate revenue are provided in Chapter 17. Examples of CC-CNSs activities in reducing cost compliment this section. The role of the CC-CNS in the changing health care delivery system is discussed in Chapter 18.

Part VII presents the professional development of the CC-CNS. Opportunities for networking, such as participation in AACN's regional CNS groups, are described in Chapter 19. Career opportunities for CNSs are discussed in Chapter 20. This will be especially useful for CNSs who have been in the role for several years and are looking for career changes that build on their knowledge and skills. Practical tools the CC-CNSs can use in role evaluation are provided in Chapter 21. Chapter 22, the final chapter, discusses current and future trends of the CC-CNS role and challenges the CC-CNS to be prepared for future changes in advanced nursing practice roles.

We believe that this book offers a perspective different from the growing body of literature on the role of the CNS. The content of this book is focused on the CC-CNS and provides actual case examples in the critical care setting. The information provided acts as a reference for CC-CNSs, as well as for staff considering CNS graduate school, graduate students, faculty, nurse managers, and nursing and hospital administrators. For all CC-CNSs this book will provide alternative strategies in role performance and rekindle and energize their efforts at excellence in practice.

Anna Gawlinski, RN, DNSc, CS, CCRN
Leslie Kern, RN, MN

Contents

Role Definition, Implementation, and Development of the Critical Care Clinical Nurse Specialist

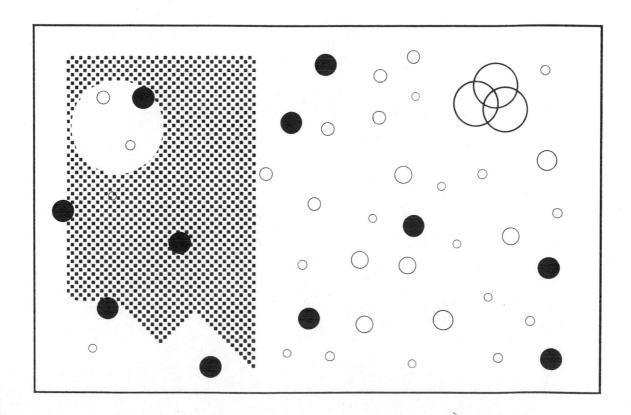

Chapter 1

Defining the Critical Care Clinical Nurse Specialist: A Collaborative Practice Model

Rochelle L. Boggs, RN, MS, CS, CCRN
Susan L. Smith, RN, MN, CCRN

The breadth of nursing knowledge, skills, and responsibilities presently required for patient care mandates the employment of nurses who are experts in a defined area of knowledge and practice.[1] In addition to needing advanced clinical knowledge, the critical care clinical nurse specialist (CC-CNS) needs collaborative skills and critical judgment to promote cost-effective quality care. Comprehensive care of critically ill patients must be patient and family centered and requires smooth collaboration among health care professionals.

The CC-CNS functioning within the framework of a collaborative practice model is the critical link among patient, physician, other health care disciplines, and the critical care environment. This chapter discusses the evolution of the CC-CNS role, the CC-CNS as content and process expert, and the CC-CNS in the context of a collaborative practice model.

EVOLUTION OF CC-CNS ROLE

The concept of specialization in nursing dates to the turn of the century,[2] when nurses who had completed specialized nursing courses were called specialists.[3] Discussions about the clinical nurse specialist (CNS) in the modern sense, however, did not appear in the nursing literature until the 1950s, when the advanced clinical nurse began to be associated with advanced educational preparation at the graduate level.

The role of the CNS evolved from the expert bedside nurse. Rieter[4] first used the term "nurse clinician" in 1943, but not until the 1960s did she define clinical practice as the absolute primary function of the profession. Rieter envisioned a nurse clinician as a knowledgeable practitioner of nursing with a high degree of discriminative judgment in solving nursing problems. The nurse clinician was a "master practitioner throughout all dimensions of nursing practice, able to provide basic and technical care based on a perceptive understanding of the patient's psychobiological needs."[4] Rieter emphasized that nurses should have complete control over nursing care and proposed that the nurse clinician was the most important means to achieving this end. The origin of the role of the CNS as we know it today was clearly conceptualized in Reiter's vision.

The evolution of the CC-CNS role parallels the historical development of the critical care unit. Critical care units evolved over the past 30 years as technology advanced. These units permit close monitoring for proper function and side effects of invasive devices. Their development played a distinct role in revolutionizing health care.[5] Predecessors to modern intensive care units (ICUs) first appeared in the United States in the 1920s to 1940s as temporary burn wards, postoperative recovery areas, shock wards, and polio wards. With the advent of cardiac resuscitation procedures and defibrillators in the 1950s, patients who had suffered previously fatal cardiac events survived. Subsequently, coronary care units were first opened in the 1960s. All of these early versions of critical care units shared a common characteristic with today's units, namely, the need for advanced nursing practice and concentrated nursing care. Thus the complexity of knowledge, technology, and services and expansion of the field of ICUs have created a demand for the CC-CNS.

DEFINITION OF CC-CNS

The *Critical Care Clinical Nurse Specialist: Role Definition Position Statement* (see below) was published in 1987 by the American Association of Critical Care Nurses (AACN). The CC-CNS is defined as "a nurse who, through study and supervised practice in nursing at the masters or doctorate level, has become an expert in the area of critical care nursing."[6] The CC-CNS functions autonomously and in collaboration with health care providers within five role components: practitioner, educator, consultant, researcher, and leader/manager. This document describes the CC-CNS as both a content and process expert. As a content expert the CC-CNS demonstrates mastery of the specific knowledge and skills required for critical care nursing. As a content expert and advanced practitioner, the CC-CNS is essential for the management of complex patient care and ensuring cost-effective nursing practice. As a process expert the CC-CNS is responsible and accountable for the development and application of standards and research to enhance the quality of care to the critically ill patient and family. The CC-CNS demonstrates rapid decision making for efficient matching of demands and resources to resolve clinical and professional issues.

Another document, the *AACN Competence Statement of the CC-CNS,* defines competence of

---

THE CRITICAL CARE CLINICAL NURSE SPECIALIST: ROLE DEFINITION POSITION STATEMENT

The American Association of Critical-Care Nurses believes the critical care clinical nurse specialist is a nurse who, through study and supervised practice in nursing at the master's or doctoral level, has become an expert in the area of critical care nursing. The critical care clinical nurse specialist (CNS) demonstrates mastery of the specific knowledge and skills required for critical care nursing. The critical care clinical nurse specialist is responsible and accountable for the development and application of standards and research to enhance the quality of care to the critically ill patient and family. As an advanced practitioner, the critical care CNS is essential for managing complex patient care and ensuring cost-effective nursing practice. The critical care CNS demonstrates rapid decision making for efficient matching of demands and resources to resolve clinical and professional issues.

WHEREAS, the critical care clinical nurse specialist is a self-directed individual whose primary function is that of the expert practitioner, with essential educator, consultant, researcher, and managerial role components, and

WHEREAS, the critical care clinical nurse specialist is vital for the application of nursing theory and research to critical care nursing practice, and

WHEREAS, the critical care clinical nurse specialist anticipates and evaluates technological, economical, social, and environmental factors to facilitate efficient health care delivery for optimal patient outcomes, and

WHEREAS, the critical care clinical nurse specialist's role implementation is contingent on individual accountability and administrative support, and

WHEREAS, the critical care clinical nurse specialist advances the nursing profession by anticipating and implementing theory based nursing practice.

THEREFORE, BE IT RESOLVED THAT the American Association of Critical-Care Nurses believes that the unique contributions of the critical care clinical nurse specialist are crucial in the management of the critically ill patient and family, critical care nursing practice, and the critical care environment, and

BE IT FURTHER RESOLVED THAT the primary focus of the critical care clinical nurse specialist's role is the management of the critically ill patient and family, and

BE IT FURTHER RESOLVED THAT the critical care clinical nurse specialist must actively participate in institutional planning and decision making to actualize the scope of the role.

THE CRITICAL CARE CLINICAL NURSE SPECIALIST: ROLE DEFINITION POSITION STATEMENT *Continued*

CLINICAL NURSE SPECIALIST ROLE IMPLEMENTATION

The critical care clinical nurse specialist exemplifies professional nursing practice. The critical care clinical nurse specialist functions autonomously and in collaboration with health care providers as a practitioner, educator, consultant, researcher, and manager. These role components include but are not limited to the following:

The Critical Care CNS as an Advanced Practitioner

* Demonstrates advanced cognitive and psychomotor capabilities in the diagnosis, treatment, and evaluation of human responses to actual and potential life-threatening health problems,
* Participates in the development, implementation, and evaluation of standards for critical care nursing practice,
* Serves as a clinical resource for the nursing staff and health care providers,
* Collaborates with the critically ill patient and family and health care providers in achieving optimal patient outcomes,
* Provides direction and support to the critically ill patient and family and to health care providers in addressing ethical and legal concerns,
* Demonstrates cost effective critical care nursing practice,
* Instills value for professional nursing practice including the utilization of standards and the nursing process and patient advocacy.

The Critical Care CNS as an Educator

* Seeks to improve patient and family outcomes through the application of educational concepts and skills,
* Assists critical care nursing staff in the acquisition of practice skills and knowledge,
* Acts as a role model of professional critical care nursing practice in the community,
* Contributes to the scientific nursing literature by publishing scholarly works,
* Contributes to the educational process and professional development of nursing students,
* Maintains current critical care knowledge and skills in a specialty area.

The Critical Care CNS as a Consultant

* Utilizes critical care nursing expertise and specialization to provide consultation services to health care providers and health care consumers,
* Incorporates the roles of practitioner, educator, researcher, and manager, and applies change theory during the consultation process,
* Facilitates the problem solving and decision making skills of the client, including the critically ill patient and family, health care providers, institutions, organizations, and legislative bodies.

The Critical Care CNS as a Researcher

* Expands the scientific base of critical care nursing practice by utilizing, facilitating, and conducting nursing research,
* Presents and publishes research findings,
* Disseminates recent innovations and research findings relevant to critical care nursing practice and patient outcomes,
* Assures ethical and legal practices in the conduct of research.

The Critical Care CNS as a Manager

* Participates in the development, implementation, and evaluation of unit, department, and institutional goals,
* Participates in the development, implementation, and evaluation of structure standards for care of the critically ill patient and family,
* Participates in quality systems relevant to the critically ill patient and family,
* Participates in formal and informal performance evaluations and professional development,
* Participates in the development, implementation, and evaluation of a realistic annual budget including revenue, personnel, supplies, and capital equipment,
* Produces direct and indirect revenues related to care of the critically ill patient and family.

Summary

The critical care clinical nurse specialist's practice encompasses the roles of practitioner, educator, consultant, researcher, and manager. High quality patient outcomes are dependent on this unique combination of roles fulfilled by the critical care clinical nurse specialist.

From American Association of Critical-Care Nurses: *The critical care clinical nurse specialist: role definition position statement,* Newport Beach, Calif, 1987, The Association.

the CC-CNS at any level of role development.[7] The differences among CNSs functioning at different levels of role development are in the degree and sophistication with which these competences are met. This document is not a job description; rather, it describes the advanced knowledge and skills of the CC-CNS. The CNS competence statements incorporate and are built on the *AACN Competence Statements for Differentiated Nursing Practice in Critical Care*.[8] The latter competence statements differentiate nursing practices of professional and technical nurses and are relevant to the CC-CNS who guides the practices of both. Differentiated competence statements are developed for the five components of the CC-CNS.

DEFINING CC-CNS ROLE WITHIN A COLLABORATIVE PRACTICE MODEL

By nature the CC-CNS role must be collaborative. The role is not structured to be independent. The CC-CNS does not choose to be collaborative; rather, collaboration is germane to the success of CC-CNS role implementation. What is fundamental practice? How does the CC-CNS function within a collaborative practice model? What does the CC-CNS do to build a collaborative practice environment? These questions are addressed in the following discussion.

Collaborative Practice

The literature defines collaborative practice in many ways. The National Joint Practice Commission defined collaborative practice as the "jointly determined relationship between the nurses and physicians, in the hospital setting, for the purpose of integrating their care regimens into a single comprehensive approach to their patients' needs."[9] Weiss and Davis defined collaborative practice as "the interactions between nurses and physicians that enable the knowledge of both professions to synergistically influence the patient care provided."[10] Stichler defined collaborative behavior as "a cooperative process, characterized by interpersonal valuing, which synthesizes and integrates the talents of two or more interdependent persons to accomplish a common goal."[11] Rubel and Thomas defined collaborating as "an attempt to problem solve with the other person and find solutions which result in higher degrees of satisfaction for both parties."[12] Thus collaboration involves coordinat-

ing, cooperating, valuing, integrating, problem solving, and sharing.

Regardless of the definition of collaborative practice, it is viewed as a critical factor in delivering quality patient care.[13] The AACN's mission statement identifies collaborative practice between nurses and physicians as one of its key values and views collaborative practice as central to optimal patient outcomes and for achieving its mission.[14] Additionally, the AACN's demonstration project selected nurse-physician collaboration as one of five fundamental values for the project.[15] The National Institutes of Health (NIH) conference on critical care recognized the value of collaborative care in stating "the organization structure should promote and require that nurses and physicians work together as colleagues at all levels."[16]

These definitions have in common the theme that successful collaborative practice depends on interdependent and cooperative decision making as well as the sharing of knowledge, goals, confidence, and mutual trust.[17] Shared decision making concerning strategies or protocols of care as well as the contribution of each member of the team is essential. The CC-CNS plays a pivotal role in the collaborative practice model and is the critical link among the patient and family, the health care profession, and the critical care environment. Figure 1–1 depicts the role of the CC-CNS within the collaborative practice model.

CC-CNS's Function in a Collaborative Practice Model

In a collaborative practice model (Fig. 1–1) the critically ill patient is the center of the critical care environment that encompasses patient- and family-centered care. The environment is a healing environment that requires the efforts of all health care disciplines. This healing environment occurs when all health care disciplines work in collaboration and care is based on recognized standards, shared processes, and measurable outcomes. In this model the CC-CNS acts as a link between the patient and other health care disciplines. This role as **linker** is vital to integrated, comprehensive care and to successful patient outcomes. The CC-CNS does this via the five role components of practitioner, educator, consultant, researcher, and leader/manager.

As practitioner, the CC-CNS contributes clinical expertise in providing care to patients with complex

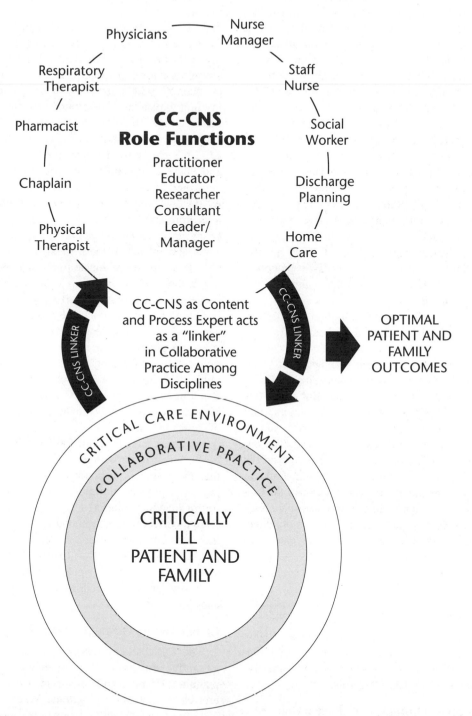

Figure 1–1 Collaborative practice model of CC-CNS. As content and process expert, the CC-CNS acts as a link between the critically ill patient and family and all health care disciplines to achieve optimal patient and family outcomes.

needs. The CC-CNS uses in-depth knowledge of critically ill patient populations to differentiate expected and unexpected responses to illness. For example, a CC-CNS's advanced clinical assessment of patients on mechanical ventilation may lead to early removal from mechanical support and earlier discharge from the critical care unit. As educator, the CC-CNS assists members of the health care team to acquire knowledge and skills to deliver care based on recognized standards. As consultant, the CC-CNS suggests approaches or resources to the health care team and facilitates communication among team members. As researcher, the CC-CNS disseminates and utilizes research to move ritual behaviors to research-based practices that help to achieve optimal patient outcomes. As leader/manager, the CC-CNS has the organizational perspective and bedside viewpoint that can help relate important information to the health team members.

This model demonstrates a unified approach to patient care. Each member of the health care team brings diverse talents and abilities to the care of the patient and family. Each member is of equal status and importance to the achievement of successful patient outcomes. As the **linker** in this model the CC-CNS coordinates, monitors, and evaluates the necessary care for the patient so that successful patient outcomes are achieved. The operationalization of this model is dependent on the interventions of each member of the collaborative practice team and on the implementation of the CC-CNS role components. In the absence of the CC-CNS as **linker** there is (1) fragmentation of patient care, (2) ambiguity in roles of health care team members, and (3) decreased flow of communication between the critically ill patient and health care disciplines.

Practice Implications

What can the CC-CNS do to build a collaborative practice environment? The CC-CNS builds a collaborative practice environment via the five components of the CC-CNS role.

Collaboration Through Practitioner Role

The advanced practitioner facilitates a collaborative practice environment through a number of activities. For example, following a caseload of patients provides an excellent way for the CC-CNS to facilitate collaboration. The CC-CNS should make it a priority to go on rounds with the physician for those patients in the CC-CNS's caseload and invite staff nurses to participate. The CC-CNS can arrange for joint practice patient care conferences on patients with interesting or unique problems, inviting physicians, respiratory therapists, pharmacists, and social workers and facilitating the staff nurses' attendance at these conferences. The CC-CNS can show interest in patient care issues and increase visibility by attending physician-generated meetings, such as mortality and morbidity reviews, trauma conferences, and coordinated telecommunication conferences. The CC-CNS can bring new and seasoned staff nurses to these sessions and introduce them to the physicians. The CC-CNS can communicate to physicians by charting in the progress notes, as well as assist staff to implement collaborative charting and encourage all personnel to chart in the same place. The CC-CNS can encourage physician review and input into new standards of care and facilitate staff-physician communication concerning standards, protocols, and guidelines governing delivery of patient care. Bringing new technologies, interventions, and ideas to the physician's attention is another activity of the CC-CNS.

As an expert clinician, the CC-CNS can facilitate clinical inquiry of staff nurses concerning actual and potential problems in patient care. During nurse and physician rounds, inquiry is an excellent forum in which the CC-CNS can initiate and facilitate collaboration. It encourages teamwork and increases communication among staff as information is gathered in an effort to provide answers and solve problems. Inquiry provides an excellent opportunity for the CC-CNS to be viewed as a leader and role model.

Collaboration Through Educator Role

The CC-CNS influences practice through collaborative efforts such as orientation, workshop planning, hospital-wide in-service workshops, and unit-based education programs. Whether learning activities are done with a group or one-on-one, they promote communication, mutual respect, and trust as well as encouragement and achievement.

Practical ways in which the CC-CNS can facilitate collaboration in the educator role include the following: Invite physicians, social workers, pharmacists, and respiratory therapists to present unit in-service topics. At the in-service workshop, provide the staff with an opportunity to network with the professionals and to get to know them personally as well as their areas of expertise. Encourage staff attendance by providing food, continuing education units, or contact hours. Market the presentation in nursing newsletters and through attractive posters, announcements at staff meetings, and personal invitations. After the in-service workshop, write a personal thank you note to the presenter. On patient rounds point out examples of research or expertise of staff members. Invite dietitians and pharmacists to work on patient education committees. Consult them when developing educational materials and community-wide health care programs.

Collaboration Through Consultant Role

The CC-CNS facilitates collaboration in the consultant role by pulling in the resources of other experts when approached by the staff with problems. This consultation process builds valuable relationships and strengthens networking ties.

For example, a staff nurse asks the CC-CNS for advice about a patient. The patient is a teenager awaiting heart transplant who is showing signs of depression and anxiety. The CC-CNS suggests to the staff nurse it would be appropriate to call a patient care conference where together the staff nurse, psychiatric liaison, social worker, and physician can discuss interventions for an appropriate care plan. A patient care conference is held, and an interdisciplinary care plan is developed for anxiety and depression.

Collaboration Through Researcher Role

The CC-CNS brings to the collaborative practice model a unique knowledge of research-based practice that is shared with physicians, nurses, and other members of the health care team to improve patient outcomes. Research-based knowledge is the foundation for CC-CNS practice. The following example shows how the CC-CNS uses this knowledge to foster collaborative practice and improve patient outcomes. During patient rounds the staff nurses identify that they are having trouble main-

taining the patency of a radial arterial line: two lines conveying heparinized flush solutions have for those patients in the CC-CNS's caseload and invite staff nurses to participate. The CC-CNS can

Collaborative Solution. In this situation the CC-CNS facilitates joint practice collaboration by presenting the result of the AACN Thunder Project to physicians and nurses. The CC-CNS states that the results demonstrated that heparin, along with patient gender, catheter length, catheter insertion site, thrombolytics, and anticoagulants, affects radial artery catheter patency.[18] Together they discuss implications of these results for practice. On the basis of this research the physician decides to put in a longer femoral artery catheter. The catheter remains patent until it is discontinued 3 days later.

Collaboration Through Leader/Manager Role

As a leader/manager the CC-CNS merges the traditional clinician's role with an administrative role. Organizational analysis, cost analysis, development of policies, procedure, standards of practice, negotiation, and conflict resolution are a few of the management skills the CC-CNS may bring to the collaborative practice team. An example of the CC-CNS working within the collaborative practice model as a leader/manager is described in the following scenario.

Residents are writing orders for radiologic tests after noon, making it virtually impossible for the tests to be done on that day and increasing the cost of care because the patient's stay in the unit is extended an extra day.

Collaborative Solution. The CC-CNS works with the staff nurses, unit secretary, and radiology department members to gather specific data regarding this issue, namely, number of times radiology tests have been ordered after noon, the increases in patient costs that occur, the specifics on which residents are writing the orders, the factors within the radiology department that affect the problem, and the stress that the situation creates on the patient and the nursing staff. The CC-CNS discusses with the residents the reasons why orders are written at this time. In a joint practice committee the CC-CNS presents the problem and the research done about the problem. Together the nurses, physicians, and radiology department members discuss suggestions for problem resolution. A solution is reached.

SUMMARY

This chapter defined the role of the CC-CNS and described how the CC-CNS functions in a collaborative practice model. Through the collaborative effort of the CC-CNS and other health care disciplines, a professional practice environment is created that provides optimal patient and family outcomes. Specific strategies and clinical examples were given of how the CC-CNS works successfully to facilitate collaboration and promote a healing environment for critically ill patients and families. Thus the CC-CNS makes a major contribution to achieving AACN's vision for "a health care system driven by the needs of patients in which critical care nurses make their optimal contribution."[19]

References

1. Nugent KE: The clinical nurse specialist as case manager in a collaborative practice model: bridging the gap between quality and the cost of care, *Clin Nurse Specialist* 6(2):106-111, 1992.
2. Smoyak SA: Specialization in nursing: from then to now, *Nurs Outlook* 24:676-681, 1976.
3. NLNE Special Committee on Post-Graduate Clinical Nursing Courses: *Courses in clinical nursing for graduate nurses: basic assumptions and guiding principles, basic courses, advanced course,* Pamphlet 2, Livingston, NY, 1945, Livingston Press.
4. Rieter F: The nurse clinician, *Am J Nurs* 66:274-280, 1966.
5. Hilberman M: The evolution of intensive care units, *Crit Care Med* 3:159-164, 1975.
6. American Association of Critical-Care Nurses: *The critical care clinical nurse specialist: role definition position statement,* Newport Beach, Calif, 1987, The Association.
7. American Association of Critical-Care Nurses: *Competence statements for critical care clinical nurse specialists,* Newport Beach, Calif, 1989, The Association.
8. American Association of Critical-Care Nurses: *AACN's competence statements for differentiated nursing practice in critical care,* Newport Beach, Calif, 1989, The Association.
9. The National Joint Practice Commission: *Guidelines for establishing joint or collaborative practice in hospitals,* Chicago, 1981, The Commission.
10. Weiss SJ, Davis HP: Validity and reliability of the collaborative practice scale, *J Nurs Res* 34:299-305, 1985.
11. Stichler J: Development and psychometric testing of a collaborative behavior scale. Unpublished manuscript. University of San Diego, Calif, 1989.
12. Rubel, Thomas, 1976.
13. Knaus WL et al: An evaluation of outcome from intensive care in major medical centers, *Ann Intern Med* 104(3):410-418, 1986.
14. American Association of Critical Care Nurses: *AACN mission statement,* Newport Beach, Calif, 1990-1991, The Association.
15. Mitchell PH, Armstrong S, Simpson TF, Lentz L: American Association of Critical Care Nurses demonstration project: profile of excellence in critical care nursing, *Heart Lung* 18(2):219-237, 1990.
16. National Institutes of Health Consensus Conference: Critical care medicine, *AMA* 250:798-804, 1983.
17. Burchell RC, Thomas DA, Smith HL: Some considerations for implementing collaborative practice, *Am J Med* 74:9-13, 1983.
18. American Association of Critical-Care Nurses (manuscript prepared on behalf of AACN and sites of the Thunder Project: Ledbetter, C., Ahrens, T., Brown, B., Gawlinski, A., Perdue, S., Quinn, A., Sechrist, K., Strzelecki, C., Walsh, S. 1993). Evaluation of the effects of heparinized and nonheparinized flush solutions on the patency of arterial pressure monitoring lines: The AACN Thunder Project. *American Journal of Critical Care* 2, (1), 1993.
19. American Association of Critical Care Nurses: Vision statement, Aliso Viejo, California, 1993.

Chapter 2

Securing and Implementing the Clinical Nurse Specialist Role in Critical Care

Ann N. Hotter, RN, MSN, CS, CCRN

A prevailing theme in both society and health care today is that one must do more with less, in a shorter amount of time, and for less cost. Every expenditure is scrutinized and critically evaluated in terms of increased efficiency or improved quality. In this environment the role of the clinical nurse specialist (CNS) has been intensely debated and in some settings either cut altogether or altered beyond recognition.[1] However, in other settings the CNS is highly valued, the number of CNSs has increased, and roles and responsibilities have expanded. What promise therefore does the future hold for the role of the CNS in critical care, and what strategies are most effective in implementing the role successfully? This chapter explores the implementation of the role of the critical care CNS (CC-CNS) as it continues to evolve and gives practical suggestions for not only getting into a system but also staying.

THEORETIC PERSPECTIVES

Rather than being cost contained out of existence, the role of the CNS is experiencing a new resurgence caused in part by the same forces that initially called it into question. The challenges facing health care today and critical care in particular are so complex that they warrant nurses who excel not only in clinical practice but also in system insight and analysis.[2] Through experience and advanced education, the CNS is in a unique position to provide these skills. Notwithstanding the knowledge and expertise of the advanced clinician, the CNS is able to provide a greater range and depth of knowledge, anticipation of patient responses, judgment about nonclinical variables, and clarity and rationale for clinical decisions.[3] For these reasons the CNS, especially in critical care, continues to be increasingly in demand despite a relatively small amount of objective and supportive research data.

Indeed, the role of the CC-CNS today is expanding in scope and complexity. Instead of limiting the application of the five role components (advanced practitioner, educator, consultant, researcher, and leader/manager)[4] directly to patients, the CNS is increasingly being asked to apply these skills to such system innovations as continuous quality improvement, case management, and product line management. In effect the CNS is recognized as an organizational specialist; as an expert change agent, the CNS can assist organizations with implementing new health care delivery systems and other innovations. A strong clinical focus combined with independence, flexibility, and advanced skills of problem solving and analysis are cardinal attributes of CNS practice. It is now no longer unusual for complex and acutely ill patients to be cared for on general care units. Critical care skills are increasingly in demand to care for these patients on general care units so that scarce critical care beds are reserved for the most severely ill or injured patients. Consequently the expectation of the CC-CNS extends beyond the boundaries of the critical care unit.

As health care reimbursement continues to shrink, CNSs are using creative techniques to generate revenue (educational programming consortiums, city-wide critical care orientation, grant-funded research) or provide more efficient care through research-based rather than ritual-based practice. As hospitals continue to search for ways to improve services, accelerate patients' progress, and capitalize on new revenue opportunities, the managerial role of the CNS is more frequently used to understand the financial aspects of inpatient care and home maintenance (i.e., cost-effective products, financially obtainable services).[5] The emerging financial component of CNS practice continues to develop in order to maintain the strong clinical focus.

Although flexibility and adaptation to changing circumstances have always been hallmarks of CNS practice, these qualities are also contributing to the future viability of the role. One's vision of the future of the CC-CNS is certainly influenced by past and present practice models.

To the casual observer the CNS may appear to "flit about," moving among projects, patient contacts, and committee responsibilities. Using a wide variety of strategies (direct patient care, interdepartmental consultation, negotiation, formal and informal teaching) the CNS operates within complex systems, draws on knowledge of many disciplines, and applies this knowledge to complex and dynamic patient situations, producing innovative solutions and helping others discover new paradigms. The CC-CNS of the future will continue to function in this manner, but the mix of information, the scope of practice, and the ability and need to quantify the outcome will expand and increase in sophistication.

Other CNSs envision a practice environment in which the CNS is "first among equals" with the staff nurse,[6] where there is a true interdependence among empowering nursing professionals. Another vision carries this concept further: since staff nurses have progressed to the point where they are considered clinical experts in their own right, the CNS of the future will be free to work at a more advanced level to advance the boundaries of professional knowledge and practice.[7] Another vision of future CC-CNS practice is one in which cost-effective patient outcomes are routinely measured and publicized and CC-CNS are used to provide program and case management leadership.[8]

RELATED LITERATURE AND RESEARCH

Implementing the role of the CNS in critical care is similar to the daunting prospect of entering any complex organization unaccompanied, with the express purpose of providing high-quality service. Although the CNS is generally not hired without some type of job description, several aspects inherent in critical care present unique challenges to successful role implementation.

For example, a CC-CNS entering an organization is expected to simultaneously belong to multiple groups such as unit staff, patient population, CNS peer group, nursing administration, hospital administration, medical staff, and ancillary staff. In addition, the CC-CNS enters at any one of a number of organizational levels somewhere between the grass roots and upper management. The new CC-CNS may therefore encounter boundaries to information and influential networks not easily penetrated by a newcomer.[9] Last, the critical care environment itself presents a challenge to successful CNS entry because of its fast pace, the combination of geographic isolation and multiple disciplines practicing within units, and the reputation of critical care practitioners as aggressive and controlling.

In this atmosphere, the CNS faces the challenges of organizational socialization and achieving role clarity. The five facets of role clarity are initiation to job tasks, definition of interpersonal roles, coping with resistance to change, congruence between self and organizational performance appraisals, and coping with structure and ambiguity.[10]

Several authors have described phases of role development or skill acquisition that can be applied to CNS practice. Baker[11] identified four phases (orientation, frustration, implementation, and reassessment) after interviewing four clinical specialists. Although applied to new graduate nurses, Kramer's stages of reality shock (honeymoon, shock, recovery, and resolution)[12] have similar characteristics and can also be used to describe CNS maturation. Oda[13] also described three phases of role development: role identification, role transition, and role confirmation. (See Chapter 3 for more information on role development.)

However, each of these authors focused primarily on the novice nurse or CNS. The question then arises of whether the experienced CC-CNS, beginning a new CNS position, experiences the same phases of role development during system integration? Based on research by Hamric and Taylor,[14] it appears that even seasoned CNSs are not immune to periods of trial and frustration. These nurses, however, seem to negotiate obstacles and pitfalls with less difficulty and with faster overall role effectiveness. In their research, which combined the opinions of both novice and experienced CNSs, Hamric and Taylor identified seven phases that the CNS goes through in successful role implementation and integration: orientation, frustration, implementation, integration, frozen phase, reorganization, and complacency. Perhaps most important, the two qualities that characterize the successfully integrated CNS are flexibility and commitment.

Covey,[15] in his book *The Seven Habits of Highly Effective People,* outlines guides toward success in CC-CNS implementation and acceptance. Covey's work is so useful to the CC-CNS because it embodies and gives direction for developing leadership skills. True leadership is seldom, if ever, conferred by rules, regulations, or academic degrees but rather by realizing and motivating others toward the achievement of a common vision. Covey's "habits" focus on values and process skills that set a framework for behaviors that can be applied to practice regardless of where the CC-CNS is on the experience continuum. Covey's habits are divided into two levels: dependence moving toward independence, and independence moving toward interdependence. First-level habits include the following: be proactive, begin with the end in mind, and put first things first. Second-level habits include the following: think win/win, seek first to understand . . . then to be understood, and synergize. Many of these habits can be integrated into successful CC-CNS practice.

Success in establishing the CNS role in the critical care environment begins long before the first day on the job. The foundation for success actually starts with analysis of one's values, strengths, personal needs, and areas for growth. Covey describes this as the habit of being proactive, or the ability to choose one's response based on values rather than feelings. With a mental self-portrait, it is not only easier to form a vision of an ideal future, but also to search for and choose the "best fit" in a work environment.

PRACTICE IMPLICATIONS
Employment: Searching for the Best Fit

Analysis of job offers and potential CNS positions includes five categories: organizational philosophy, hierarchic and political structure, expectations of the CNS, reporting mechanisms, and organizational support. Much of this information can be gathered by reviewing hospital literature or during a telephone interview. Preparing before the face-to-face interview increases the likelihood of success through each step of the hiring and orientation process and may minimize or even prevent difficulties once the CNS is established in the system. Factors such as salary, benefits, facilities, or reputation will only be temporarily satisfying, both for the CC-CNS and the organization, if a good fit is not an initial priority.

Organizational Philosophy

Because hospital and nursing department philosophies are written in philosophic terms, it is necessary to "read between the lines" to identify organizational values and financial priorities. Beside reviewing the hospital and nursing department philosophies, several other aspects may provide some insight into the organization's value system. For example, is the role of the CNS a new one or already well established? Does the creation of the role herald a new direction in the nursing department or its perceived relationship with the medical staff and other disciplines? What model of nursing care delivery is practiced throughout the institution and particularly in critical care? Is the current model satisfactory, or is there a desire to change? How does administration view the role of the CC-CNS contributing to the patient population and the hospital's mission both now and 5 years in the future?

Organizational Support

Either before or during the personal interview, it is useful to ask some preliminary questions about organizational support. In other words, what resources are available to help the CC-CNS remain current and knowledgeable (conference and educational support), as well as efficient (secretarial support, computer and library access)? A question on where CNS salary falls within the nursing department pay scale may reveal how the CNS is organizationally valued (top of the clinical ladder or equal to nurse manager, assistant nurse manager, or clinician). Although these aspects of organizational support may not be critical initially, they may increase in importance as one's tenure in the organization increases.

Hierarchic and Political Structure

Initially, information on organizational life may not be easy to glean. Reviewing the organizational chart provides structure to assess nursing's scope of authority, reporting mechanisms, and the position of the CNS. For example, was the hospital established by the community, a government agency, a religious community, or a group of physicians? What is the composition of the board of directors or the highest decision-making body? What position does the highest member of the nursing department hold, to whom does she or he report, and who reports to this person? The answers to these questions provide understanding of how decisions are made in the organization and the political power base of various groups.

Specifically investigate the history of the role of the CNS. How long has the role been established in the organization and in critical care? Has it changed or evolved since its inception and in what way? Did others apply for the CC-CNS position (especially in-house candidates), and will you be working with them? What has been the past relationship of the CC-CNS with the nurse manager, and what are the administration's expectations for this relationship in the future? Are these expectations clearly communicated or assumed? Is there a need for strong team-building skills, or will the CC-CNS be entering an already established team?

Expectations of CNS

Expectations of the CNS are probably best gathered face-to-face during the interview process, because they often go well beyond what are apparent in the job description. Groups to survey include (but should not be limited to) staff nurses, physicians, and administrators. The results of these interviews help establish some practice priorities, facilitate acceptance into the system, and set the

foundation for long-term effectiveness. Interviewing other CNSs already in the system on their expectations of a new colleague may provide a perspective on group and system norms. This is particularly true if there was a predecessor in the CC-CNS position. By recognizing the discrepancy between the expectations of various groups and one's own learning needs, the CC-CNS is better prepared to mitigate some personal reality shock.

Reporting Mechanisms

Reporting mechanisms may determine expectations or practice priorities. In other words, to whom the CC-CNS reports may influence which role component will take precedence. For example, if the CC-CNS reports to the director of education, activities may be heavily influenced by an educational perspective. If the CC-CNS reports to a product line manager, administrative, consulting, or marketing activities may take priority. Whether the CC-CNS's reporting senior is a nurse or someone from another discipline, it is crucial that a mutually acceptable balance be established between administrative support and CC-CNS autonomy on such issues as CC-CNS practice, schedule, and shift options. Certainly if the CNS role has line rather than staff authority, the reporting mechanisms and level of accountability will be much more explicit. Line authority in the CNS role may thus decrease some ambiguity but may also reduce some of its spontaneity and flexibility. Regardless of whether the CC-CNS role is line or staff, fluid, open, and clear communication in both directions of the chain of command is indispensable to smooth CNS integration.

The Interview

The same level of preparation that goes into getting invited to interview should be applied to the interview itself. It is reasonable to expect that all the people participating in the interviews will have reviewed a candidate's resume beforehand and either consciously or unconsciously will focus on the elements most important to them (variety or type of experience, research interests, publications, etc.). Although the list of people that a CC-CNS candidate interviews with is fairly standard (nurse administrators, nurse manager, director of nursing, other CNSs), the CC-CNS should seek interviews with important groups such as staff nurses, unit medical director, key physicians, and patients. These groups can provide valuable and often unpredictable perspective into the actual quality of patient care. The information gathered from such a marathon interview process is well worth the effort. Plan your time accordingly to avoid a very long day or request several days of shorter interview periods if possible.

The interview should never be totally one-sided. Before the interview, anticipate and prepare questions for each type of audience you will encounter. For example, in explaining the role components of the CC-CNS or the particular skills you have to offer, show evidence of a clinical protocol, a multidisciplinary consultation project, or a patient education program you have helped develop. This strategy is particularly helpful if the role of the CNS is new to the organization.

Above all, exude quiet but enthusiastic confidence! It must be clearly evident that you not only love being a nurse, but also are capable of enkindling that passion in others. Medley[16] describes the categories of selling oneself in an interview as enthusiasm, sincerity, tact, and courtesy. Each of these qualities is necessary to create a favorable impression and convey interest on the part of the prospective employer.

Orientation
Structured vs. Nonstructured

Once an offer of employment has been accepted, the structure of orientation should be explored. Invite suggestions for people to include in orientation and thus begin building the foundation for your future network. The structure of orientation will vary according to the history of the role in the organization. For example, there may be a well-structured orientation with a CNS preceptor or mentor, a self-directed unit orientation, or a program somewhere in between. A structured CNS orientation may be available if the role is already established in the institution or if the nurse administrator is familiar with the role. Structure offers the advantages of less ambiguity and a known, controllable pace but the disadvantage of less opportunity for spontaneity or depth.

If the organization has never had a CNS previously, orientation may be very loosely organized because no one is quite sure what the CNS needs. Whereas this can be quite frustrating, it becomes

necessary for the incoming CNS to state explicitly to what activities and people she or he would like to be introduced. It is helpful to make these requests during orientation, especially as it relates to patient care on the unit, to maximize the learning opportunities available when new to the organization. For example, if you are hired as the cardiac care unit CNS, it would be useful to meet the cardiac rehabilitation nurse or discharge coordinator; a neurology/trauma CNS might include the head of physical therapy or the emergency department. In this way the CC-CNS can both establish a link with key people in the organization with whom she or he will be working and use the opportunity to explain the CNS role and how other departments can use it. These "people links" are actually seeds of a network that should begin to blossom and expand by the end of the orientation year.

In the final analysis the structure of orientation is not as important as ensuring the CC-CNS has someone to confide in, discuss issues with, and gain insight. This confidant may be either a CNS who can serve as a mentor or preceptor or a nurse in another role, but ideally one who has more experience in the organization. Above all, this person must be "safe," one who will both listen and respond uncritically, empathetically, and honestly.

To make the orientation period as educational as possible and set a strong foundation for the future, several groups and strategies should be included. Meet again with some of the same groups encountered during the interview process (nursing staff, nurse managers, key physicians, department heads), but this time to elicit more specific information as to what these people do and what they expect you can offer to them.

Orienting with Staff

It is very important during the orientation period to make time to demonstrate clinical proficiency. This strategy serves several purposes: first, patient care provides a familiar frame of reference to the CC-CNS who is often in a new environment. Providing direct patient care clearly demonstrates that the role of the bedside nurse is valued by the CC-CNS. In addition, the high visibility provided by direct care allows the CC-CNS to identify and observe informal staff leaders, clinical experts, and group norms.

A second advantage of providing direct patient

care during orientation is that it allows the CC-CNS to experience the strengths and weaknesses of the orientation program firsthand. By using the tools already in place (such as clinical checklists), the CC-CNS can better judge their validity, practicality, and effectivness.

Third, and perhaps most importantly, orientation with the staff to patient care allows the staff the opportunity to see that the CC-CNS is clinically competent and not above "getting hands dirty." Although the CC-CNS generally possesses greater depth of knowledge in a particular area or a broad perspective on professional practice, not every CC-CNS comes to a particular unit as a clinical expert. For example, the unit may accept pediatric patients or want to expand or create a new program such as open-heart cardiac surgery or transplantation. By acknowledging a lack of personal expertise, the CC-CNS can use and learn from the experienced clinical staff nurse already in the system. The strategy of professionally "hanging around" (not devoting all time on a unit to professional activities but more informal or social ones) allows the staff to get to know the CC-CNS as a person rather than just an authority figure. This human connection is very important while the CNS works to clinically get established in a new area.

Orienting with Nurse Manager

Only second in importance to orientation with the staff is orientation with the appropriate nurse manager and administrators responsible for the area the CC-CNS will practice in. The success of the relationship between CC-CNS and nurse manager can have long-range implications. For example, it is not unusual for the CNS to be at a higher educational level than either the nurse manager or administrator. This discrepancy can potentially cause a communication barrier unless clear, effective communication is a priority.

Probably more important than reviewing "rules" of management is the sharing of insights, perspectives, and priorities in as open a manner as possible. During orientation, explore with the nurse manager what she or he sees as needs of the unit, patients, staff, and administration. How are decisions made? How are things communicated? What does the nurse manager see as acceptable methods for the CNS to communicate with staff (i.e., attending staff meetings, unit rounds, memos)? Is the nurse

manager willing to set aside time for regular meetings such as over coffee or at lunch or only on an as needed basis? What does the nurse manager view as the major strengths and areas for growth for the unit, as well as major sources of frustration?

Obviously these issues are fairly complex and thus not able to be fully explored in a few sessions, particularly if a sense of trust has not had an opportunity to develop. Yet by explicitly exploring the nurse manager's concerns for the unit, these concerns can become areas of mutual support. The beginning foundations for the nurse manager/CNS team are established.

Orienting with Physicians

Establishing a relationship with key physicians and the long-range opportunity of educating them to the CNS role probably begins best on the clinical unit. The CNS/physician relationship is important for three major reasons. First, by establishing a productive team, each member contributing from a unique perspective, the CNS can demonstrate the benefits of collaborative practice. Second, the sophistication and scope of nursing practice are interrelated with the sophistication of medical practice. By establishing a good working relationship with key physicians, both CNS and physician mutually enhance and stimulate advances in their own fields. Third, the political reality is that physicians can also be powerful gatekeepers throughout the larger organization. By cultivating the CNS/physician professional relationship, the CNS may be in a better position to have system-wide impact.

However, since the CNS role is still something of a mystery to many physicians, a variety of strategies may be necessary to get one's foot in the door. If possible, inquire about participating in physicians' morning rounds. Ask for or seek out articles on areas of the physician's expertise (especially if he or she is the author). Attend monthly conferences or morbidity and mortality reviews.

Finally, the most eloquent graduate school description of the CNS role pales beside evidence of clinical expertise, accompanied by short but perfectly timed explanations of what the CNS can offer the patient population. In this way the above activities may also strategically position the CNS to positively impact physicians' practice.

Orienting with Key Administrators

The administrative component of orientation should not be neglected and indeed should receive special care and preparation. Meeting key administrators provides the CNS with the unique opportunity to understand the broader perspective of the organization's direction and priorities, as well as subtle forces that may have a major impact at the unit level. Come prepared with both general and specific questions about the department's concerns/issues related to critical care. Meetings of this type can provide a wealth of information!

If necessary, use the meeting as an opportunity to explain who you are and what a CNS can do. Rehearse your message in advance, or use examples that are meaningful to professionals from other disciplines.

The process of CNS orientation conceptually extends well beyond the usual 3-month probationary period. The effective CNS requires a working knowledge of not only how things work (policy/procedure, lines of authority, etc.) but also why they work that way (communication patterns, group process, etc.). For this reason it is not unrealistic to consider the orientation period to actually consume the first 6 months on the job. Many CC-CNSs feel self-imposed or external pressures to begin concrete projects or committee work soon after employment. It is absolutely vital that the CC-CNS has support to take time to get to know the staff and their strengths, weaknesses, and communication patterns in order to develop effective strategies for change.

STRATEGIES FOR SUCCESSFUL ROLE IMPLEMENTATION

Unit-Based Practice

The limits and boundaries of CC-CNS practice are becoming increasingly blurred. Although the CNS title (CNS-pulmonary, CNS-trauma, CNS-ICU) may provide potential users of CNS services with a frame of reference, it can be artificially limiting. For the CNS who is new to the institution or to the role, it may be easier to become integrated into the system if practice is initially circumscribed to one unit or a few smaller units. Over time and with successful assimilation, the CC-CNS will be increasingly consulted for the critically ill patients on general care units or to collaborate on projects that involve a variety of departments.

Initially, within a unit-based practice, a large proportion of CNS energy is spent in meeting people, maintaining high visibility, explaining the CC-CNS role, and beginning involvement in projects. The recurring challenge for the CNS is to maintain a balance between clinical involvement and visibility, and professional growth.

At the completion of orientation, the CNS should be ready to set first-year goals for practice. Goal setting helps to provide both structure and measurable outcomes. Goals should combine a mixture of professional practice-oriented and professional role-oriented statements to address personal growth and satisfaction. Realistically, goals may require several years for achievement and may be broken down into annual objectives. In addition, realistic goals may require acknowledging that certain systems or practices must be established first before direct action on the major goal can begin. For example, before a model for primary nursing can be implemented, the CNS might need to work on systems that promote accountability such as documentation.

Another way of establishing goals is by categorizing them according to CNS role components (see p. 18). This method helps the CC-CNS specifically address each component as well as monitor how the proportion of time and energy devoted to each will fluctuate as the CC-CNS gains experience. In addition to setting specific role-oriented goals, the new CC-CNS may have secondary goals such as increased visibility or expertise, which could also be considered benefits. These secondary goals thus serve as catalysts for future consultation, ideas for researchable problems, and, of course, direct patient care. Combining the Covey habits of "begin with the end in mind" and putting "first things first," the CC-CNS is better able to remain proactive, forward thinking, and focused on goals rather than reactive, harried, and ineffective. The resulting flexibility allows the CC-CNS to react to crises such as sudden staffing shortages or accreditation visits without losing sight of progress toward the goal.

Day-to-Day Activities

Particularly during the first year, CC-CNS activities have several major purposes: increased clinical visibility, increased expertise, and improvement of patient care and outcome. In this way staff

---

GOALS AND OBJECTIVES OF THE CRITICAL CARE CLINICAL NURSE SPECIALIST—YEAR 1

Clinical Practice
- Establish nursing rounds incorporating ICU staff on a biweekly basis.
- Attend house officer rounds at least three times per week.
- Provide direct patient care to a critically ill patient at least twice per month.
- Act as role model to staff in applying the nursing process to patients and families by contributing to the nursing care plan.
- Increase the frequency of allied health disciplines consultation.

Educator
- Assist critical care nurse educator in updating and teaching critical care course.
- Provide ACLS review courses to staff to increase number of certified nurses.
- Develop programmed instruction on intracranial pressure (ICP) monitoring.
- Provide monthly education and hands-on experience with peripheral nerve stimulator (PNS) to critical care residents.
- Establish liaison with local nursing school program.

Consultant
- Act as coordinator for development of critical care flow sheet.
- Act as consultant to staff in family crisis intervention.
- Consult with emergency department to develop standards of care for patients with hemodynamic monitoring.
- Consult with pharmacy to establish guidelines for administration of neuromuscular blockade.

Researcher
- Initiate review of the literature for research on nitroprusside toxicity.
- Provide staff with research articles or critiques related to common diseases or procedures.
- Develop a list of possible researchable clinical problems.

Personal
- Maintain involvement in local chapter of AACN.
- Write an outline for one manuscript for publication by end of first year.

---

members get to know the CNS as a person and are more likely to initiate consultations simply because of increased accessibility. The most obvious strategy is that of clinical rounds, since it puts the CC-CNS in close and immediate contact with patients, families, and staff.

For the CC-CNS, no ideal method of making rounds exists, since it must be individualized to integrate with unit activities (family visits, physician rounds, postoperative admissions, etc.), or other preset commitments (committee meetings, ongoing courses). The CC-CNS may choose to do rounds alone or with the nurse manager or charge nurse, also depending on availability or the need to focus on a particular aspect of care from both a clinical and management perspective.

Making rounds at the bedside offers the advantage of combining subjective and objective patient data as a basis for discussion (one picture is worth 1000 words). Questions can explore admitting diagnosis, significant past medical history, course of disease, therapies used, potential for complications, patient and family dynamics, and common patient needs (nutrition, skin condition, sleep, activity, education). The manner of questioning should include an implicit assumption of the nurse's good judgment and caring attitude until proven otherwise. This approach avoids unnecessary accusations and defensiveness. Obviously, all the above information does not have to (and often cannot) be obtained at one pass through the unit! Some can be gleaned through chart review; however, over time staff members become able to anticipate common questions and act on them without being prompted.

Clinical rounds also help the staff nurse to develop oral presentation skills and thus be better prepared to interact with physicians and peers. Ideally, formal rounds are frequent enough to elicit the necessary information and assess patient progress, yet not so frequent as to be a burden to both the staff and the CC-CNS.

Another benefit of high clinical visibility and the use of clinical rounds is the continued increase in expertise of both the CC-CNS and staff. Few CC-CNS come to new positions as clinical experts in every aspect of their specialty. When the CC-CNS encounters a new population or technology it is imperative to seek resources to quickly address one's knowledge deficit. For example, an adult-focused CC-CNS may start in a unit that begins to admit pediatric patients or employs unfamiliar technologies. In this case, it is important to first acknowledge a lack of specific knowledge or experience and seek out the information from the literature, colleagues in other settings or disciplines, or nursing experts who may already be on the unit.

Clinical experts present on the unit can be identified by simple observation and conversation. However, a significant time investment by the CC-CNS early in the first year through the use of individual appointments can reap huge rewards. One CC-CNS used 15-minute appointments to meet one-on-one with staff members to get to know them as individuals and their experiences and perspectives on how the CC-CNS could help the unit. Although initially time consuming, this interview strategy gave the CNS valuable insight and exposure to begin building lasting relationships.

Committee Commitments

The key to keeping committee involvement as an activity that enhances the role is selectivity. It is often tempting to get involved in committees or task forces to solve nagging problems, because CNS involvement can provide the committee with meaningful clinical perspective as well as group process skills. However, if clinical practice and visibility suffer, the CNS eventually loses credibility both on the unit and the committee.

Initially, choose committees that introduce the CC-CNS to a large group of key people, as well as provide opportunities to learn how things work (orientation, policy and procedure). Gradually, as the CC-CNS becomes more familiar with organizational process and has established credibility with formal and informal leaders, other more complex, high-profile, or politically charged committee assignments can and should be sought.

Nurse Manager and CC-CNS as a Team: Synergy at Its Best

Perhaps the single most important relationship to cultivate for long-term CC-CNS acceptance and effectiveness is one with the nurse manager. A strong and dynamic CC-CNS/nurse manager team is very productive, since it uses the unique strengths and perspectives of each role. As a team both CNS and nurse manager use the resources both inside and outside the organization to provide quality patient care and advance nursing practice, jointly set unit goals, and demonstrate colleagueship and collaborative practice.

The nurse manager can be both a powerful (positive or negative) resource gatekeeper and role model. Particularly in the early stages of CC-CNS integration, the nurse manager sets the tone for staff, physicians, and other disciplines, thus heavily influencing both the frequency and type of consultation, as well as support for innovation. The key to the synergy of the CNS/nurse manager relationship is not so much complete agreement on all issues but that there is mutual sharing of individual strengths, viewpoints, and energies and that solutions to problems are addressed from different perspectives but with a common vision.

To state that open communication is fundamental to the CNS/nurse manager relationship borders on being a cliche, since its truth is so obvious. However, establishing this type of rapport is not easy. A simple first step is for both CNS and nurse manager to develop a general appreciation of the other's role, authority, *and* limitations. Begin these discussions during weekly meetings, informally over lunch outside the building, or even while attending conferences together. In this way, expectations are not as likely to exceed capabilities.

A practical strategy to achieve this insight is to make patient rounds together. Often while looking at the same picture, each nurse focuses on different but complementary aspects (assessment data/documentation, interdisciplinary consultation/discharge planning). Through open patient-focused discussion, the CNS and nurse manager complement rather than compete with each other and thus are exposed to each other's perspectives.

Another cornerstone of clear, positive communication is that the perception of what is said is consistent with what is intended. How often has a colleague said, "Oh, I didn't mean it *that way* . . . !" after realizing that remarks have been misinterpreted. Take a mental millisecond to review *beforehand* how something will sound. Meet regularly to share perceptions and strategies. Plan a retreat or mutual unit goal setting meeting away from the hospital. These types of sharing activities broaden understanding beyond the job description to include motivations, emotions, and perceptions.

This type of understanding of another's frame of reference is the essence of empathetic listening according to Covey and is one of the most important ways of building trusting relationships.[18] This form of empathetic listening is also the basis for the habit of "seek first to understand, then to be understood."

All of the above activities also need to include assistant nurse managers because these nurses are often most knowledgeable of the day-to-day needs of staff and serve as role models of leadership skills. By investing time and energy in building the CC-CNS/nurse manager relationship, it is easier to deal with inevitable periods of conflict or the need for staff counseling, since both parties will not feel that either is working in isolation but rather from a common frame of reference.

Dealing with Conflict

The Covey habit of "think win/win" relates best to the interpersonal rather than the strategic process of goal attainment. This habit or paradigm is actually the frame of mind and heart that constantly seeks mutual benefit in all human interactions.[15] As the CNS begins to get deeply involved in clinical issues and develop change agent skills, it is inevitable that conflict in varying degrees will occur. Therefore conflict management is not only a process but a survival skill for the CC-CNS! The win/win paradigm is important for the CC-CNS to develop early, because it may help to temper some potentially overaggressive enthusiasm in the process of goal achievement. By investing the time and energy in a win/win attitude rather than a win/lose one, the CC-CNS builds a reputation as a diplomatic team player and sets the foundation for a long-term productive network of colleagues.

It is readily apparent that good communication skills are essential to conflict management *and* prevention. However, other ingredients include assertive skills, the appropriate use of humor, and the ability to negotiate, as well as the willingness to apologize when wrong. Without an established support network or a repertoire of past CC-CNS experiences to relate to, it is not uncommon for the new CC-CNS to begin a cycle of increasing self-doubt. Conflict management is a learned skill; tactic identification with a trusted mentor, role playing, sincere efforts to seek information to understand the context of issues, and the commitment to avoid emotional games are all strategies that will increase the chances for CNS satisfaction and success.[17]

Communicating CC-CNS Role

In addition to the strategies described earlier that are designed to increase visibility and utilization of the CC-CNS, two theoretic concepts based on marketing theory assist the new CC-CNS to optimize the impact of activities. These concepts are marketing goals and target markets. In other words, who are the people that the CC-CNS wishes to influence to utilize her or his services (physicians, staff nurses, families, administrators)? What are the specific goals the CC-CNS wants to promote with each group, such as decreased complication rates or length of stay, increased depth of clinical knowledge, improved understanding and coping skills, and increased cost savings?

Identify target markets and develop short repetitive messages using phrases relevant to each market, describing what the CC-CNS does.[18] For example, a marketing message to patients/families might be "I assist the nursing staff to develop new ways of solving complex problems" or "I help patients and their families adjust to the challenges of this illness, so they can function at their best after discharge." A marketing message to physicians might be "I help to prevent complications by not only individualizing my patient care according to the patient's unique needs, but also observing for trends in our patient population to better anticipate complications should they occur." A marketing message to an educator could be "One of my contributions to education is to build on core knowledge and apply it in new ways to help solve recurring clinical problems." A marketing message to an administrator might be "I work with the nurse manager and staff nurses to identify efficient ways of providing nursing care, and working toward care that is based on research rather than tradition."

Each message contains key words or phrases that support rather than threaten the audience. If possible, include examples from practice to further illustrate these points. The new CC-CNS may not have developed a repertoire of examples, but these will quickly multiply if the CC-CNS is alert to recognizing them in practice.

SUMMARY

Establishing the role of the CNS in critical care requires careful analysis, patience, a high tolerance for ambiguity and frustration, a sense of humor, and enthusiasm! Time for orientation and goal setting is essential to survive the first year in the role or in a new CC-CNS position. A patient and long-term perspective allows the CC-CNS to carefully evaluate the system and patiently craft an ever-widening network of multidisciplinary collegial support. Using meaningful communication and timely examples of what an advanced nursing role has to offer both patients and an institution, as well as supporting these actions with measurable outcomes, CC-CNSs will establish the role as a permanent, viable component of nursing practice.

CASE STUDY 1

Noreen K (NK) was hired as a CC-CNS in a multipurpose 24-bed ICU in a 1000-bed level I trauma center. She had 2 years' experience as a CC-CNS at a rural community hospital; the trauma center ICU had a CNS, but this person left this newly created position after 6 months to relocate.

In addition to going through hospital orientation, NK asked to be assigned to a preceptor in the unit and complete unit orientation, in order to not only assess the orientation program from a staff nurse perspective, but also to observe communication patterns among staff and with physicians and to demonstrate to staff that she was competent in patient care. Added benefits of this slower approach to CC-CNS system integration was that NK was able to introduce herself to physicians in a familiar, nonthreatening context (patient care) and to get a good idea of the specific department heads she would like to meet more in depth.

Initially, NK sensed that the staff (and even the nurse managers) were a little wary of her, even though outwardly friendly and polite. She realized that there was an uneasy sense that she was there to change everything or to be a "spy" for the nurse manager. The challenge before NK as the CC-CNS was to get a true sense of patient progress or lack of it and make suggestions for improvement, yet not intimidate anyone in the process!

Following orientation, NK started a pattern of listening to reports in the morning or touching base with the charge nurse to identify problem areas where she could have some impact. She would make rounds several times per day in the unit, sometimes "quickie" rounds that focused only on the patients' needs identified earlier in the day. Questions on these rounds were specific and to the point: "How did your patient respond to the diuretic you gave earlier?" "Did the dietitian come by today to see Mrs. S?" or "Were you able to get the order for the low air-loss bed?" Sometimes longer rounds took 1 hour or more as NK took time to read charts, review histories, or talk to patients and families. While on the unit, she made a point of learning people's names and greeting them, going into patients' rooms to answer call lights or alarms if everyone was busy (a quick and easy way to assess patient acuity), and trying to answer physicians' questions if the primary nurse was unavailable. If NK noted something in a patient room (dampened hemodynamic waveforms, new vasoactive medications begun) or in the patient's condition (confusion, respiratory changes) that needed to be addressed, she would attempt to talk with the assigned nurse first, to explore what had already been tried or what observations the nurse had made.

Progress was slow at first, as staff nurses and physicians varied from small acts of kindness to suspicion ("What are you doing in my room?") and outright hostility ("I don't care what big university you went to, the physicians want it this way, so if it ain't broke, don't fix it.") NK tried to respond with a mixture of assertiveness, approachability, humor, and occasionally brutal honesty ("Even big universities sometimes have good ideas." "Even though the physicians like things this way, have you found this therapy to be effective?" "Maybe we could share some of the newest studies available with Dr. K, that might make him reconsider."). A key support during this first year was the relationship she built with both the critical care educator and nurse manager. NK had the luxury of being able to speak freely with these two nurses, neither of whom had a graduate degree or experience as a CC-CNS but who both had great experience in the system, as well as a shared vision of what the future could look like.

One strategy that NK successfully used in addressing particularly sensitive clinical issues was diversionary deflection. If she had an idea or suggestion regarding patient care, depending on the volatility of either the suggestion or the physician, she would decide on an approach that would maximize the chances of success. For example, if it was a suggestion that she felt reasonably certain that the physician would accept, she would be in the room for rounds and state something like "Sue and I were discussing Mrs. Jones's ABGs, and we felt that she might be able to tolerate . . . . Does that sound reasonable to you, Doctor?" If on the other hand, the suggestion was a little riskier, NK was careful to either use the first person or take the physician aside to address the issue herself in order to absorb any potential flak. In this way the staff learned to trust NK, since as the CC-CNS, she was willing to share credit with the staff for their problem-solving abilities yet would not set them up for failure or humiliation to achieve her own goals or force her own will on others.

CASE STUDY 2

Ten months ago, Delores K. (DK) was hired as the CC-CNS in a midsize community hospital. The unit is almost exclusively devoted to adults, but hospital administrators had decided to expand its cardiac surgery program to include pediatric patients in order to avoid referrals to a distant tertiary center and to increase its market share.

DK has no pediatric open-heart experience, but

the nurse manager does; because of this, the nurse manager states that she will take care of the orientation and clinical experience of the staff. As the CNS, DK feels strongly that she should not be excluded from this new program but realizes that without sufficient clinical expertise, her ability to contribute is significantly limited.

After analyzing her own emotions and motives, DK begins to realistically discuss her concerns with the nurse manager, including not only her need to increase her own knowledge base and practical experience, but also the impact that her total exclusion will have on the staff's perception of the CC-CNS role. DK is careful to recognize the nurse manager's expertise in a nonthreatening way, often over lunch or at coffee, asking her to share past experiences. DK explores the possibility of seeking clinical experience either by going outside the institution or as the nurse manager's student.

By exploring with the nurse manager the many aspects of this new program, DK is able to identify those activities in which she could participate after she has gained the necessary experience (skills check-offs, care plan development, lectures). Together the CC-CNS and nurse manager create an action plan with 3-, 6-, and 12-month evaluation points, with the ultimate goal of full CNS participation.

References

1. Williams O'Rourke M: Generic professional behaviors: implications for the clinical nurse specialist role, *Clin Nurse Specialist* 3(3):128–132, 1989.
2. Sparacino PS: Strategies for implementing advanced practice, *Clin Nurse Specialist* 4(3):151–152, 1990.
3. Spross JA, Baggerly J: Models of advanced nursing practice. In Hamric A, Spross J, editors: *The clinical nurse specialist in theory and practice,* Philadelphia, 1989, WB Saunders Co.
4. American Association of Critical Care Nurses: *The critical care clinical nurse specialist: role definition,* Newport Beach, Calif, 1987, The Association.
5. Norris MK, Hill C: The clinical nurse specialist: developing the case manager role, *Dimen Crit Care Nurs* 10(6):346–353, 1991.
6. Gross J: Personal communication, 1992.
7. Palmer C: Personal communication, 1992.
8. Gross D: Personal communication, 1991.

9. Krcmar CR: Organizational entry: the case of the clinical nurse specialist, *Clin Nurse Specialist* 5(1):38–42, 1991.

10. Wanous JP, Reichers AE, Malik SD: Organizational socialization and group development: toward an integrative perspective, *Academy of Management Review* 9:670–683, 1984.

11. Baker V: Retrospective explorations in role development. In Padilla GV, editor: *The clinical nurse specialist and improvement of nursing practice,* Wakefield, Mass, 1979, Nursing Resources.

12. Kramer M: *Reality shock: why nurses leave nursing,* St Louis, 1974, C.V. Mosby.

13. Oda D: Specialized role development: A three-phase process, *Nursing Outlook* 25:374–377, 1977.

14. Hamric AB, Taylor JW: Role development of the CNS. In Hamric AB, Spross JA: *The clinical nurse specialist in theory and practice,* ed 2, Philadelphia, 1989, WB Saunders Co.

15. Covey S: *The seven habits of highly effective people,* New York, 1989, Simon & Schuster.

16. Medley A: *Sweaty palms: the neglected art of being interviewed,* Belmont, Calif, 1978, Lifetime Learning Publications.

17. Beare PB: The essentials of win-win negotiation for the clinical nurse specialist, *Clin Nurse Specialist* 3(3):138–141, 1989.

18. Hall-Johnson S: Marketing techniques for critical care nursing, *Crit Care Nurs Currents* 4(1), 1986.

Chapter 3

Critical Care Clinical Nurse Specialist: Novice to Expert

Deborah Goldenberg Klein, RN, MSN, CS, CCRN

Implementing the clinical nurse specialist (CNS) role in the critical care setting is a challenge even for the most experienced CNS. The complexity of the role can be frustrating and overwhelming. Understanding the different phases of CNS role development can be helpful to both the novice and experienced critical care CNS (CC-CNS). This chapter discusses the phases of CC-CNS role development, strategies to enhance role effectiveness, and two case studies.

THEORETIC PERSPECTIVES

Role theory is a collection of concepts and hypotheses that suggest how people behave in a particular societal role. A role is composed of functions performed while a person occupies a certain position in society.[1] The CNS role consists of five components: practitioner, educator, consultant, researcher, and leader/manager. Anyone entering a new role experiences a process of role development before being able to function with maximum effectiveness. CNS role development is a complex process because of the expanded boundaries and responsibilities of the position.

Both novice and experienced CC-CNSs go through a process of role development. However, the experienced CC-CNS's path varies from that of a neophyte CC-CNS. Understanding the development process is important if educators are to adequately prepare nurses for the expanded role and for both CC-CNSs and administrators to set realistic performance expectations. Role development is a dynamic process. The role is continuously defined as it changes and the individual CC-CNS develops within the role. In addition, priorities in

the role must be determined in relation to the clinical situation and the development of the staff. It is crucial that CC-CNSs provide clear definitions of their role functions to help prevent role conflict.[2]

RELATED LITERATURE AND RESEARCH

The process of role development in nurses has been conceptualized by several authors. Benner[3] identifies five stages of skill acquisition in clinical nurse practice based on the Dreyfus model: novice, advanced beginner, competent, proficient, and expert. Although Benner's work did not focus specifically on the CNS, the process of role development and skill acquisition that she describes can be applied to the developing CC-CNS.

Benner describes the *novice* as a beginner with no experience in the situation in which she or he is expected to perform. Behavior is governed by rules determined to be necessary to guide performance. However, it is difficult for the novice to be successful because the rules cannot give the most relevant tasks to perform in an actual situation. For example, a CC-CNS with graduate work and in-depth experience in adult critical care would be at the novice stage were she or he to transfer to a neonatal intensive care unit.

In the second stage, *advanced beginner*, the nurse demonstrates marginally acceptable performance. The nurse has been involved with enough situations to recognize, either alone or with a mentor or preceptor, recurrent meaningful patterns. However, the nurse still focuses on the rules and tasks that have been taught. Assistance from a preceptor is needed to help set priorities. For example, a new CC-CNS is often enthusiastic and eager to make change. Without experience in the components of the CC-CNS role, the new CNS may attempt to implement all role components simultaneously (e.g., start a unit-based research project, develop and implement a new intraaortic balloon pump [IABP] course, and implement weekly patient care conferences), without the support of the nurse manager or the critical care staff. A preceptor or mentor would be helpful in assisting this new CC-CNS in setting priorities and focusing on strategies that would facilitate timely implementation and enhance role development.

The third stage of skill acquisition is *competent* nurse. Competence develops when the nurse begins to see actions in terms of conscious goals or plans. The plan establishes perspective and is based on conscious, abstract, and analytic thought of the problem. Deliberate planning helps achieve efficiency and organization. The competent nurse lacks the speed and flexibility of the proficient nurse (the next higher stage of development) but can manage more complex patient situations. In addition, competent nurses have enough experiential knowledge to recognize incompetence. They may become anxious and take on more responsibility than they can handle.[4] A CC-CNS at this stage would be able to identify a clinical need, develop a plan to address that need, and successfully implement and evaluate the plan with the support of the nurse manager and nursing staff (e.g., a family support group or a hemodynamic monitoring review class).

The *proficient* nurse perceives situations holistically based on experience. This nurse knows what events to expect in a given situation and how plans need to be modified in response to these events. The proficient nurse recognizes when the expected normal picture does not occur. For example, she or he is able to recognize deterioration in a patient before explicit changes in vital signs and is able to respond appropriately. Decision making is more precise. The proficient CC-CNS is a recognized, trusted, clinical expert who is consulted by the critical care nurse manager and staff as well as other departments within the institution. For example, a CC-CNS with expertise in wound management may serve as a consultant to the institution. A CC-CNS with expertise in cardiac transplantation may move from the competent stage with a strong clinical, consultation, and education

focus to the proficient stage with a focus on new program development and research related to cardiac transplantation patients.[5]

The fifth and final stage is *expert* nurse. The expert nurse has an extensive background of experience and an intuitive grasp of each situation because of an understanding of the total situation. Clinical performance is highly proficient. Analytic problem-solving methods are used only when faced with a new situation or when the initial grasp of the problem proves to be incorrect. Expert nurses are not just engaging in knowledge utilization; they are developing clinical knowledge.[6] Expert nurses provide consultation for other nurses. They recognize early clinical changes in a patient and can effectively make a case for further medical evaluation. In the intensive care unit (ICU), nurses have the opportunity to compare their observations and develop consensus about conclusions with other nurses to further enhance performance. CC-CNSs move into the expert stage when they can describe clinical situations where their interventions made a difference. For example, a CC-CNS recognizes that certain physiologic conditions appear to be present in critically ill patients with skin breakdown. A research study is developed to determine these physiologic variables. Based on the results of the study, patients at risk for skin breakdown are identified (e.g., low cardiac output conditions, elderly, obese, immobile) and interventions implemented to prevent skin breakdown (e.g., turning schedules, pressure relief devices, skin care protocol). As a result of this planned intervention, the CC-CNS is able to demonstrate a significant decrease in skin breakdown, a significant cost savings in supplies to treat skin breakdown, and a decrease in ICU length of stay.

Although other models for CNS role development have been developed (Table 3–1), Baker's phases have additional validity for CC-CNS role development.

Baker's Model

In phase 1 the new CNS is fresh from a graduate program or new to the institution. Time is spent becoming familiar with a new work situation, including the institution's functioning, the personnel, and the policies. The CNS is often enthusiastic and optimistic with feelings of anxiety and confusion. These feelings sometimes interfere with conceptual

TABLE 3–1 Phases of CNS Role Development

Phase	Baker[7]	Kramer[8]	Oda[9]	Hamric and Taylor[10]	CNS Characteristics
1	Orientation	Honeymoon	Role identification	Orientation	New CNS; optimistic, enthusiastic, anxious, confused; eager to prove self as clinically competent and to make change; clarifying role to self and setting
2	Frustration	Shock/ rejection	—	Frustration	Overwhelmed with responsibilities and priorities of role; conflict between graduate school values and real-world values, unrealistically high performance expectations; feelings of confusion, anger, depression, isolation, and frustration; resistance encountered
3	Implementation	Recovery	Role transition	Implementation	Rethinking and reclarifying role to self and setting; modifying activities in response to feedback; implementing specific projects with tangible results; perspective returns; secure in role; consultation role expanded
4	Reassessment	Resolution	Role confirmation	—	Mutual respect between CNS and staff; role functions evaluated, reorganized, or further developed; enthusiasm and optimism renewed; risk taking, creative, challenged
				Integration	Self-confident; wide recognition and influence in specialty area; challenged; congruence between personal and organizational goals and expectations
5				Frozen phase	Self-confident; conflict between personal goals and organizational goals and expectations; angry, frustrated
6				Reorganization	Organization experiencing major changes; pressure to change role that is incongruent with own concept of CNS role and goals
7				Complacent phase	Settled, comfortable in role; questionable impact on organization; practice constructed to meet selected, narrowly focused needs

knowledge.[11] The CNS is eager to prove herself or himself as clinically competent and hopes to bring about change by being a role model.[7] One of the major tasks of this phase is to clarify the role, to oneself first and then to others in the setting.[9] The phase may be shortened in an institution where CC-CNSs have been effectively used or if the CC-CNS is experienced in the CNS role.

In phase 2, CNSs are often shocked by the overwhelming multitude of responsibilities and the anxiety that resistance to change evokes. New CC-CNSs often have unrealistically high performance expectations. They begin to realize that one person cannot perform all role functions described in the literature, much less simultaneously. Conflict between graduate school values and real-world values becomes apparent. These conflicts may be due to adjustment to change, territoriality, interpersonal differences, or the way a particular CNS implements the role.[12] Role confusion may affect CC-CNS performance and impede integration into the system. Feelings of confusion, anger, depression, isolation, and frustration may temporarily freeze the CC-CNS in this phase. The CC-CNS wonders about personal worth and feels that perhaps an impostor will soon be discovered.

Other factors may complicate the CC-CNS's sense of frustration, including role ambiguity, lack of authority, resistance from staff nurses, lack of support, lack of role models, and role competition.[13-15]

Role ambiguity occurs when there is a lack of consistency in describing the roles and responsiblities of the CC-CNS. Clearly defined goals, role responsibilities, and mutual agreement about role expectations are essential. Lack of authority for the CC-CNS is an area of concern because the CNS role has historically been envisioned as purely clinical without administrative responsibilities. The CNS has been expected to be a change agent by virtue of advanced knowledge, skill, and expertise. As a result the CC-CNS is usually assigned a staff position without direct authority. The power base of the CNS is expert power. This means that by virtue of the CC-CNS's knowledge and skill, she or he has the ability to affect the behavior of others. The CC-CNS must be highly skilled in interpersonal relationships and in developing and maintaining channels of communication. Cultivating working relationships will help establish credibility and increase consultation referrals.[16] Resistance from the nursing staff and the nurse manager occurs when they perceive that the CC-CNS is needed to improve care. Establishing credibility can be done by focusing on the role of expert practitioner and acting as a role model and patient advocate during the early phases of the CC-CNS role.

Lack of authority may be amplified by lack of visible administrative support for the CC-CNS role. Lack of recognition such as no appointment to clinical evaluation committees and no recognition of CC-CNS contributions to quality patient care could significantly limit the CC-CNS's range of influence and potential.

The lack of role models for the CC-CNS can limit job satisfaction and role development. Peer support can help by providing a way to exchange ideas, share experiences, and give feedback.

Baker describes phase 3 as a period of organization and reorganization and of rethinking and clarifying one's position to the staff and health care team. Oda discusses this phase in a similar manner and emphasizes that as the CNS interacts with others, she or he begins to modify approach in response to feedback received from the nursing staff and other health care professionals. Trust may be substituted for the pervasive feeling of constantly being tested. The CNS is able to effectively implement and balance new subroles. The consultant role is increasingly used and may surpass the more tangible role of educator. Consultation for clinical expertise is more frequently received if the CC-CNS remains patient oriented and highly visible on the patient units. Focusing on specific projects and visible tasks with tangible results can be rewarding. The desire to be all things to all people decreases as the CC-CNS becomes more comfortable directing others to more appropriate resources. Enthusiasm and optimism return as positive feedback is received and expectations realigned. This security is a sign of developmental progression enabling the CC-CNS to feel that the role is finally gaining cohesiveness.[12] Lack of structure or self-goals, time management, and evaluation of progress may be stressful for those who are used to teamwork or following the direction of a leader.[11] This phase is critical, because it can lead to either positive or negative resolution.[17]

In phase 4 the energy and time spent in building relationships and learning the system decrease, allowing for the exploration of new and stimulating areas of interest. According to Baker, role functions are evaluated, reorganized, or further developed. Mutual respect between the CC-CNS and staff has developed, and administration supports the role. New directions and goals are formulated. Kramer believes this final phase can have a negative or positive result. Negative outcomes leave the CNS unsettled in the job, performing poorly or no longer functioning as a change agent in the system. Kramer describes positive resolution as those CNSs who are highly functional with high job satisfaction, who are risk takers, and who are creative.

Hamric and Taylor's Model

Hamric and Taylor[10] found in their study that CNSs with more than 3 years of experience used descriptors that fell outside of Baker's phases. They identify four additional phases of role development: integration, frozen phase, reorganization, and complacency. CNSs in the integration phase rated themselves at an advanced level of practice. There was congruence between personal and organizational goals and expectations. CNSs were either moderately or very satisfied with their present positions. They were self-confident and assured in the role. They continuously felt challenged by the clinical problems confronted; by changes in technology; by new projects within the institution; and by greater involvement in professional activities, research, and publishing. These findings are consistent with Holt's premise[18] that the focus of development of the experienced CNS is to improve the care of all patients within the specialty by enlarging the sphere of influence beyond the immediate workplace.

CNSs in the frozen phase reported major conflicts between their goals and the organization's goals. Although these CNSs were confident, self-assured, and at an advanced level of practice, administrative support for programs or goals valued by the CNS was generally lacking. These CNSs believed they were not achieving their maximum potential and were in a frozen state because of factors beyond themselves and the CNS role. Feelings of anger and frustration were apparent. Reassessment and renegotiation of both the role and position within the organization are necessary to resolve conflicts and further role development.

The reorganization phase is typically experienced by CNSs in organizations that are involved with major changes in nursing or hospital administration and financial constraints. These changes often require a reorganization in CNS practice that is incongruent with the CNSs' concept of role and goals. If the role change is expected to be permanent, the CNS must decide whether this new role is adaptable or whether it can be renegotiated to incorporate elements that preserve the integrity of the CNS role, allow for job satisfaction, and meet the new needs of the organization. For example, in some hospitals, CNSs are focusing on

new patient care delivery systems such as case management. If no compromise can be found, a career move for the CNS may be indicated.

Hamric and Taylor found a small number of CNSs in a complacent phase. They were settled and comfortable with varying degrees of job satisfaction. Although these CNSs were not necessarily negative, Hamric and Taylor question the extent to which complacent CNSs influence institutions. CNSs in this phase for long periods are not seen as change agents but have constructed their practices to meet selected, narrowly focused needs. For example, the CNS who does all the preoperative education instead of empowering and developing the staff nurses to do this activity is not moving forward. CNSs in this phase need to reenergize by changing some aspect of practice or focus on a new population or new institutional need. The CNS role must change to allow for growth.

• • •

Movement of the CC-CNS through any of these phases occurs at varying rates and is impossible to predict. The length of time it takes to progress through each phase varies, depending on individual CC-CNSs and the system in which they are practicing. Regression often occurs, especially if the system is experiencing major changes.[19] Girard[11] describes CC-CNS role phases as cyclic rather than interacting in a circular way. A CNS does not move completely from one stage to another as experience progresses. Rather, a CNS alternates between effective and ineffective functioning with adequate functioning occurring along a continuum. This cyclic model allows for the continual fluctuating of performance along a continuum of adequate performance.

The evolution of the CNS role is characterized by continued defining, redefining, and refocusing. Because the role is designed to meet changing needs of patients and institutions, role expression must change. For example, the CC-CNS should develop the staff nurses to do what the CC-CNS has done before as the CNS develops new activities, such as chairing unit patient education and continuous quality improvement committees. CC-CNS role development must be an ongoing, dynamic process for the CC-CNS to be effective.

PRACTICE IMPLICATIONS
CC-CNS Developmental Activities

Although exact time periods cannot be attached to each phase of role development, Benner's framework can be used to present CC-CNS role development and strategies that can enhance successful role implementation. Table 3–2 describes progressive role development of each of the five role components of the CC-CNS.

Novice CC-CNS

The first year of practice as a CC-CNS is crucial in establishing credibility and laying the foundation for future development.[20] Developmental tasks include learning about the formal and informal organization, establishing relationships, building a power base, identifying influential individuals in the organization, and clarifying the CC-CNS role to self and others. Role conflict can arise if the CNS's preconceived role expectations do not conform to how the role is expected to be enacted. To learn this new role the CNS must relinquish previous roles such as student and staff nurse.

Whether a novice or an experienced CC-CNS, the newly employed CNS needs a thorough orientation (see Chapter 2). A comprehensive orientation and a job description defining specific skills help to promote role integration.[21] A competency-based orientation offers the CNS a method to demonstrate the proficiencies that are of central importance to the CC-CNS role. A competency-based orientation focuses on the integration of knowledge, skills, and attitudes necessary for the role of the CC-CNS. The CC-CNS job description should be developed based on the competencies required to implement the role. CNS competencies may differ between institutions; however, they should be based on the CNS role components of practitioner, educator, consultant, researcher, and leader or manager.[21,22]

The CC-CNS needs time to become familiar with the organizational structure, philosophy, goals, policies, and procedures of the institution and critical care unit. At the institutional level the CC-CNS supervisor identifies key individuals for the CC-CNS to meet, shares departmental objectives, and helps the CC-CNS identify skill deficits that need attention. Role expectations are discussed with a focus on short-term goals. The goals developed should pertain to the enhancement of the individual CC-CNS performance as well as to program objectives of the institution. For example, one goal for a novice CC-CNS could be to communicate to the ICU nursing staff the findings of one published study monthly if the CC-CNS supervisor wanted to develop nursing research in the ICU. The CC-CNS's goals should be shared with others whose roles interface with the CNS so they will know what to expect and what not to expect of the CC-CNS. For example, goals can be shared at staff meetings with the nurse manager and unit director. Goals can be posted in the unit for the first few months. This classification of priorities can help prevent misunderstandings and conflicts.

Novice CNSs need feedback frequently during the first year, preferably at least every 3 months.[10] For example, the administrative supervisor of the CC-CNS may wish to give feedback and encouragement to the new CNS at weekly meetings. Setting limits, addressing problem situations, and maintaining a sense of perspective are areas where a new CC-CNS may need assistance. Assigning a more experienced CNS as a preceptor to act as a role model and advocate is important. Meeting with other CNSs in the institution is helpful in learning how the CNS role is implemented and in assessing for a possible mentor. If there are no other CNSs or if all the CNSs are novices, the new CNS may be encouraged to meet with other CNSs in other institutions in the community.

Within the intensive care unit, it is imperative that the new CC-CNS demonstrate clinical competence. During the first 6 months, the CNS's clinical knowledge and skills are constantly tested by the staff. The CC-CNS cannot affect change unless critical care expertise is established. This expertise can be demonstrated through consistent involvement in direct patient care on the units for which the CC-CNS is responsible. The CC-CNS can either assign oneself to patient care or work with other nurses as they provide care. Time scheduled for direct patient care should never be cancelled.[12] During this time the CC-CNS can demonstrate clinical skills and assess the skills and educational needs of the nursing staff. The CC-CNS can begin role modeling direct patient care. In addition, the CC-CNS can become familiar with the culture of the unit as well as the protocols, standards, and

TABLE 3–2 Progressive Development of Five Roles of CNS

Stage	Characteristics
PRACTITIONER ROLE	
Novice	Purpose: Orientation to organization
	Caseload: Critically ill patients with complex needs (few)
	Other: Establish role expectations and goals with supervisor
	Consult mentor or preceptor regarding patient goals
Advanced beginner	Purpose: Orientation to CC-CNS role
	Caseload: Critically ill patients with complex needs
	Other: Less consultation with mentor
Competent	Purpose: Maintain and enhance exposure to new situations
	Caseload: Larger caseload of critically ill patients with complex needs
	Other: Functions independently
	Prioritizes caseload
	Effectively resolves problems and recognizes needs of others
Proficient	Purpose: Extend influence beyond ICU
	Caseload: Critically ill patients with complex needs
	Other: Independent
	Faster, more flexible and efficient
	Anticipates problems and complications and intervenes to manage
	Self-assured
	Greater team coordination
Expert	Purpose: Plan and implement strategies to meet "routine" clinical needs; move beyond to stretch clinical practice of staff; move into new arenas to maintain CNS interest and facilitate CNS growth
	Caseload: Critically ill patients with complex needs
	Other: Intuitive grasp
	Teaches others to identify needs and works with them to meet needs
RESEARCHER ROLE	
Novice	Familiarize self with research-based interventions in area of specialty
	Implement research findings into own practice
	Present or publish thesis
Advanced beginner	Present or publish thesis
	Incorporate research findings into standards and protocols
	Share research findings with staff
	Identify clinical issues needing research
Competent	Identify clinical issues needing research
	Join hospital nursing research committee
	Develop research study with nursing staff
	Promote incorporation of research findings into practice of staff through journal clubs and in-service workshops
Proficient	Provide leadership in hospital research committee
	Identify doctorate-prepared nurse researcher mentor
	Conduct clinical research study
	Seek funding for research
	Publish or present research findings
Expert	Conduct clinical research on a larger scale, building on previous work
	Seek national funding for research
	Continue to publish or present research findings

TABLE 3–2 Progressive Development of Five Roles of CNS *Continued*

Stage	Characteristics
EDUCATOR ROLE	
Novice	Identify and prioritize educational needs of nursing staff through direct patient care or working with staff at bedside
Advanced beginner	Develop and present formal and informal patient and staff educational programs based on identified needs
	Assist staff in development of patient, family, and staff educational materials and programs
Competent	Develop self-instructional modules or videos for staff, patients, and families
	Present programs locally and regionally
Proficient	Develop and facilitate formal programs
	Present programs nationally
	Publish
Expert	Assist other CNSs in program development
	Continue to publish
CONSULTANT ROLE	
Novice	Establish credibility clinically
	Identify key people who later may serve as source for consultations
	Clarify CNS role to self and others
Advanced beginner	Cultivate working relationship at all levels of organization
	Develop patient referral patterns and communicate to appropriate individuals (nurse manager, staff, physicians)
Competent	Demonstrate flexibility in responding to priorities
	Provide consultation to health care professionals in area of expertise
Proficient	Serve as clinical consultation in critical care to external agencies
	Provide consultation to all levels of organization
Expert	Formalize mechanism for making services and expertise available to larger audience
LEADER OR MANAGER ROLE	
Novice	Assess environment
	Learn organization
Advanced beginner	Role model professional behavior and patient advocacy
	Establish credibility
	Cultivate professional relationships
Competent	Serve as change agent in nursing service
	Demonstrate skill in problem solving, decision making, and interpersonal relationships
	Identify mentor for self
	Explore role as mentor for others
	Develop staff experts in specific areas of patient care (wound care, family crisis)
Proficient	Serve as change agent within institution
	Establish leadership role locally and regionally through presentations and consultation
	Consider doctoral study
	Become a mentor
Expert	Recognized nationally as nursing leader through relevant publications, research, consultation, presentations, and clinical practice
	Develop, implement, and evaluate innovative approaches to care delivery
	Doctoral study

level of practice. Part of the assessment includes identifying the perceived nursing leaders in the ICU, the method of new staff orientation, the relationship between the nursing staff and physicians, and the leadership style of the nurse manager. In addition, the CC-CNS can spend time in the outpatient setting working with physicians to learn more about the patient population cared for in the ICU. This experience will also promote positive relationships with the physicians. All these factors are strategies the CC-CNS will use in implementing the different CNS role components.

The CC-CNS may further substantiate the clinical role by wearing attire similar to the staff nurses and by exhibiting flexibility in scheduling self.[17] Working off shifts increases CC-CNS visibility and influences acceptance by staff. Off shifts may be scheduled in 1-week blocks or 10- to 12-hour shifts in an effort to overlap shifts. After this initial orientation period, the CC-CNS should maintain a flexible schedule to come in early or stay late to continue contact and enhance utilization by the evening, night, and weekend nursing staff. Although this type of flexibility may not be required by other nurse manager roles, flexibility and clinical visibility are essential to CNS role success.

The CC-CNS must identify and clarify the role to self and others, especially if the role is newly created. Appointments with nursing administrators and physicians are scheduled to introduce the role and discuss implementation. Attending staff meetings on all shifts to discuss the CC-CNS role and placing the CNS job description in the unit communication book for the nursing staff to review will also enhance communication of the role.

Integration into the system may be further aided by being accessible to nursing staff by beeper and distributing business cards to professional contacts (Fig. 3–1). These techniques enhance exposure of the CNS role. During this stage, information should be absorbed and judgment on issues reserved until the CNS role is accepted.[12] Keeping a log or a list of needs or ideas for future projects is helpful. Opinions of the CNS will be valued at a later time when the CC-CNS has become more knowledgeable and entrenched in the day-to-day operations of the system.

Once the baseline assessment of the units and the institutional system is completed, the CNS can formulate specific goals and action plans. This pro-

Sara Jones, RN, MSN
Critical Care Cardiac Clinical Nurse Specialist
Extension 1234, Beeper 7890
Leave message at 1233, 1232

Offers assistance in:

- **Patient Care:**
  - Care of the hemodynamically unstable patient
  - Psychosocial support for the critically ill patient and family
  - Skin care and wound management
  - Patient education concerning heart disease and implications for life-style
  - Cardiac risk factor modification
  - Activity progression for the cardiac patient
  - Low cholesterol dietary management

- **Nursing Education:**
  - In-service workshops
  - Patient care conference

ABC Medical Center

Figure 3–1 Sample business card.

cess is helpful in providing structure and direction, both of which are important for performance evaluation and for a sense of accomplishment. The CC-CNS during this stage must begin to internalize self-worth in the role.[10]

Advanced Beginner CC-CNS

The focus of activities during this stage is establishing and implementing the CC-CNS role. The CC-CNS increases visibility and credibility by spending a majority of time as an expert practitioner, role model, and patient advocate. For example, the CC-CNS can serve as a patient advocate by broadening the understanding of the nursing staff about the experience of a family with a loved one in the ICU. As an example, the CC-CNS can have one family member write down what she perceives as problems encountered in meeting the needs of her critically ill mother. By sharing this list with the ICU staff and promoting discussion, a better understanding of the ICU experience by the nursing staff may be achieved. Establishment of these aspects of the CNS role is important as the CC-CNS begins to implement change and promote education.

The CC-CNS can develop the practitioner role by implementing walking rounds to increase visibility, establish the consultant role of the CC-CNS, and develop patient referral patterns. Walking rounds provide the opportunity to identify patient care problems, suggest problem-solving strategies, and assist the staff in providing patient care, all of which help to increase credibility and enhance staff nurse acceptance. Walking rounds are best done with the nurse manager at a time of day that is selected by the nurse manager, CC-CNS, and ICU staff. Nursing staff should be encouraged to participate in walking rounds so that it does not appear that the CC-CNS is "policing" care. Participation in interdisciplinary patient care conferences provides an opportunity for the CC-CNS to function as a role model, an expert practitioner, and an advocate of the nursing staff. The interaction with other team members also helps to establish role identity and patient referrals.

Strategies that promote education of the nursing staff, patients, and families are best implemented at this time. Copies of interesting articles or pertinent clinical research can be made available through the patient chart or bulletin board. The CC-CNS should always sign her or his name with a "for your information" notice to promote the role of the CC-CNS as a resource person. Providing an opportunity for the nursing staff to identify topics is one strategy that can be used in developing a staff education program including in-service and patient care conferences. Patient education is becoming more important as changes in reimbursement policies result in earlier patient discharge. The CC-CNS can serve as a resource for the nursing staff in patient education content and can assist in the development of patient and family educational materials.

Family support by the ICU staff may not be effectively provided in the intensive care unit because of time constraints on the ICU staff. The CC-CNS can serve as a liaison for the family. The CC-CNS can often find ways to make a bureaucratic system more responsive to family needs. For example, a family member from out of town has been told there are no accommodations for her at the hospital late Friday afternoon. The CC-CNS discovers that the lack of accommodations is due to unavailability of housekeeping services to clean the room until Monday morning. A telephone call to the housekeeping supervisor results in the room being cleaned and available to the family within a short time. The CC-CNS can also promote staff nurse involvement with families by offering to "cover" the staff nurse's patient assignment so the staff nurse can participate in family conferences. However, if the CC-CNS has a relationship with the family, the CC-CNS may also need to attend the family conference.

During this period of role development, the CC-CNS is typically performing tasks that are requested from a variety of different sources. Directors may request management coverage on units without nurse managers. Nurse managers and supervisors may solicit assistance for units inadequately staffed, and staff nurses may request patient assignment coverage for a variety of reasons. These requests place the CC-CNS in a difficult situation where requests for involvement are being initiated but are often inappropriate for the CC-CNS role. The CC-CNS must decide how to cope with this dilemma without alienating management and staff. For example, if inadequate staffing is an issue, the prudent CC-CNS can facilitate care by assisting in direct care 1 day per week and creating or supporting efforts to create long-term solutions to staffing dilemmas. This strategy can reconfirm the clinical expertise of the CC-CNS, enhance role modeling to promote change, and reestablish clinical credibility in a CC-CNS who has been in the position for several years.

Because of the need to establish clinical credibility and concentrate on direct care activities, clinical research activities during this period are directed at implementing research findings of others into practice, presenting research findings at staff in-service meetings, and incorporating research findings into standards of care. Presenting or publishing one's graduate work can be useful as a starting point. Identifying potential research problems can serve as the basis for future research.

Providing concrete examples of when to call the CC-CNS will enhance role acceptance and utilization. For example, in one community hospital a CNS consultation is automatic if the patient is in the unit for more than 3 days. Recognition and positive reinforcement are powerful motivators of human behavior. They can be effectively used to develop close associations. A crucial task during this period is to develop a support system with other CC-CNSs. This provides a mechanism for communication, collaboration, and feedback regarding role development. In addition, the CC-CNS needs to develop a reality-based perspective of the setting in which she or he works and begin to work toward short-term goals or projects that can provide immediate gratification.

Competent CC-CNS

By this stage a successful CC-CNS should have established a strong power base and should be ready to focus on the role of change agent. Planned change involves competence in the skills of problem solving and decision making as well as skill in interpersonal relationships. If the CC-CNS does not have the administrative authority to implement change, credibility becomes a key element. The CC-CNS can best bring about change in clinical practice through collaboration with the nurse manager and nursing staff. This involvement may take the form of committee work with a focus on quality improvement. Beginning steps include identifying a problem, collecting relevant data, and formulating a written proposal for accomplishing the desired outcome. Inclusion of the nurse manager and staff in the process fosters the feeling of involvement and commitment to the planned change.[23]

An increase in the number of patient consultations from nurses and physicians is often seen during this period. A fee for consultation can be explored as a mechanism for generating income for the nursing department. Because of the rapidly changing population and physiologic changes in patients that occur in the ICU, the CC-CNS should be able to demonstrate flexibility in responding to priorities. If a crisis arises, the CC-CNS should be able to respond appropriately whether it be serving as a resource to the nursing staff, working with the staff, solving problems, or directing resources.

The role of the CC-CNS in patient care conferences has moved from facilitator to that of developing the staff nurse as facilitator. The development of a patient care work sheet containing relevant information (e.g., pertinent history, psychosocial assessment or problems, current status, medical assessment and plan, nursing plan, and recommendations) will enhance this process. The CC-CNS should be able to identify educational programs that are consistent with staff needs based on knowledge gained from walking rounds, communication with other health team members, and identified problem areas. The CC-CNS can facilitate

staff education by developing self-instructional modules or videos, coordinating workshops, and expanding personal development to include topics outside the ICU. The credibility and expertise of the CC-CNS have usually expanded beyond the institution, and there may be requests to present programs locally and regionally. The CNS should consider publication of clinical experiences in professional journals.

Working relationships with colleagues and professional networking are usually well established. The CC-CNS is able to participate in more leadership activities within the hospital (chairperson of a committee) and the community (AACN chapter officer). Serving as a preceptor for graduate students provides the CNS an opportunity to contribute to the professional growth and development of others. These experiences, although satisfying to many CC-CNSs, also stimulate self-evaluation and reassessment of the role. The CC-CNS can also serve as a mentor to nursing staff members.

Research efforts during this period focus on identified clinical issues. The CC-CNS may coordinate a small study or assist the staff in a research project. The formation of a journal club to disseminate research findings that may impact practice in the ICU helps to promote the implementation of research into practice.

Proficient CC-CNS

The role of the consultant is the major focus of the CC-CNS in this stage.[24] A significant amount of time is spent on consultation beyond the ICU. The CC-CNS must ensure that the nursing staff have been developed to handle clinical issues and problems the CC-CNS once handled in order to successfully move beyond the ICU. This may include clinical consultation outside the hospital or as a member or chairperson of interdisciplinary committees or involvement in projects that impact clinical practice in the ICU. However, the opportunity to provide direct patient care and to function as a role model for nursing staff in the ICU must still be integrated. This ensures that clinical expertise and credibility are maintained and enhanced, lines of communication are kept open, and opportunities to identify potential problems are maintained.

The CC-CNS with more than 5 years' experience has demonstrated competence and problem-solving ability so that she or he is able to serve as a consultant for all staff levels. Nursing administrators may seek advice about handling difficult situations or personalities, program development, or strategies to improve existing services as the CC-CNS has become management's link to the bedside. Staff nurses may consult the CC-CNS in the development of patient educational materials, in the revision of patient care forms, or in patient-focused projects. Physicians may consult the CC-CNS for system- or patient-related concerns. The CC-CNS serves as an organizational specialist and change agent because of her or his knowledge of organizational change theory.

Presenting at national meetings is an appropriate goal for this period. Collaboration with an experienced researcher or with other CNSs is realistic and rewarding. Cooper[25] suggests consideration of doctoral study at this point.

Many CNSs perceive themselves at this stage as autonomous, highly motivated, self-directed professionals.[10] Continued role development may become frozen if the goals of the institution or supervisor are seen as restrictive or incompatible or if conflicting or competing demands are made for the CC-CNS's time and attention. When such circumstances arise, even the most experienced and integrated CC-CNS needs visible administrative support and advice as well as objective, constructive counsel from a trusted mentor.

Role maturity has been achieved along with acceptance and reciprocity. Oda et al[26] describe the determinants of role maturity as proficiency, position, recognition, and reciprocity. Proficiency refers to competence in the CNS subroles of clinical practice, education, consultation, and research. After some experience in the role, a CC-CNS moves in a hierarchic or lateral manner on the organizational position ladder. Over time a CC-CNS receives recognition as an expert by others on the interdisciplinary team. Reciprocity is present between CC-CNSs as the need for testing each other disappears. Trust has been developed over numerous collaborative experiences, and role integration has occurred within the system.[1]

Expert CC-CNS

What are the role options for career advancement for the experienced CNS who has achieved a level of role maturity? Oda et al[26] found in their study of CNSs that a move to an administrative position was not considered role advancement. Their data suggest that some experienced CNSs perceive a lack of satisfaction with their current role and would benefit from role stimulation and creative challenges. Such strategies for role enhancement may be beneficial for CNS retention. Examples of such incentives are sabbaticals for self-renewal,[27] monetary recognition for clinical excellence,[28] and entrepreneurship.[29]

Wolf[30] recognizes the need of the experienced CNS to help hospitals move from quality focus to a quality–cost balance by changing the focus of the CNS from the patient and nurses to systems. Examples of this "second generation" of CNSs include identifying and correcting system-wide factors contributing to problematic patient outcomes such as length of stay or hospital-acquired complications, identifying and correcting system-wide factors contributing to inefficient and ineffective nursing practice, developing strategies to modify nursing practice while maintaining quality outcomes, evaluating new technologies and supplies for cost control effectiveness, developing innovative approaches to care delivery systems that positively affect the quality–cost balance evaluation of care through research, and developing strategies that support a resource-driven model of care.

Another strategy that may further challenge the CC-CNS is formalizing a mechanism for making services and expertise available to others, for example, forming a small company that offers educational programs. Continuing to publish clinical research, developing new research studies based on previous work, and seeking external funding for research offer new challenges. Doctoral study may be reconsidered during this period.

Strategies to Successful Role Development

Two other strategies that can enhance CNS role development are long-term goal setting and mentoring.

Setting Long-Term Goals

Goals provide a purpose, direction, and focus. The setting of goals between the CNS and supervisor provides a framework for measuring CNS effectiveness, decreases role ambiguity, fosters purposeful activity, and ensures CNS development. Through goal-setting dialogue, the organization (represented by the supervisor) and the CNS find the mutuality of purpose that binds them together.[31]

In setting a 5-year goal of professional critical care nursing practice, it is useful to list qualities that exemplify that practice, followed by activities that foster those qualities. For example, utilizing nursing research as a basis for practice and active investigation are professional nursing attributes. If the staff and institution have not been exposed to much nursing research, it may be unrealistic to expect to conduct a study during the first year. However, rather than let the research component lie dormant, the CC-CNS may develop strategies such as posting pertinent studies in the unit, exposing staff to the research basis for proposed practice innovations, critiquing a sample study to assist staff in recognizing its merits, or involving staff in small pilot studies. Once possible strategies are listed, arrange them along a loose time line based on the unique needs of the unit. This process is then repeated for other problem areas or aspects of professional practice that the CC-CNS identifies, such as accountability or continuity (establishment of primary nursing, evaluation of documentation system) and communication skills (assertiveness, conflict management skills, improved family support). After the list is completed, all aspects are arranged along a 5-year steplike time line (Fig. 3–2). The yearly deadlines are somewhat fluid, since some projects are so complex that they cannot be accomplished by a fixed date.

By creating this mental time line, the CC-CNS develops the Covey habit of "first things first"[32]; this habit involves effective self-management and the ability to organize and execute around priorities. Combined with "begin with the end in mind," this habit also helps the CC-CNS remain proactive, forward thinking, and focused on goals rather than reactive and harried. In daily practice the CNS mentally asks, "Does this activity relate to my goals?" Priority setting and decision making about time use become easier. The resulting flexibility allows the CC-CNS to react to crises such as sudden staffing shortages or accreditation visits without losing sight of progress toward the goal.

Mentoring

Mentoring can be effectively used in the development of the novice CNS. A CNS mentor can help the novice CNS clarify the role of the

Goal: Integrate nursing research as a basis for nursing practice.

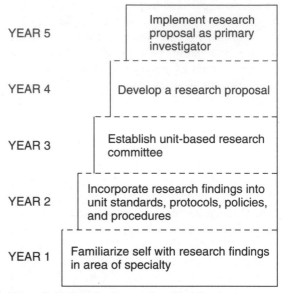

Figure 3–2 Sample 5-year plan. Timelines are approximate, and areas of focus and strategies are based on individualized unit needs.

CNS in the institution and decrease confusion, frustration, and anxiety. In addition, a CNS mentor can enhance the skills and interpersonal behaviors of the novice CNS through encouragement, guidance, sharing, and caring. The novice CNS may bring new knowledge and an unbiased perception of the CNS role. Through mutual sharing of experience and knowledge, both the mentor and the novice may benefit by enhanced self-esteem, professional productivity, and value to the institution.[33]

Mentoring is defined as a patron-protege relationship where one who is more experienced (mentor) serves as a guide, role model, counselor, teacher, and sponsor for a newer, less experienced person (protege).[34] Mentoring promotes professional development, career satisfaction, and success. Only recently has the nursing literature stressed the importance and necessity of mentoring in the development of CNSs.[33]

Mentorship is an intensely personal, active, long- or short-term relationship. Both the mentor and protege can benefit considerably from a mentorship. The mentoring relationship requires careful thought, planning, and matching of mentors and proteges.[33]

Darling[35] has identified three elements that are vital in a mentoring relationship: attraction, action, and affect. Attraction refers to the admiration or desire to emulate the mentor in some way. Action means the mentor is willing to invest time and energy in a mentoring relationship. Affect refers to the positive respectful feelings generated by a satisfying mentoring relationship.

Seeking a Mentor

Selecting a mentor requires careful matching of mentors and proteges. Not all experienced CNSs are appropriate mentors. The first step in seeking a mentor is to identify what one needs assistance with and who can specifically help. For a novice CC-CNS the logical choice is a more experienced CNS. However, the choice should also be based on admiration, affection, respect, and trust and should outweigh feelings of envy or being threatened. Mentoring relationships take time to develop, and therefore, as the novice CC-CNS is learning about the role and seeking advice and guidance, potential mentors can be evaluated. A novice CC-CNS looks for someone who can communicate knowledge and skills effectively, is creative, collaborates, and demonstrates entrepreneurship. In addition, someone who is effective with conflict resolution, is assertive, empowers, and is respected may be a potential mentor. Once a potential mentor is identified, the protege should start sharing ideas. By sharing ideas one can see if there is compatibility. Another way to select a mentor is to ask for help. By asking for help, one can tap that source and begin to establish a relationship. As a mentoring relationship develops, both the mentor and protege gain from ongoing reciprocal communication. For example, a newer CC-CNS may approach a more experienced CNS regarding a clinical issue that the newer CC-CNS has been unable to resolve. The ensuing discussions may bring into focus the newer CC-CNS's inability to work effectively with the nurse manager. The more experienced CNS, through teaching, coaching, and role modeling, can demonstrate more effective behaviors to assist in enhancing the CNS/nurse manager relationship. To facilitate a good match between a mentor and protege, congruence must exist between the mentor's and protege's perceptions

about the mentoring relationship. The best match occurs when mentors demonstrate empathy and provide concreteness, genuineness, and self-disclosure while the proteges seek to understand themselves and the roles of the CNS. Mentors must be willing to assist proteges in facing the realities of the CNS role and at the same time help them achieve the highest level of functioning possible.[33]

SUMMARY

The CC-CNS has many unique challenges in role development. Although significant barriers may exist, such as limited administrative support and guidance, limited understanding of the CC-CNS role, resistance to change, and unrealistic expectations, the CC-CNS may strive to be successful in the role. Because the CC-CNS is a nontraditional role, she or he may be viewed with suspicion. In addition, it is common with new roles that people consider one's personality as much as one's activities. Consequently, considerable responsibility is placed on the individual CC-CNS to sell the role. Specific strategies for role development have been discussed throughout this chapter. However, personal characteristics that a CC-CNS has or can acquire help with successful role development.

A CC-CNS must be flexible and open. The CC-CNS must listen to the staff's point of view, examine the constraints of the environment on the staff, and have realistic expectations of what the staff can do. An effective CC-CNS can prioritize *with* the staff, not prioritize for them. A successful CC-CNS can admit mistakes or shortcomings and be willing to look at more than one approach to solving a clinical issue. The ability of a CC-CNS to incorporate these personal characteristics is the foundation for successful CC-CNS development.

CASE STUDY

Caroline P (CP) has been the CNS for a 12-bed cardiac care unit (CCU) and 13-bed medical intensive care unit (MICU) at a large medical center for 4½ years. Her previous experience was as a staff nurse in a combined surgical intensive care unit (SICU)/MICU and later clinical instructor at a community hospital. She was then a staff nurse (full-time evenings) for 1½ years in a CCU before being promoted to the CNS position for the MICU and CCU.

During her first year in the CNS role, CP maintained a clinical focus. She spent time working with staff in the MICU to demonstrate her clinical competence. She offered several clinically focused in-service workshops in both units. Quality assessment and improvement activities focused on the measurement of QT intervals in the MICU. This project offered a way to evaluate one skill of the nursing staff, to educate the nursing staff, and to feel successful about implementing a change in practice. She used other experienced CNSs as role models and identified a mentor.

By CP's fourth year of practice, she had successfully proven her clinical competence. Her focus had shifted to include other CNS role components. Educational programs had been developed, implemented, and evaluated, such as a basic critical care course and a basic ECG course. CP has been able to identify bedside clinical issues and offer appropriate resolutions. Her consultation role had moved from nurse-to-nurse consultation at the bedside to that of a recognized expert, for example, developing a protocol for weaning from mechanical ventilation. Based on her observations of pressure ulcer development, a research project had been developed to identify variables influencing pressure ulcer development in critically ill adults. In addition, because of CP's interest in critical care nurse development, a research study was developed in collaboration with a nurse manager focusing on clinical decision making in critical care nurses.

CP identifies several barriers to her role as a CC-CNS. The first is the lack of authority. She believes that she has power only through influence and knowledge. Another barrier is the amount of energy that is devoted to maintaining communication and rapport with the nursing staff. Misperception of the CC-CNS role by others and the inability to effectively manage time are also seen as barriers.

One positive event that took place during this past year was the recognition she received from the MICU staff for her efforts. During a 4-month interval between nurse managers, CP was able to provide lead-ership, give support to the assistant nurse manager, help the staff resolve problems and work with MICU staff as a team. In recognition of her efforts, the MICU staff sponsored a catered lunch and gave her a gift. In addition, she was recognized at the annual clinical excellence in nursing award dinner for her efforts.

CP has a mentor who she uses for a clearer understanding of issues and to bounce off politically correct strategies. She identifies that she has difficulty saying "no" and has a tendency to overcommit. Her goals for the next year include expanding the consultation role, publishing, and completing her research studies.

Commentary. CP has effectively moved into the more advanced CNS role. She has learned that she has a strong power base and clear goals for the next year. She has identified her areas of weakness and effectively uses her mentor.

References

1. Biddle BJ, Thomas EJ: *Role theory: concepts and research,* Huntington, NY, 1979, Robert E Krieger Publishing Co.
2. Topham DL: Role theory in relation to roles of the clinical nurse specialist, *Clin Nurse Specialist* 1(2):81-84, 1987.
3. Benner P: *From novice to expert,* Reading, Mass, 1984, Addison-Wesley Publishing Co.
4. Villaire M: Patricia Benner: uncovering the wonders of skilled practice by listening to nurses' stories, *Crit Care Nurs* 12(6):82-89, 1992.
5. Grady KL: Evolution of a cardiac transplantation program: role of the clinical nurse specialist, *Focus Crit Care* 16(2):130-134, 1989.
6. Benner P, Tanner C, Cheslac C: From beginner to expert: gaining a differentiated clinical world in critical care nursing, *Adv Nurs Sci* 14(3):13-28, 1992.
7. Baker VE: Retrospective exploration in role development. In Padilla GV, editor: *The clinical nurse specialist and improvement of nursing practice,* Wakefield, Mass, 1979, Nursing Resources.
8. Kramer M: *Reality shock: why nurses leave nursing,* St Louis, 1974, Mosby–Year Book.
9. Oda D: Specialized role development: a three phase process, *Nurs Outlook* 25(6):374-377, 1977.
10. Hamric AB, Taylor JW: Role development of the CNS. In Hamric AB, Spross JA, editors: *The clinical nurse specialist in theory and practice,* ed 2, Philadelphia, 1989, WB Saunders Co.
11. Girard N: The CNS: development of the role. In Menard SW, editor: *The clinical nurse specialist: perspectives on practice,* New York, 1987, John Wiley & Sons.

12. Page NE, Area DM: Practical strategies for CNS role implementation, *Clin Nurse Specialist* 5(1):43-48, 1991.
13. Harrell JS, McCulloch SD: The role of the clinical nurse specialist: problems and solutions, *J Nurs Admin* 16(10):44-48, 1986.
14. Ball GB: Perspectives on developing, marketing, and implementing a new clinical specialist position, *Clin Nurse Specialist* 4(1):33-36, 1990.
15. Aradine CR, Denyes MJ: Activities and pressures of clinical nurse specialist, *Nurs Res* 21(5):411-418, 1972.
16. Clark S: The clinical nurse specialist in critical care, *Crit Care Q* 5(1):51-59, 1982.
17. Hamric AB: Role development and functions. In Hamric AB, Spross J, editors: *The clinical nurse specialist in theory and practice,* New York, 1983, Grune & Stratton Inc.
18. Holt FM: Executive practice editorial, *Clin Nurse Specialist* 1(3):116-118, 1987.
19. Tierney MJ, Grant LM, Cherrstrom PL, Morris BL: Clinical nurse specialists in transition, *Clin Nurse Specialist* 4(2):103-106, 1990.
20. Baker PO: Model activities for clinical nurse specialist role development, *Clin Nurse Specialist* 1(3):119-123, 1987.
21. DiMauro K, Mack LB: A competency-based orientation program for the clinical nurse specialist, *J Contin Educ Nurs* 20(2):74-78, 1989.
22. Fenton MV: Identifying competencies of clinical nurse specialists, *J Nurs Admin* 15(12):31-37, 1985.
23. Martin JP: From implication to reality through a unit-based quality assurance program, *Clin Nurse Specialist* 3(4):192-196, 1989.
24. Burge S et al: Clinical nurse specialist role development: quantifying actual practice over three years, *Clin Nurse Specialist* 3(1):33-36, 1989.
25. Cooper DM: A refined expert: the clinical nurse specialist after five years, *Momentum* 1(3):1-2, 1983.
26. Oda DS, Sparacino PSA, Boyd P: Role advancement for the experienced clinical nurse specialist, *Clin Nurse Specialist* 2(4):167-171, 1988.
27. Mayberry MA: Objective sabbatical: a time for self-renewal, *Nurs Admin Q* 11(2):9-12, 1987.
28. Hesterly S, Sebilia AJ: Recognizing clinical excellence, *J Nurs Admin* 16(10):44-48, 1986.
29. Strasen L: Promoting entrepreneurship in the acute setting, *J Nurs Admin* 16(11):9-12, 1986.
30. Wolf BA: Clinical nurse specialists: the second generation, *J Nurs Admin* 20(5):7-8, 1990.
31. Brown SJ: Supportive supervision of the CNS. In Hamric AB, Spross J, editors: *The clinical nurse specialist in theory and practice,* ed 2, Philadelphia, 1989, WB Saunders Co.
32. Covey SR: *The seven habits of highly effective people,* New York, 1989, Simon & Schuster.
33. Caine RM: Mentoring the novice clinical nurse specialist, *Nurse Specialist Clin* 3(2):76-78, 1989.
34. Levinson DJ: *The seasons of a man's life,* New York, 1978, Alfred A Knopf.
35. Darling LW: What do nurses want in a mentor? *J Nurs Admin* 14(10):42-44, 1984.

Part II

The Critical Care Clinical Nurse Specialist as Practitioner

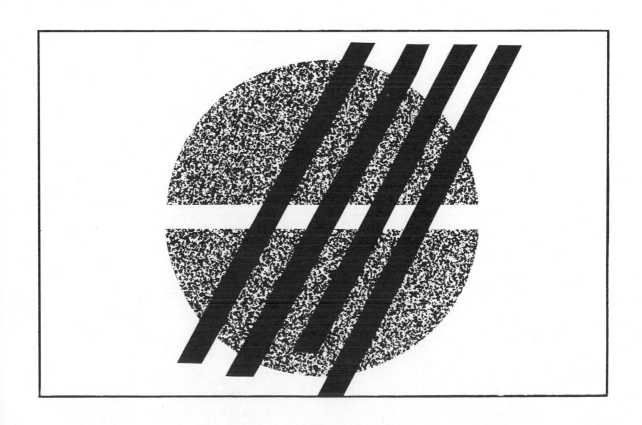

Chapter 4

The Unit-based Critical Care Clinical Nurse Specialist

Teresa Halloran, RN, MSN, CCRN
Anne Padwojski, RN, MSN, MBA, CCRN

The creation of critical care units for acutely ill patients, coupled with the increased use of technologic innovations, necessitated the development of a clinical nursing expert who could direct clinical practice and mentor new nurses. Paralleling other clinical areas, the unit-based critical care clinical nurse specialist (UB-CNS) role evolved. The evolution of the unit-based role also correlated with changes in critical care practice. As critical care units became more highly specialized, so did the UB-CNS. Now, in a health care environment focused on cost containment, the UB-CNS is again evolving. Some institutions are moving toward generalization, with the UB-CNS covering more areas than in the past. In other institutions the UB-CNS role is evolving into newer roles of case manager and director of new programs. What are the unique contributions of the UB-CNS? What does the future hold for this generic CC-CNS role? These are some of the many issues addressed in this chapter.

THEORETIC PERSPECTIVES

The UB-CNS can be defined as a master's-prepared nurse with an area of expertise related to critical illness whose practice is geographically limited to a specific patient care unit within a hospital. The UB-CNS is a formal member of the nursing team for one or more critical care units. The expertise of the individual should match most of the patients seen within the unit; however, an individual CNS may not have expertise regarding all populations but rather will develop this expertise with time in the role. For example, a pulmonary CNS

may decide to take a position in a medical intensive care unit (ICU) where the predominant population has respiratory disorders but where a number of patients have sepsis, renal failure, and diabetic complications. This UB-CNS would develop expertise in the care of the other patient populations over time.

The specific UB-CNS role is in contrast to the population-based CC-CNS (PB-CNS) described in Chapter 5 who specialized in the care of a specific patient population defined by a medical or nursing diagnosis or a disease-specific problem. The PB-CNS may follow patients to many geographic locations and generally is not part of any one nursing unit as a team member. This individual has developed expertise with a specific patient population, and her or his work focuses on meeting the population's needs.

The way in which the UB-CNS defines her or his relationship with other nursing team members is crucial to the role's success. A requirement for the successful implementation of the UB-CNS role is the development of a collegial relationship with the nurse manager, to be discussed later in this chapter.

RELATED RESEARCH AND LITERATURE

An extensive amount of literature is available about the theory and practice of the CNS. However, little literature is available regarding the practice of the CC-CNS and even less regarding the UB-CNS. Authors have attempted to clarify the role of the UB-CNS by defining their functions and competencies, such as those incorporated in

43

AACN's position statement, The Critical Care Clinical Nurse Specialist: Role Definition Position Statement.[1] Other methods have involved time delineation with the role components.[2] Arford and Olson[3] suggest that clarity of the role is best achieved by analysis of the organization goal, and identification of these goals can best be met by the UB-CNS or nurse manager. This requires an analysis of the organization's needs as well as the roles involved. A basic premise of this approach is that both the CNS and nurse manager are master's prepared.

PRACTICE IMPLICATIONS

The UB-CNS role is unique in how the role components are operationalized. This section looks at each role component and the activities that distinguish the UB-CNS from other CNS roles.

The UB-CNS Practitioner

The UB-CNS has a practice that is rooted in care of the patients in a particular critical care area. The patient population often represents a broad-spectrum. The UB-CNS will carry a caseload of patients, but usually this caseload consists of patients or families with special needs beyond the staff nurse's knowledge or experience. In addition, the UB-CNS's influence on this patient or family is usually limited to the time the patient is in critical care. When it is time for a patient from the UB-CNS's caseload to move out of critical care, the UB-CNS provides a report of the patient's critical care course and nursing diagnoses to the receiving unit. The UB-CNS's sphere of influence is therefore short-lived and geographically limited.

The physical presence of the UB-CNS on the unit facilitates collaboration between CNS and staff members. Open communications with staff regarding patient problems, conflict resolution, and troubleshooting of equipment are part of the UB-CNS's everyday activities. This vignette provides a glimpse of a UB-CNS's typical morning:

When I arrived, the night shift informed me that they again had difficulty reaching Dr. Davidson during an emergency. The nurse manager is off today so they asked if I would call and speak to him. Next, I checked the intraaortic balloon pump waveform on a heart failure patient and found dangerous timing; the night nurse had not observed the change. The charge nurse came to me at 8:15 and said that Mr. Eisen's wife was hysterical last

night and would be here at 8:30 to discuss her husband's care with us. Another patient, who was to be discharged home from the unit today, is in need of discharge teaching. (His day nurse had another very sick patient and felt he would not have time to teach the patient.) A patient care conference was scheduled for 10:00; the primary nurse caring for the patient informed me at 9:30 that she was not prepared and would not have time to prepare for it. At 11:00 a representative from the company who makes our monitoring equipment presented himself unannounced and said we had to schedule in-service programs for the equipment upgrades. In the meantime a patient arrested unexpectedly, and the family is extremely anxious, standing in the hallway crying.

In the practitioner role the UB-CNS uses the skills of negotiator, problem-solver, knowledge expert, and caregiver on a daily basis while episodically fighting fires on the unit. Within a collaborative nurse manager/UB-CNS structure the UB-CNS is accountable for quality improvement (see Chapter 7), feedback into performance appraisals, and clinical standards for nursing practice.

Establishing and Maintaining Standards of Practice

In collaboration with the nurse manager the UB-CNS is accountable for establishing and maintaining standards of care. Both parties guide and coach staff to develop unit standards. This can be accomplished through meetings with a staff-appointed committee or a unit clinical practice committee.

The UB-CNS can use AACN's outcome[4] and structure[5] standards as starting references on the unit. Another good starting point is the Agency for Health Care Policy and Research's clinical practice guidelines.[6] From this foundation, staff can develop population- and unit-based standards. Standards should be research based whenever possible or reflect expert opinion when a research base does not exist. Care standards are then incorporated into quality improvement studies and revised as nursing practice changes or new research is published.

To ensure a smooth standard implementation process the CC-CNS uses a number of strategies: (1) involvement of several staff in writing standards, (2) multimedia approaches to informing staff of changes in standards, (3) increased CC-CNS visibility on the nursing unit when new standards are implemented, (4) bedside rounds to evaluate if standards are in use and if they are being accurately interpreted, and (5) evaluation of staff performance based on their compliance with written standards of care.

The UB-CNS should be responsible for ensuring that new personnel are oriented to unit standards through critical care classes, unit skills checklists, one-on-one education, and mentoring of new nurses at the bedside. The UB-CNS may not be the person who teaches the standards but is responsible for ensuring that a mechanism is in place.

Patient Care Conferences

The patient care conference is a valuable learning tool that provides opportunities for staff to share knowledge and experiences. It also promotes group problem solving, group cohesiveness, and creativity. Other benefits of patient care conferences include reinforcement of practice standards, incorporation of research findings into the care plan, discussion on application of current nursing diagnoses, and staff development as clinical leaders.

Setting up the patient care conference requires planning and direction from the UB-CNS. The conference should be presented by staff; however, the UB-CNS may present the first conference with staff assistance as a model for future conferences. In future conferences the UB-CNS would serve as a consultant.

Staff can benefit from a simple form that outlines the topics for the conference and allows space for the nurse to make notes about the patient (see box).

Patient case studies can include unusual or challenging nursing diagnoses or common patient diagnoses with critical evaluation of routines and ideas for improvement. The conference may be at a mutually set time, or it may be presented on each shift. It is also beneficial to involve other health care personnel as appropriate to the care plan (i.e., social work, physical therapy, respiratory therapy), because this reinforces a team approach to patient care. Conferences may be held weekly at a specific time or may be decided on informally on a shift basis.

Patient care conferences can be formal or informal. Formally planned conferences can be advertised with flyers or during unit meetings. Advantages to formally planned meetings are advanced staff awareness and increased preparation time. Disadvantages to formal conferences are that

---

WORKSHEET FOR PATIENT CARE CONFERENCE

Date _____

Patient Name _____

Hospital Number _____

CONDENSED PERTINENT HISTORY:

PSYCHOSOCIAL ASSESSMENT/ PROBLEMS:

MEDICAL PROBLEMS, CURRENT ASSESSMENT, AND PLAN:

NURSING DIAGNOSES/NURSING PLAN:

CONCLUSIONS/RECOMMENDATIONS/ FOLLOW-UP:

---

patient problems may change by the time the conference is held, whereas informal conferences address current problems. Informal planning can be rushed, and staff and ancillary personnel may be unable to attend at short notice.

Once the conference is completed, the care plan should be changed to reflect conference results. The conference should be formally written or summarized for the entire staff to read. A conference book is helpful to document patient care conference results and allow absent staff members an opportunity to review the discussion. Patient care conferences are also a quality monitoring tool that can be shared on hospital accreditation visits.

The UB-CNS as Educator

Unlike the PB-CNS the UB-CNS is accountable for education and orientation of staff members. In some hospitals this responsibility is shared with an educational specialist assigned to the unit. Details of the CC-CNS staff education role are covered in Chapter 8.

Patient education is one of the features of the PB-CNS and the UB-CNS. The basic difference is in the amount of time spent in this activity. Whereas the PB-CNS spends a significant amount of time in this direct patient care role, the UB-CNS is more of a coordinator of patient education activities on the unit. As described in Chapter 9, the critical care setting presents unique barriers to patient education. These barriers require the UB-CNS to be creative in patient education programs.

The UB-CNS as Manager/Leader

Successful implementation of the UB-CNS role requires collegial relationships with the nurse manager. An informal survey by one of the authors (TH) showed that UB-CNS role conflicts occurred most often with physicians and nurse managers. The common factors for role conflict are authority over clinical practice decision and policy decisions regarding clinical practice activities. It is imperative for the UB-CNS to outline role responsibilities with the nurse manager and to understand and appreciate the specific contributions of the nurse manager to unit functions. The new UB-CNS meets with the nurse manager to discuss the role of the UB-CNS within the unit and how the two roles will interface to meet mutually set goals. The nurse manager is vital to the success of the role, because the manager is the key support for implementation and can assist in developing and reinforcing the role in the unit. Effective utilization of both roles can result in better patient outcomes and a more efficient unit. The UB-CNS role must be clearly defined by both the UB-CNS and the nurse manager so that mutual goal achievement is recognized and role conflict avoided.

The UB-CNS and nurse manager team begins with common goal setting. On an annual or biannual basis the UB-CNS and nurse manager meet to set up annual goals. During this planning session the UB-CNS can outline where the nurse manager can assist. Once these goals are defined, regular meetings are established to review goal achievement. Other strategies for establishing and building the team include (1) weekly meetings on current issues; (2) joint consultation on issues specific to

expertise; (3) joint planning of unit-based activities, such as education courses and negotiating joint projects and individual responsibility; (4) open communications in resolution of conflicts and role confusion; and (5) mutual support during times of high stress (e.g., the UB-CNS offers to assist the nurse manager with performance evaluations during budget time).

The UB-CNS Researcher Role

Research knowledge is vital to content expertise and validation of practice at an advanced level. A research-based practice differentiates the UB-CNS from the experienced staff nurse and distinguishes the UB-CNS as an advanced practitioner. Anderson and Hicks[7] have stated that the CNS at the very least should be able to interpret, evaluate, and communicate to nursing staff research findings relevant to their clinical specialty.

A detailed discussion of research generation and utilization is presented in Chapters 13 and 14. This section briefly focuses on the UB-CNS's role in research.

The UB-CNS must first have access to current nursing research journals and critical care nursing literature. If an institution does not have a library, the UB-CNS can get subscriptions to journals through the nursing department. Access to computers with library search capabilities is also helpful.

Second, the UB-CNS must schedule time for reading research articles. It is now relatively easy to have a search program within the UB-CNS's office computer. (The National Library of Medicine's program, Grateful Med, is available for $29/yr, and the user then pays for time spent running a search, which on the average is 30 cents per search.[8]) Within minutes a subject can be thoroughly searched using any number of search programs and information readily obtained to be discussed with staff at the bedside.

Third, the UB-CNS can develop a research-based foundation by (1) attending nursing programs with a research component, (2) attending local nursing organizational meetings where networking opportunities exist, (3) participating in physician rounds and questioning physicians about innovations in patient care, and (4) attending research-based medical meetings.

A fourth way the UB-CNS can promote research-based practice is to replicate a pertinent study from the nursing literature to further validate or refute research findings as a foundation for a change in practice. Gaits et al.[9] described a unit-based research forum in which the research on accuracy of coagulopathy results drawn from venous vs. arterial lines was reviewed for application in clinical practice. The staff developed a research utilization protocol based on these findings and evaluated the results of their study. Consequently, the unit policy was changed and staff members now obtain their coagulopathy specimens from an arterial line.

Last, research can be incorporated into rounds and patient care conferences by the UB-CNS. As the patient's progress is reviewed at the bedside, the UB-CNS can use this time to review pertinent research findings and explore alternative interventions for patient management.

The ability to generate, disseminate, and use research is essential to the UB-CNS. The UB-CNS incorporates research into practice to improve patient outcomes, delete unnecessary nursing rituals, and provide cost-effective care.

The UB-CNS as Consultant

The UB-CNS role as a clinical expert promotes consultation with nursing staff, physicians, other departments, and the nurse manager. Since the position is unit based, consultation outside of the unit may be limited; however, other nursing units or departments may periodically require the assistance of the UB-CNS. For example, a gastrointestinal laboratory supervisor who has purchased a new defibrillator and monitor may approach the UB-CNS about providing an in-service workshop on the new equipment or for help to develop a policy for its use.

Variations in UB-CNS Role Implementation

The UB-CNS does not practice nursing in the traditional manner of staff nurses. One of the earlier components of CNS practice was as a primary care practitioner for a specific patient caseload. The emphasis seems to have changed from direct caregiver to a more integrated, broader approach of consultant, teacher, and researcher. This changing emphasis has occurred as a result of nurses and institutions examining how to attain maximum utilization of a nurse prepared at the master's level.[10]

Various surveys have found that neither administrators nor CNSs view direct routine patient care as a function of the CNS. The UB-CNS must identify and define the target group that requires the CNS's services. The target group could be physicians, nurses, or select patient populations. Thus a variety of utilization patterns for the UB-CNS is available.

The traditional focus of unit-based practice is based on geography and the types of patients admitted to the specific unit. Depending on the type of unit, the UB-CNS would work with organ-specific critical care patients (e.g., open heart surgery) or a broad spectrum of critical care patients (e.g., medical-surgical unit). The traditional focus of the UB-CNS has evolved, paralleling the evolution of critical care units. Unit-based practice in smaller community hospitals may not be possible because of limited resources. The CC-CNS may be expected to have multiple roles involving a variety of units or patient services. In larger urban teaching institutions with multiple disease- or organ-specific critical care units, unit-based practice may be the norm. For the UB-CNS to be successful, the realities and constraints of the setting must be taken into account.[11]

Current and Future Trends Impacting UB-CNS Role

A number of trends in critical care have impacted or will impact the UB-CNS. Reduction in health care reimbursement and increased acuity have spurred the development of innovative utilization patterns for the CC-CNS, such as case management. Some UB-CNSs are transitioning into a pure case management role (see also Chapter 6). In this role the CC-CNS may have increased administrative responsibilities and potentially less emphasis on clinical management, particularly in working with nursing staff. In turn, the UB-CNS gains authority and accountability for patient care outcomes, which can be a source of personal satisfaction.

Many hospitals are downsizing and combining smaller critical care units under one manager. For some the setting will remain organ specific. Combinations include cardiac medicine and surgery or neurologic medicine and surgery. Other units will have patients with multifactorial diseases. Instead of creating new units for newly developed critical care programs (e.g., transplant surgery), these patients will be incorporated into an exisiting system. This will require a more global focus of the UB-CNS, or it may create opportunities for a PB-CNS or case manager within a multipurpose unit, such as a bone marrow transplant PB-CNS in the setting of a larger surgical ICU with pre-hospitalization and post-hospitalization responsibilities.

Managers may not be able to hold the traditional position of clinical expert and manager in large multicombination units. The manager will rely on the UB-CNS to oversee implementation of unit goals and projects and to take full responsibility for quality patient care.

As the capabilities of the UB-CNS are recognized, the institution will seek to broaden this individual's scope of influence. The UB-CNS may have multiple requests for guidance in program development and patient management outside the normal practice setting or target population. This has the potential to dilute the effectiveness of the role within the unit. It is therefore important for the UB-CNS to keep constantly aware of the institution's goals and ever-changing philosophy. Formal committees of all hospital-based CNSs should be developed to provide an opportunity for networking, sharing information, and reacting as a whole to issues related to role implementation.

CASE STUDY

Mr. K. is a 53-year-old man admitted to the cardiac care unit with ischemic cardiomyopathy and refractory ventricular tachycardia. This is not his first admission for this condition. He has previously undergone ablation on three occasions over the past 2 years; all three were unsuccessful. He has been evaluated for a heart transplant and is now on the waiting list. Because at this admission he is quite ill with pneumonia as well as heart failure, an intraaortic balloon pump (IABP) is inserted.

His wife is a very dependent woman who relies primarily on her husband as a source of support. She is particularly anxious because of Mr. K.'s declining condition. While at the bedside, she is constantly questioning the nurse about the care she is giving Mr. K. Mrs. K. also keeps making suggestions for his care that are not particularly appropriate. For ex-

ample, she feels that exercise of his extremities is very important, and she continues to lift up his leg with the IABP present when when the nurse has explained why this should not be done.

The nursing staff approached the UB-CNS, Linda Stevens, regarding Mrs. K.'s behavior. They told Linda that they felt Mrs. K. was very manipulative and that she made them feel very uncomfortable. The nurses are starting to "pull straws" in morning report to decide who will care for Mr. K., because no one is comfortable working with his wife.

Linda decided that a patient care conference was indicated. She spoke with the nurse caring for Mr. K. and decided on a good time for the conference that day. The nurse was asked to complete the care conference worksheet (see opposite page) and to bring this with her to the meeting. Linda contacted the heart transplant coordinator and the heart transplant social worker to invite them to participate in the conference.

All the staff working that day attended the conference while the nurse manager and assistant nurse manager observed the patients. The conference was held in the unit, in an area out of hearing of patients and families but close enough for staff to be available in an emergency. The nurse caring for Mr. K. presented his history and current nursing and medical problems. Some of the other staff members joined in to add their observations about Mrs. K.'s behavior. Linda inquired as to whether Mrs. K. had every received formal psychologic support or evaluation. The heart transplant social worker said that Mrs. K. had undergone the usual evaluation with her husband and that she had seemed all right at the time (3 months ealier), In their discussion the group determined that Mrs. K.'s behavior was situational and that a consistent approach by nursing staff might be all that was needed to support her.

An action plan was developed (Fig. 4–1) that included interventions by the social worker (who had a relationship with Mr. K.) and the UB-CNS who represented the unit as a manager and who could also be a source of support to Mrs. K.

Date 4-29-94

Patient Name Mr. K.

Hosp. Number 163-22-47

CONDENSED PERTINENT HISTORY: 53 yr. old male with ischemic Cardiomyopathy, ventricular aneurysm and refractory v. tachycardia. Unsuccessful ablation x3. Admitted with pneumonia and heart failure.

PSYCHOSOCIAL ASSESSMENT/PROBLEMS: Patient's wife not coping well with loss of control over patient's illness; this is making patient care difficult for nurses. Pt. is coping well; but has expressed fears of dying.

MEDICAL PROBLEMS, CURRENT ASSESSMENT, AND PLAN: Pt. currently on Bretylium at 5mg/min. and lopressor. IABP on 1:1. Ventricular tachycardia is associated with emotional excitement; e.g. bad dreams and anxiety. Pt. is on list awaiting heart transplant.

NURSING DIAGNOSES/NURSING PLAN:

1. Ineffective family coping secondary to patient's illness and high risk for sudden death.
   Plan: a) Take wife away from bedside to discuss her perceptions about what the patient needs.
   b) Have CNS meet with wife in private to discuss her concerns about the nursing care and pt's. condition.
   c) Assign consistent caregivers as much as possible.

CONCLUSIONS/RECOMMENDATIONS/FOLLOW-UP:

1. Patient care conference to be repeated in 4 days to assess wife's response to interventions.
2. Nursing care plan to be revised by primary nurse with assistance from the CNS with suggestions for how to approach Mrs. K.
3. CNS to arrange for daily reports to wife on patient's condition by the house staff.

Figure 4–1 Work sheet for patient care conference

The plan was implemented and evaluated 1 week later. Although some of Mrs. K.'s behaviors improved, others did not change. It was decided that a formal psychologic consultation was indicated. The UB-CNS, in collaboration with the staff nurse, spoke with Mr. K.'s cardiologist regarding the need for this consultation. The cardiologist agreed, and a psychologist was contacted.

One week later, as Mr. K.'s condition was improving, Mrs. K. began to show signs of improvement in her response to his illness. She was still quite anxious but had taken control of her anxiety. The staff had now all been made aware of Mrs. K.'s behavior and had been given strategies by the psychologist for working with her. They felt a sense of accomplishment in being able to better manage this difficult family member.

SUMMARY

The nursing leaders who first envisioned the CNS role most likely pictured the unit-based CNS position. From this generic concept the CNS role has germinated into many variations. Although this book is directed toward all CC-CNS roles, this chapter has focused on the implementation of the UB-CNS. The discussion here is brief, since many of the UB-CNS's responsibilities are covered throughout this book. This chapter has defined the UB-CNS role and demonstrated some of the ways this role is distinct from other CC-CNS roles.

References

1. American Association of Critical Care Nurses: *Competence statements for critical care nurses,* Laguna Niguel, Calif, 1989, The Association.
2. Robichaud A, Hamric A: Time documentation of clinical nurse specialist activities, *J Nurs Admin* 16(1):31-36, 1986.
3. Arford P, Olson M: A structural perspective of nurse manager and clinical nurse specialist collaboration, *Clin Nurse Specialist* 2:119-126, 1988.
4. American Association of Critical Care Nurses: *Outcome standards for nursing care of the critically ill,* Laguna Niguel, Calif, 1990, The Association.
5. American Association of Critical Care Nurses: *Standards for nursing care of the critically ill,* Laguna Niguel, Calif, 1989, The Association.
6. U.S. Department of Health and Human Services: *Clinical practice guideline: acute pain management: operative or medical procedures and trauma,* Rockville, Md, 1992, The Department.
7. Anderson G, Hicks S: The clinical nurse specialist—role, overview, and future prospects, *Austr Nurses J* 15(8):36-38, 1986.
8. U.S. Department of Health and Human Services: *National Library of Medicine fact sheet on grateful med,* Bethesda, Md, August, 1992, National Institutes of Health.
9. Gaits V et al: Unit-based research forums: a model for the clinical nurse specialist to promote research, *Clin Nurse Specialist* 3(2):60-64, 1989.
10. Montemuro M: The evolution of the clinical nurse specialist: response to the challenge of professional nursing practice, *Clin Nurse Specialist* 1:106-110, 1987.
11. Stark P: Factors influencing the role of the oncology clinical nurse specialist, *Oncol Nurs Forum* 10:54-58, 1983.

The Critical Care Clinical Nurse Specialist in Joint Practice with Physicians

Diane K. Dressler, RN, MSN, CCRN, CCTC

A major health care trend affecting critical care delivery systems is that of increasing specialization. Major medical centers have multiple critical care units with increasingly specialized patient populations. For example, units may be designated as medical, surgical, cardiovascular medical, cardiovascular surgical, respiratory, pediatric, neurologic, trauma, or transplant. Expert clinicians with advanced educational preparation are a necessary component of this system, which aims to provide high-quality care for these highly specialized, high-risk, high-cost patients. The population-based CC-CNS (PB-CNS) is valued more than ever as an individual who can provide continuity in patient care and who can educate the health care team about specialized patient needs. This chapter explores the PB-CNS role, using the example of a CC-CNS in joint practice with a cardiothoracic surgeon.

THEORETIC PERSPECTIVES
PB-CNS Framework and Definitions

PB-CNS specializes in the care of a specific patient population defined by a medical or nursing diagnosis or a disease-specific problem. For example, a PB-CNS may specialize in diabetes, pediatric cardiology, pulmonology, thanatology, pain management, body image disturbances, or crisis intervention. In critical care this specialization has followed the specialization of critical care units and may include CC-CNSs with expertise in areas such as cardiovascular surgery or transplantation. The

PB-CNS role has several characteristics that distinguish it from the unit-based CNS (UB-CNS). Whereas the UB-CNS is hired by the nursing department and is an employee of the hospital, the PB-CNS may be employed by the hospital, by a clinic, or by physicians. The PB-CNS operates within the five CNS role components (see Chapter 1) but spends more time in the practitioner, consultant, and educator roles than in other roles.[1] Compared with the UB-CNS, the PB-CNS spends little time in staff development and education and more time in primary patient care. Patient interventions by the PB-CNS may be acute (as in the diabetes CNS who educates patients about their insulin) or long term (as with the joint practice CNS who sees patients in an ongoing manner with a physician). The PB-CNS often works within a wide geographic distribution in critical care and non–critical care areas and is therefore viewed as a resource for all nurses caring for patients within the PB-CNS's area of expertise.

The PB-CNS who is hired by the hospital or by the nursing department often holds departmental responsibilities, such as participation in hospital committees. This individual may also be expected to teach nursing courses along with the UB-CNSs. In contrast, the PB-CNS who is hired by a physician or physicians (i.e., joint practice CC-CNS [JP-CNS]) is accountable only to the practice and the patients within that practice. Although the JP-CNS communicates with nursing staff within the hospital setting, the link with hospital nursing is informal and the degree of involvement with hospital nursing depends on how the JP-CNS operationalizes the role.

The JP-CNS

Physicians have recently recognized the value of expert nurses and have come to rely on them for consultation with special patient populations. As interactions between CNSs and physicians have increased, liaisons have resulted in physician-nurse teams. An increasing number of physicians and nurses are seeking professional arrangements with the goal of ensuring high-quality care for a specific group of complex patients.[1-4] These associations have been referred to as associated practice, collaborative practice, and joint practice.

The terms "associated practice" and "collaborative practice" are applied broadly to describe a setting where nurses, physicians, and other health care providers work together cooperatively. These relationships are characterized by open communication, shared responsibility, problem solving, decision making, and the carrying out of mutually agreed on plans for patient care.[5] The term" joint practice" refers to a formal arrangement where a nurse and physician work together in a peer relationship. Typically both will be employed by a practice corporation or institution. Because they mutually share responsibility for patients, they each contribute unique skills and perspectives, increasing the quality of care and their own role satisfaction.

The joint practice movement began approximately 20 years ago. The National Joint Practice Commission was established in 1972 by the American Nurses Association and the American Medical Association with funding from the W.K. Kellogg Foundation.[6] The purpose of the commission was to study nurse-physician relationships and make recommendations regarding collaborative practice. The commission worked for 10 years, increasing trust and cooperation between nurses and physicians. Their goal was to see nurses and physicians working together to provide improved patient care.

The development of the nurse practitioner role in the 1970s further advanced the concept of joint practice. A nurse practitioner can be defined as "a registered nurse who holds a certificate entitling her/him to provide primary health care under the direction of a physician."[1] Nurse practitioners implemented joint practice in primary care settings and began moving into the hospital setting in the 1980s.[7] During this same period, advanced practice nurses in the form of CNSs increased in numbers. Hospital-based physicians began to recognize and respect the competency of these advanced practice nursing roles.

A number of factors have influenced the advancement of these expanded roles for nurses. Stereotyping of nurses as subservient to physicians persists despite the current social changes in women's roles.[8] Many still view the advanced practice nursing role as a physician substitute and fail to see nursing's unique contributions.[9] Institutional barriers face the joint practice nurse who wishes to obtain clinical privileges. In some areas advanced practice nurses have been forced to obtain licensure as physician assistants to gain practice privileges. It is fortunate that these situations have diminished and nurses are overcoming these barriers and assuming increased responsibility for health care delivery through these expanded roles.[10]

Successful joint practice recognizes and utilizes each discipline's different areas of expertise. There is general agreement that nursing and medical services are complementary but not usually interchangeable either in responsibility or accountability.[11] Nursing's expertise relates to psychosocial assessment and intervention, patient teaching, counseling, health maintenance, caring, and comforting.[6] Physician expertise relates to disease identification, treatment plans, and medical management. Blending this care and cure process provides a level of care that could not be provided by either discipline alone.

In joint practice, physician and nurse expertise begins to mesh. The nurse in advanced practice has skills in areas that overlap the medical domain, such as physical examination, diagnostic testing, and therapeutic management. Since the nurse does not abandon the role of caring, comforting, and guiding, the nurse and physician roles continue to be complementary. Conversely, physicians may demonstrate increased involvement in areas previously considered to be within the nursing domain, such as health promotion and patient education. The overlap of these areas increases mutual understanding and leads to optimal patient care, as together the nurse and physician provide more comprehensive care than either can provide alone.

RELATED RESEARCH AND LITERATURE

Although numerous articles describe the PB-CNS, few articles have been written on the joint practice collaborative practice CNS role.[1] One of the most comprehensive and enlightening studies was conducted by Riegel and Murrell.[1] In this descriptive study the authors investigated perceptions of competency behaviors of JP-CNSs and sought to describe the subroles that make up this expanded CNS role.

Fifty-four JP-CNSs participated in this study. Of interest is that nine (17%) were dual qualified as CNSs and nurse practitioners. About one third (35%) were invited by the physician into the collaborative practice. Forty-four percent felt physicians hired them to implement the CNS role (e.g., patient/family education, nursing perspective in practice), and 42% felt that physicians had low, vague, absent, or unrealistic expectations. Some physicians expected the JP-CNS to save them time and increase the number of patients the practice could handle. Others expected the JP-CNS to work as an assistant, secretary, or office nurse.

Geographically, the JP-CNSs spent the majority of their time in the office or hospital, with some making home visits. Only 36% of JP-CNSs had formal hospital privileges. These privileges included permission to visit patients and access to medical records. Only 37% had permission to dictate; 48% wrote medical orders; and 31% admitted or discharged patients.

Twenty-one percent of JP-CNSs billed insurance companies for reimbursement. None of these reimbursed were both CNSs and nurse practitioners, but seven were medical-surgical CNSs.

Figure 5–1 shows time spent in various activities. About half of the JP-CNS's time was spent in the practitioner role, with the rest of time divided among research, education, and consultation. The researchers sought to explore differences between the JP-CNS and the CNS/nurse practitioner but found no significant differences between the two roles. This may have been in part because of the small sample sizes.

Essential competencies for the JP-CNS were identified (Table 5–1). As the authors note, "These

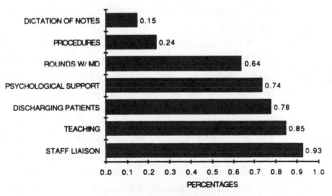

Routine hospital duties (N = 46).

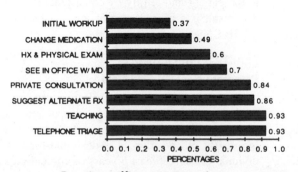

Routine office practice duties (N = 45).

Figure 5–1 Time spent by joint practice clinical nurse specialists in hospital and office practice duties. (From Riegel B, Murrell T: CNS in collaborative practice, *Clin Nurse Specialist* 1(2):63-66, 1987.

TABLE 5-1 Essential Competencies of CNS Respondents (N = 53)

	Mean	Standard deviation
Demonstrates clinical expertise in selected area of practice	5.82	0.43
Continues to develop in-depth knowledge base to promote patient care	5.78	0.55
Accepts personal accountability for patient care	5.75	0.52
Serves as role model for advanced nursing practice	5.63	0.63
Provides consultation to patients	5.62	0.73
Functions within laws affecting advanced nursing practice	5.62	0.75
Promotes individualized patient care that reflects depth, breadth, and continuity	5.53	0.70
Works collaboratively to facilitate interdisciplinary health care	5.50	0.71
Assumes leadership to facilitate interdisciplinary collaboration	5.44	0.70

From Riegel B, Murrell T: CNS in collaborative practice, *Clin Nurse Specialist* 1(2):63-66, 1987.

priorities reflect a focus on expert interdisciplinary clinical practice and professional responsibilities. The low priority items appear to reflect many of the constructs deemed essential by the profession, e.g., nursing diagnoses, theory, and research."[1] The authors suggested several reasons for this finding: (1) JP-CNSs may lack time to commit to theoretic nursing ideals; (2) physician partners may not value these competencies; and (3) the JP-CNS may feel these are skills that are already mastered.

Other studies on the JP-CNS role have supported the result of Riegel and Murrell. Littell[3] described an office-based collaborative cardiology practice. The JP-CNS role focused on patient management from initial office visits to hospitalization, posthospitalization care, and even home visits. Specific activities included history taking, physical examination, test and treatment collaborative decision making, patient education, telephone triage, independent treatment of minor conditions, and office management.

In another cardiology collaborative model, Burke[2] assisted with office procedures such as treadmill tests and interpreted test results. Nursing-specific activities included patient counseling on cardiac risk factor modifications (weight loss, stress reduction, diet, and exercise).

Nowicki[4] worked collaboratively with a plastic surgeon. In this JP-CNS model, she focused on nursing issues, including psychosocial support, continuity of care, coping disorders, body image changes, and impaired skin integrity.

The literature describes advanced nursing practice models where the nurse practices in an outpatient setting, an inpatient setting or both.[12] The JP-CNS is an example of such an individual. In collaboration with a physician, the JP-CNS develops guidelines that define the scope of her or his practice. The hospital where the JP-CNS will see patients must also develop guidelines for defining the scope of practice for this role. The specific duties may change as the nurse's skills increase, but the JP-CNS always practices within these guidelines.

In the critical care setting, the JP-CNS evaluates patient's needs, assessed for nursing care problems, and anticipates and plans for future needs. In addition, the JP-CNS serves an important liaison role with families, communicating with and counseling them in the absence of the physician. Often the JP-CNS is able to provide data obtained in the outpatient setting that facilitates individualized care. Briding the gap between outpatient and inpatient care enhances the quality of care and provides a unique opportunity for emotional support to the patient and family by consistent caregivers. The result is a high degree of job satisfaction for the JP-CNS.[1]

PRACTICE IMPLICATIONS
Preparation for JP-CNS Role

Graduate education is necessary to prepare for entering joint practice in a specialty area. Although a new master's-prepared nurse can enter into a JP-CNS position, it is desirable for this individual to have at least 5 years of clinical nursing experience with the specific patient population.

Previous CNS experience is not necessary but is helpful.

When exploring the possibility of a joint practice association, a number of things should be considered. The joint practice concept will most likely be successful in a physician practice with practitioners able to collaborate effectively and delegate professional tasks. This may follow naturally with physicians who routinely interact with critical care nurses, since collaborative practice has often already been established.[8]

In meeting the physician, the JP-CNS must come prepared to articulate the advantages of nurse-managed care from the physician's perspective. Suggested topics include (1) crisis intervention skills, (2) patient education, (3) management of complicated patients' needs, (4) telephone triaging and counseling, (5) independent management of minor patient problems, (6) improved continuity of care, (7) an ability to work with hospital nursing staff to solve patient care issues, (8) potential increased patient and family satisfaction, (9) potential reduced patient complications and length of hospital stay, and (10) potential time savings for the physician. It is important to know in advance if you will be able to generate any independent income or how this could be accomplished. It is equally important to come to this meeting with knowledge of the salary range for JP-CNSs in your community.

Job expectations should be clearly defined and negotiated to ensure the JP-CNS is not taking on nonnursing responsibilities. The time commitment, especially pertaining to weekend time and call time, should be clarified. Other employment issues to be addressed include malpractice insurance, attendance to professional meetings, and coverage for time off. Much thought, discussion, and trust needs to go into the planning of a successful joint practice relationship.

Organizational support is another component of a successful joint practice. The scope of physician activities is defined by the medical staff of an institution, but that of a JP-CNS is less easily defined.[1] The JP-CNS may be openly opposed, merely tolerated, or effectively integrated into the health care team. For the first JP-CNS within an institution, mechanisms for granting practice privileges will need to be developed. The new JP-CNS can facilitate this process by meeting with key individuals from within the institution: director of nursing, medical staff committee chair, unit-based CNSs within the institution, and the nurse managers of areas where the JP-CNS will see patients. It may be necessary to "sell" the joint practice concept. All of these individuals will want to know exactly how the JP-CNS will interact with patients and staff, how interventions will be communicated, and how their role will interface with UB-CNSs. Early on, the JP-CNS should meet with staff in patient care areas and discuss her or his role. Once staff members recognize the value of the JP-CNS's knowledge and skills, they quickly accept and utilize this individual.

Nurses in joint practice relationships recognize that over time medical and nursing activities may begin to mesh, resulting in some degree of professional role diffusion.[13] Examples of typical physician responsibilities that a JP-CNS may take on include ordering of diagnostic tests (echocardiograms, computed tomography [CT] scans of the brain, 12-lead electrocardiograms [ECGs]), and removal of invasive lines or tubes (eg., chest tubes, pacing wires, femoral sheaths, pulmonary artery catheters). In reverse, the physician, learning from the JP-CNS, may begin to think about continuity of care needs earlier in patients' hospitalization and may call for a visiting nurse consultation several days before discharge.

The impact of joint practice activities on patient outcomes needs to be examined. It would also be of value to examine JP-CNSs' knowledge and ability to manage medical ailments. This knowledge could provide further evidence for CNS management of primary health problems and a rationale for expansion of reimbursement of CNS interventions.

JP-CNS in a Cardiothoracic Surgery Practice

Through education and extensive clinical experience, the CC-CNS is uniquely qualified to assist with the management of patients with unusual and complex problems. One such patient group who benefits from the specialized skill of the CC-CNS is the cardiothoracic surgery patient. A number of characteristics of specialty practice require nurse management and may prompt the addition of a CC-CNS to the cardiac surgery practice.

Cardiac surgery, like many specialty practices,

is a field of high technology and continuous innovation. The many high-risk patients currently undergoing cardiovascular surgical procedures require nursing care management throughout the hospitalization and transition into the home. Patients who receive thoracic organ transplants, mechanical circulatory assist devices, and investigational drugs require intense nursing management that can be facilitated by joint practice teams. The research aspects of these complex procedures require a clinical coordinator who is often an advanced practice nurse. The increased technology also increases the need for humanizing the care and providing consistent emotional support to the patient and family. The JP-CNS works with staff nurses as an educator and resource who is available to assist with the management of these patients.

Because of the complexity of patient problems and therapeutic procedures, attention to detail is necessary in both the preoperative and postoperative periods to ensure safe patient care. Preoperative patients are interviewed and screened by the JP-CNS for physical or emotional problems that may complicate the surgery. Appropriate intervention is carried out to ensure that the patient is in optimal condition for surgery. For example, medical management in patients with poorly controlled diabetes is intensified before surgery, and these patients require planned nursing interventions after surgery to prevent blood sugar abnormalities and wound complications.

Postoperatively, numerous problems are identified by staff nurses, patients, family members, and community health nurses that require nursing management, such as problems with wound care, sleep disturbance, elimination medication side effects, pain control, and ineffective coping. The JP-CNS is the person who provides continuity for patient care through the various phases of illness and ensures ongoing communications with all health care providers. In a busy surgical practice the JP-CNS can be called on to help prioritize and facilitate rapid medical intervention for emergent situations.

Components of the JP-CNS Role

The JP-CNS operates within the five CNS role components, with emphasis on the practitioner, educator, and consultant roles.

Practitioner

The JP-CNS works with patients in both inpatient and outpatient settings. Cardiovascular surgical patients, for example, are preoperatively in settings that vary from the physician's office to the critical care unit. Patients are observed daily, with special attention and time given to medically complex patients or patients with multiple nursing diagnoses. The role is one of communication and coordination of patient care. Communications are with patient, family, consulting physicians, bedside nursing staff, and other patient care providers. A major part of the JP-CNS role includes problem identification and management.

Over time the JP-CNS becomes astute at identifying problems associated with the cardiovascular surgical patient and works with others to prevent problems or to intervene early in their management. Observation of numerous patients with similar illness trajectories yields practical wisdom on how to manage problems such as poor wound healing, pulmonary complications, and physical deconditioning. Interpretation of individual problems is simplified by knowledge regarding the patient's health history and whether the problem existed preoperatively (e.g., the patient with history of a focal neurologic deficit preoperatively develops the same postoperatively). When problems occur, emotional support is facilitated by the CNS's established relationship with the patient and family. For example; when a complication such as wound infection occurs in the critical care unit, the JP-CNS works with the critical care nurses to devise a care plan that meets the patient's and family's need for information as well as the patient's physiologic needs.

Although research has demonstrated that many JP-CNSs do not function within a nursing framework,[1] I have found a nursing diagnosis–based practice to be useful in guiding interventions. Following cardiac surgery, the universal problems of ineffective airway clearance, decreased cardiac output, and potential for ineffective family coping occur. Using a nursing diagnosis framework facilitates nurse-to-nurse communications and collaborative problem solving.

Working with families of critically ill patients is an important part of the JP-CNS practitioner role. In addition to the information provided by physicians, families may need detailed explanations of patients' progress and continuing problems. The JPCC-CNS provides information in terms families can understand and in a supportive manner. In the critical care unit families may need a daily report, depending on the complexity of the patient's medical condition and the family's need for information. When family members are unable to visit, they may need a daily telephone call.

I make rounds each morning to see the hospitalized patients, who may number from 20 to 30 patients on any given day. Time is spent primarily with those patients falling out of the usual recovery trajectory. During these initial rounds, patients are assessed and nursing and medical problems identified. If immediate interventions are indicated, the JP-CNS can order needed tests and contact the surgeon for further instructions. Later in the day, the JP-CNS makes rounds with the surgeon and reviews the morning assessment and interventions. Approximately 75% of my time is spent in the inpatient setting. In the surgeon's office, only patients requiring nursing follow-up are seen. For example, the patient who requires follow-up with a special diet, wound healing, or compliance with medication taking would be seen as an outpatient by the JP-CNS.

The practitioner component of the JP-CNS role is the most time consuming but often the most rewarding. It has been noted that the only group of nurses with graduate education who have remained exclusively involved in direct patient care services are nurse practitioners.[7] Population-based JP-CNSs clearly belong in this category.

Educator

The JP-CNS may provide formal or informal education to patients, families, and clinical nurses. Informally, the JP-CNS performs bedside education to explain new surgical procedures, rationale for medical management directions, and interventions to prevent complications of cardiac surgery. On a more formal basis, the JP-CNS performs hospital- or community-based nursing education on new technology or treatment innovations. At times, students may become part of the surgical practice and the JP-CNS may become involved in teaching students of nursing, medicine, physician assistant, or perfusionist programs.

The JP-CNS may also write about experiences with new technology and treatment innovations for the nursing literature. For example, my experience with innovations in surgical treatment for end-stage heart disease prompted an article on how to introduce new technology to staff nurses.

Patient and family teaching is a major part of my role. The educational process is ongoing, from the prehospitalization through the posthospitalization period. In preparation for discharge, the JP-CNS provides patient and family with instructions or works with nursing staff to ensure discharge education is completed. The JP-CNS is available by telephone for questions by patients and families on discharge.

Researcher

The daily practice for the JP-CNS is a potential laboratory for clinical nursing research. The JP-CNS's extensive clinical experience leads to the identification of relevent clinical nursing research problems. For example, I was involved in a clinical study to evaluate the effect of antiembolism stockings on the development of deep venous thrombosis, pulmonary emboli, and leg edema in postoperative coronary artery bypass patients. This study revealed that in most patients these stockings became constrictive (because of rolling down) and actually impaired wound healing. In another study I worked with nursing staff to evaluate adverse reactions to autotransfusion and found an increase in febrile responses in patients who were autotransfused vs. those who were not.

Assisting with medical research is also within the JP-CNS's realm.[11] Data collection for new surgical procedures for investigational drugs and devices can be complex and is facilitated by a research assistant who is knowledgeable about the research process. The JP-CNS may be in charge of securing patient consents, data collection, chart reviews, or patient interventions. The JP-CNS may also serve as a resource to staff nurses and assist in surveying and managing complications related to the research. With the physician team, I facilitated a study of the safety of autotransfusion, looking at the risk of infection and blood hemolysis with this procedure. This research resulted in a joint publication of results.[14]

Consultant

The JP-CNS works closely with staff nurses and primary nurses to provide care for patients with complex needs. Care conference are conducted and recommendations implemented in consultation with the joint practice physician. For example, the JP-CNS attends rehabilitation conferences on patients with neurologic complications following cardiac surgery. The JP-CNS provides information related to the patient's history and cardiac care plan and facilitates communication and coordination of care among consulting physicians, rehabilitation personnel, and staff nurses. In patients with unusual complex needs such as a transplant patient admitted to the hospital with acute rejection, the JP-CNS consults with critical care nurses to plan nursing care. The JP-CNS is a resource to staff regarding the complex needs of these immunosuppressed patients and is available for staff questions and concerns.

Evaluating Effectiveness of the Population-Based JP-CNS

Little research has been conducted to evaluate the effectiveness of a JP-CNS arrangement. More of the literature has focused on nurse practitioners in joint practice with physicians. Early studies noted that the main difference between the nurse practitioner and physicians was that the nurses included more "caring" functions such as support and comfort measures in their treatment plans.[9] McLain[10] studied nurse practitioners and physicians in joint practice to evaluate their degree of collaboration. Despite the nurse practitioners' clinical competence and willingness to assume responsibility, physicians remained in the authoritarian position, and understanding and respect were limited. Campbell et al.[15] carried out an extensive analysis of 400 nurse practitioner patient interactions in a joint practice. Patient responses to the joint practice arrangement were very positive. Nurses were observed to exhibit more concern with psychosocial issues, but overall little difference appeared between physician and nurse patient interactions, since many nurse practitioners appeared to follow a medical behavior model. Conversely, the physicians in joint practice displayed more sensitivity than those in solo practice. Campbell et al. concluded that professional convergence occurs and providers tend to develop similar styles over time.

Evaluation of the effectiveness of population-based JP-CNSs can be carried out in a number of ways. Patient feedback and family feedback are very important, since the consumers of this health care approach may have the most information pertaining to its effectiveness in providing high-quality care. Feedback from physicians and interdisciplinary team members is also valuable, because a major focus of the role is to communicate with and coordinate the efforts of these providers. Analysis of the patient population's length of stay and number of complications can objectively document the advantages of the JP-CNS role.[16]

The Chronically Critically Ill Patient and the Role of the JP-CNS

Long-term critically ill patients are a growing segment of the critical care population.[17] Principal diagnoses vary, but frequently these are cardiovascular surgical patients who have suffered complications. The complications may be related to the surgery or exacerbations of other chronic conditions precipitated by surgery, such as postoperative respiratory failure caused by chronic pulmonary disease.

These patients are usually ventilator dependent and may spend weeks to months in a critical care unit. Typical nursing diagnoses include impaired pulmonary gas exchange, decreased cardiac output, alteration in level of consciousness, alteration in nutrition, potential for infection, fluid volume disturbances caused by renal insufficiency, impaired physical mobility, and ineffective patient or family coping.

Intensive and effective management of these patients is particularly important in view of current costs of health care and limited reimbursement for prolonged hospitalization. The JP-CNS works collaboratively with multiple disciplines to plan care. Collaboration is carried out with staff nurses, hospital-based CNSs, respiratory therapists, physical therapists, occupational therapists, speech therapists, dietitians, and multiple consulting physicians.

CASE STUDY

Mrs. R. was a 77-year-old woman admitted to the hospital with the diagnoses of severe tricuspid valve regurgitation, mild to moderate mitral regurgitation and stenosis, and mild aortic regurgitation. Before admission, the patient had been experiencing dyspnea with minimal exertion, decreased exercise tolerance, abdominal distention, liver enlargement, peripheral edema, and excessive fatigue. Other pertinent history included one transient ischemia attack 2 years ago with no residual effects, an inferior myocardial infarction 10 years ago, and a previous smoking habit of one pack per day, which she quit 3 years ago.

Preoperatively the JP-CNS evaluated Mrs. R. and made the following observations: (1) a history of recent onset of dysphagia; (2) malnutrition as evidenced by low serum albumin levels and a 50-lb weight loss over the past year; (3) evidence of hypoxemia and hypercarbia on blood gas results, possibly related to undiagnosed lung disease; and (4) dry skin and mucous membranes with little subcutaneous tissue and poor skin turgor. Mrs. R's heart failure was so severe now that there were no options left except surgery. In preparation for possible complications the JP-CNS developed a postoperative care plan that focused on prevention of complications (see box).

Mrs. R. underwent a mitral valve replacement with a Carpentier-Edwards valve and a tricuspid valve annuloplasty. Following surgery, Mrs. R. did not awaken from anesthesia for 24 hours. During this time the surgeons feared that she had suffered an intraoperative stroke. The JP-CNS worked closely with the family members, who were extremely upset. The family asked the JP-CNS about the need to make a decision on cessation of life-support equipment. The JP-CNS shared with the family that it was too soon to determine that Mrs. R. had suffered irreversible brain injury and that loss of consciousness after heart surgery was often temporary. In the meantime the JP-CNS worked with the nursing staff to ensure that Mrs. R. received passive exercise and that aspiration precautions were followed.

On the second postoperative day, Mrs. R. awakened and was clearly able to express her wishes to the nursing staff. The JP-CNS worked with the nursing staff to explain to Mrs. R. about her recovery

---

CARE PLAN FOR MRS. R.

Problem 1: Potential for pneumonia and/or difficulty weaning from mechanical ventilator.
Action Plan: (1) Maintain restricted fluid intake to prevent fluid overload and pulmonary congestion. (2) Turn patient every 2 hours beginning the hour after return from the operating room. (3) Begin chest physiotherapy when patient is hemodynamically stable. (4) Suction patient as needed using sterile technique.

Problem 2: Potential for aspiration of food or fluids related to dysphagia.
Action Plan: (1) Follow aspiration precautions at all times. (2) Before initiation of oral intake, have patient perform swallowing tests according to protocol. (3) Observe patient for 30 minutes following first intake of oral fluids for signs of aspiration or respiratory distress.

Problem 3: Potential for impaired skin integrity and poor wound healing caused by malnutrition and poor skin condition.
Action Plan: (1) Assess skin condition every 6 hours for signs of pressure or breakdown. (2) Turn patient every 2 hours. (3) Place a special support mattress on the patient's bed in the operating room. (4) Call for a dietary consultation on postoperative day 1.

---

from surgery and to assure her that she was doing well.

On the fourth postoperative day, Mrs. R. was weaned from the mechanical ventilator. She remained quite weak and needed much assistance to generate an effective cough. The JP-CNS worked with the nursing staff to develop an individualized plan for pulmonary care, a plan that would allow rest periods for Mrs. R. The danger of aspiration remained. The JP-CNS was so concerned about this potential problem that she arranged for a swallowing consultation from a speech therapist who specialized in this area. The speech therapist recommended a special swallowing test, which would be performed with a dye under fluoroscopy. Because Mrs. R. was too weak to travel to radiology for this test, the JP-CNS, in consultation with the surgeon, decided to meet Mrs. R.'s nutritional needs through the tube feedings. The swallowing test was performed on the sixth postoperative day, and the cause of dysphagia was identified. Based on this result, a special menu was developed for Mrs. R. that included soft, solid foods and limited liquids.

Mrs. R. remained in intensive care for the first 6 postoperative days because of continued problems with mucous clearing, poor blood gases, and concerns for possible new neurologic deficits. Mrs. R.'s weakness prevented her from generating a strong cough, and therefore she was at great risk for pneumonia. She began to show signs of depression as her weakened condition overwhelmed her. The JP-CNS spent many sessions with Mrs. R. to assist her to work through these feelings.

Mrs. R. gradually regained her strength and began to get out of bed. Again, the JP-CNS worked with the nurses in the telemetry unit in developing a program for Mrs. R.'s gradual rehabilitation. At this point in Mrs. R.'s recovery, the JP-CNS focused on Mrs. R.'s nutritional needs and began to plan for discharge. On daily rounds the JP-CNS examined Mrs. R.'s wounds for signs of infection and her skin for signs of breakdown. The JP-CNS also evaluated Mrs. R.'s response to exercise, observing heart rate and blood pressure changes. Mrs. R. continued to progress uneventfully and was discharged home on postoperative day 14.

The preceding case study demonstrates how the expertise of the JP-CNS can be used to implement preventive measures in a patient who was a candidate for major postoperative complications. This patient had been critically ill for an extended period but, with the close observations of the JP-CNS, was able to leave the hospital in a reasonable amount of time.

SUMMARY

Following the trend toward increasing specialization in critical care units, CC-CNSs have also specialized in the care of specific patient populations. Physicians have recognized the expertise of nurses in advanced practice, facilitating collaborative efforts. Some PB-CNSs have entered into joint practice arrangements with physicians where each contributes unique skills and perspectives, increasing the quality of patient care and enhancing role satisfaction.

According to Fawcett and Carino[18] the future hallmarks of successful nursing practice will be the development of alternative systems of nursing care delivery and the refinement of nurse-physician collaborative practice. Joint practice is a mechanism by which both these concepts are advanced. The achievement of both desired patient outcomes and practitioner satisfaction can result from formal partnerships between physicians and nurses across all health care settings, including the critical care unit.

References

1. Riegel B, Murrell T: CNS in collaborative practice, *Clin Nurse Specialist* 1(2):63-66, 1987.
2. Burke LE: The clinical nurse specialist in collaborative practice, *Momentum* 1:3-5, 1983.
3. Littell SC: The clinical nurse specialist in private medical practice, *Nurs Admin Q*, pp 77-85, Fall 1981.
4. Nowicki CR: The plastic surgical clinical nurse specialist and the plastic surgeon: a model for collaborative practice, *Plast Surg Nurs* 5:50-56, 1985.
5. Weinstein R: Hospital case management: the path to empowering nurses, *Pediatr Nurs* 17(3):289-293, 1991.
6. Hughes AM, Mackenzie CS: Components necessary in a successful nurse practitioner-physician collaborative practice, *J Am Acad Nurs Pract* 2(2):54-57, 1990.
7. Brown SJ: The clinical nurse specialist in a multidisciplinary partnership, *Nurs Admin Q* 8(3):36-46, 1983.
8. Trueman MS: Collaboration: a right and responsibility of professional practice, *Crit Care Nurs* 11(1):70-72, 1991.
9. Mauksch HO, Campbell JD: The nursing presence examined by assessing joint practice. In *Perspectives in nursing 1987-1989*, New York, 1988, NLN Publication.
10. McLain BR: Collaborative practice: the nurse practitioner's role in its success or failure, *Nurs Pract* 13(5):34-38, 1988.
11. King MB: Clinical nurse specialist in collaboration with physicians, *Clin Nurse Specialist* 4(4):172-177, 1990.
12. Elpern EH: Associated practice: a case for professional collaboration, *J Nurse Admin* 13(11):27-35, 1983.
13. Davis LL: The politics of interdisciplinary collaboration in professional practice, *J Prof Nurs* 2(4):206, 266, 1986.
14. Tector AJ, Dressler DK, Glassner-Davis RM: A new

method of autotransfusing blood drained after cardiac surgery, *Ann Thorac Surg* 40(3):305-307, 1985.

15. Campbell JD et al: Collaborative practice and provider styles of delivering health care, *So Sci Med* 30(12):1359-1365, 1990.

16. Weiland AP: Physician and nurse joint practice: a descrip-

tion of nurse practitioners on a cardiac surgery service, *Heart Lung* 12(6):576-580, 1983.

17. Daly BJ et al: Development of a special care unit for chronically critically ill patients, *Heart Lung* 20(1):45-51, 1991.

18. Fawcett J, Carino C: Hallmarks of success in nursing practice, *Adv Nurs Sci* 11(4):1-8, 1989.

Chapter 6

The Critical Care Clinical Nurse Specialist as Case Manager

Sandra L. Tidwell, RN, MN

CURRENT HEALTH CARE CHALLENGE

Nursing as a science and an art has its foundation in quality and excellence. Current changes in the health care environment threaten that foundation. Rising costs and decreasing availability of health care dollars are just two factors driving change in our health care environment today. The advent of diagnostic-related groups (DRGs) and managed care has altered the pattern of reimbursement from fee-for-service to prospective payment, resulting in reduced occupancy, revenues, and available work force for health care institutions.[1] Managed care, or "contract medicine," is the predominant reimbursement system for the 1990s. It has been predicted that by the year 2000, 75% to 85% of hospital inpatients will be covered by fixed-price managed care systems.[2]

A shift to outcome-oriented evaluation has attained nearly universal acceptance in the health care field. Quality of care is an area of competition not only for medical centers, but also for third-party payors. "Blue Cross and other payors are developing extensive data bases on quality performance. Quality is measurable and will be monitored closely in the 1990s."[3] Hospitals and clinics increasingly focus on continuous quality improvement processes.

An increase in patient acuity has lead to an increase in the number of intensive care beds. "Although more than 30,000 short-term general hospital beds were eliminated between 1980 and 1987, nearly 20,000 beds have been converted to intensive care beds to accommodate the increase in pa-

tient acuity and the demand for critical care."[4] The formation of more intensive care and intermediate care units has lead to frequent transfer of patients from one area of care to another. This, with the increase in subspecialties, has resulted in fragmented patient care.[5] Fragmented care causes patient and family confusion and can decrease accountability for cost and patient outcomes at the nursing and provider level.

An increase in patient acuity, the aging population, and advances in biomedical technology have spawned a greater demand for nurses, especially critical care nurses. The average registered nurse vacancy rate in 4500 United States hospitals is reported at 15.6% in the intensive care unit and 13.8% in medical and surgical units.[4]

The need for patient and family education has increased because of more knowledgeable consumers and earlier discharges from the hospital. With the decrease in hospital length of stay, patients are leaving the hospital sicker and spending more of their convalescence at home.

Prospective payment has changed health care's focus from a "day of care" to an episode of illness. Hospitalized patients are more acutely ill, require a greater number of care providers, and are discharged to home earlier. A major challenge currently facing nursing is how to provide safe, effective quality patient care within our ever-changing health care system.[6] Health care delivery models must be adapted for today's challenging health care environment.[7]

Case Management

A major barrier to the balance of quality and cost containment has been the lack of control over the care delivery process.[8] Howard et al.[9] state that the first critical step in controlling costs is to identify variables that influence costs in specific patient populations. Case management is a system that allows for identification of these variables. Restructuring the patient care delivery system to include case management of high-risk, high-cost patient populations has been identified as the most promising solution.[5,6,10] Zander[7] describes nursing case management as a restructuring of the clinical production processes at the provider-consumer level to resolve the cost/quality puzzle.

Nursing case management was initially designed with the nurse at the bedside as the patient's case manager.[11] Studies have demonstrated the added benefits of the clinical nurse specialist (CNS) in the role of case manager. This chapter begins with a discussion of how the CNS can interface within a case management framework: (1) working with a staff nurse who is the case manager, (2) working with a master's-prepared case manager, and (3) as a case manager. The remainder of the chapter focuses on an example of a critical care CNS (CC-CNS) who now operates as a case manager. The development of a case management system is described with emphasis on the CC-CNS's role as coordinator of case-managed care for cardiac surgery patients.

THEORETIC PERSPECTIVES
Definitions

Case management and managed care are confusing broadly used terms in health care today. At times they are used interchangeably by insurance companies, in the social welfare field, in community health, and in acute care settings. In all of these settings the common application describes balancing limited resources with quality patient care. Zander[12] describes both managed care and case management as "clinical systems which structure and design the care-giving process at the provider-client level to better achieve cost and quality outcomes." She differentiates them in how they affect nursing care delivery, stating that managed care can be used with any nursing care delivery model but that case management changes the level of authority and accountability for specific

categories of patients from the nurse manager to a designated group of non–line management nurses.

Managed care in this chapter, however, will refer to "those health care delivery and reimbursement arrangements in which the buyers actively manage the use and costs of covered health services by plan enrollees."[2] In this chapter, *case management* refers to a collaborative, patient-based system that involves planning, organizing, coordinating, and monitoring outcomes and resources to achieve quality, cost-effective patient care within a defined time frame. *Case manager* refers to the person with accountability and authority for daily implementation of the case management process in a specific DRG group.

Features

All nursing case management models differ somewhat in their design. However, basic to any case management system are the goals of cost savings and improved quality of care within an acceptable length of stay. Nurse, physician, and patient satisfaction is another common added goal. Most models have expected or standardized clinical outcomes, typically referred to as the critical pathway.[10,11] The critical pathway is an abbreviated outline of the daily physiologic and functional steps that a patient of a specific diagnostic group would routinely follow for a course of treatment. Many models involve a multidisciplinary group in planning and monitoring the system. Charges, length of stay, staff and patient satisfaction, and patient deviation from the care plan are common outcome criteria analyzed in case management.

RELATED RESEARCH AND LITERATURE
Roles of CNS in Case Management

In its publication *Nursing Case Management*, the American Nurses' Association (ANA) recommends that a baccalaureate in nursing (BSN) plus 3 years of experience be the minimum level of preparation for a nurse case manager.[13] The ANA recognizes that although this recommendation is the minimum, many case management programs prefer a master's-prepared CNS with experience in areas related to the target population and one who has experience in settings the case manager is most likely to use. In addition, the ANA cites that most nursing programs lack adequate theoretic preparation for a nurse to successfully function in the role of case manager.[13]

The CNS can be involved in case management in one of three roles: (1) CNS working with a staff nurse who is the case manager, (2) CNS working with a master's-prepared case manager, and (3) CNS as a case manager. Table 6–1 lists areas of CNS involvement in case management in each of these roles. The role of the CNS in a specific case management system is determined by the needs of the agency, the number and availability of CNS, salary costs, and the level of nursing staff skills.[14]

Harper Hospital, in Detroit, Michigan, piloted case management using BSN-prepared nurses as case managers. A study was done following the pilot that revealed both positive and negative as-

TABLE 6–1 Three Roles of the CNS in Case Management

CNS with Staff Nurse Case Manager

Available as a resource to staff nurse case manager

Assists in identification of case types to case manage

Assists in development of critical pathways

Enhances planning and clinical decision making

Analyzes variances from critical pathway

Assists in hospital-wide communication

Assists in modification of critical pathways for individual patients

Evaluates patient and financial outcomes

Develops educational programs

CNS with Master's-prepared Case Manager

Consults with case manager on complex cases in CNS's area of expertise

Develops education programs for staff or patients when need identified

CNS as Case Manager

Monitors individual patients for ongoing care planning and variance analysis

Identifies case types to case manage

Develops critical pathways

Audits quality of care

Acts as resource to staff nurse

Educates patient and family

Follows patient throughout system

Coordinates discharge planning

In-service staff

pects of BSN nurses as case managers. An increase in quality of care was noted along with an increase in job satisfaction of the nurses. These case managers expressed frustration with the difficulty in case managing while delivering direct patient care. They felt a lack of preparation for instituting change and lacked confidence in their ability to collaborate and delegate. Harper Hospital has since switched to using the CNS as the case manager.[1] Initially, there was some fear that using the CNS as the case manager would interrupt the primary nurse-patient relationship and dilute the primary nurse role. Maklebust et al.[15] state that most staff nurses found it a great benefit to have a master's prepared CNS to consult with, and they reported many benefits, such as (1) a decrease in the stress of the staff nurse by CNS functioning as a nurse advocate, (2) the ability of the CNS to keep the team focused on discharge planning and patient education, (3) development of teaching strategies, (4) realistic goal setting in difficult patients, (5) an increase in patient readiness for discharge, and (6) increased patient satisfaction.

Many authors describe the CNS as being the ideal case manager.[15-22] In their paper "CNS Leadership Opportunities in Case Management," the Clinical Nurse Specialist Special Interest Group of the American Association of Critical Care Nurses states: "By education and expertise, the CNS is well suited to play a central role in the implementation of a case management system."[16] They describe two ways that institutions may involve the CNS in case management: (1) as the case manager and (2) as a resource to the staff nurse case manager. As a resource to the staff nurse case manager the CNS directly consults with and supports the case manager throughout the patient's episode of care.[16]

Gaedeke Norris and Hill[21] state that the CNS is in a unique position to implement case management to achieve both cost reduction and improved quality of care. The role of case manager is noted to be both an enhancement to and an area of potential growth for the CNS.[17,18] Schroer[19] describes case management as a model to use in integrating the roles of the CNS and nurse practitioner. Rudy and Grenvik[23] describe such a role in their article "The Future of Critical Care" and foresee an expansion of the roles of critical care nurse practitioners and case managers.

Components of CC-CNS Role and Case Management

Today's health care environment also has impacted the CC-CNS role. Because of constrained resources, the CC-CNS needs to balance quality improvement with the ability to contain costs. Cost containment is no longer purely an administrative role but has been synthesized into the traditional clinician role of the CC-CNS.[24]

The role of case manager incorporates and enhances all five components of the CC-CNS role: practitioner, educator, consultant, researcher, and manager/leader. Several authors describe how these role components are demonstrated in case management.[16,18,19] Below are outlined each of these components with suggested applications in the role of case manager.

1. Of Practitioner
   a. Prioritizes diagnostic groups of critically ill patients to be case managed
   b. Develops protocols and critical pathways for each diagnostic group
   c. Develops discharge planning programs
   d. Selects critically ill patients to case manage
   e. Assesses patient care planning and technology used for optimal cost savings and quality outcomes
   f. Provides individualized care of critically ill patients
   g. Acts as role model for critical care staff nurses
2. Educator
   a. Educates critically ill patient and family
   b. Educates critical care staff on clinical issues, DRGs, reimbursement, resource utilization, and admission and discharge criteria
   c. Coordinates educational programs and materials development
3. Consultant
   a. Using a collaborative model approach, collects information from and communicates with all members of health care team to ensure optimal patient outcomes
   b. Coordinates collaborative practice group meetings
   c. Consults with physicians on advanced practice issues
   d. Coordinates discharge planning
   e. Generates referrals to social services, chaplain, home health care agencies, and extended care facilities
   f. Acts as a resource to staff nurse on individual patients
   g. Consults on standard development and protocols and revision of patient acuity and classification system
4. Researcher
   a. Analyzes variance from critical pathways
   b. Identifies system problems
   c. Conducts retrospective and concurrent monitoring of quality of care
   d. Identifies critically ill patients and diagnostic groups in need of case management
   e. Evaluates and compares products and technology to identify cost and quality effects
   f. Investigates new or existing nursing interventions and techniques for cost effectiveness and patient benefit
   g. Facilitates research-based nursing practice through the dissemination and utilization of new knowledge on care of the critically ill patient/family system
5. Manager/Leader
   a. Monitors and evaluates patient and cost outcomes
   b. Allocates human and material resources required for care of critically ill patient and family
   c. Attempts to balance financial and regulatory aspects of care with clinical aspects
   d. Negotiates with various hospital departments on cost containment strategies
   e. Assists in design of cost-effective critical care nursing systems

The components of the CC-CNS role add tremendous depth to the role of case manager. "The CNS, who has advanced expertise in pathophysiology, human responses to both actual and potential illness, health care resources, and other elements impinging on care is best prepared to coordinate and direct care as a case manager."[21]

Outcomes

When Harper Hospital restructured their case management system to use the CNS as case manager,[1,25] positive results included a reduction in overall length of stay by 1 full day, development of educational programs and discharge instructions, conferences with nursing staff to strengthen clinical knowledge and assistance in care planning on complex patients, identification of systems problems, and retrospective and concurrent auditing of quality.[25]

Parkland Memorial Hospital in Dallas, Texas, studied the impact of the CNS case manager on cost and quality outcomes in three patient populations. They were able to document reductions in length of stay and readmission rate and an increase in appointment compliance.[20]

Hillcrest Medical Center in Tulsa, Oklahoma, analyzed their newly developed case management program and cited not only cost savings but also an improvement in quality of care. An increase in satisfaction of both physicians and nurses was also observed.[10]

The CNS is of great benefit to case management, and case management offers a unique opportunity to document the cost effectiveness of advanced nursing practice.[26] Cronin and Maklebust[1] state that the CNS is cost effective as a case manager. Cost savings are seen through the CNS's expertise in in-depth assessments, early interventions, and effective, timely discharge planning. They noted that documentation of case management services assisted in gaining third-party reimbursement and that research-based evaluation of new products aided in reducing charges.

Costs and patient and provider outcomes of case management have been analyzed; however, few studies have analyzed the tools used in case management. Strong and Sneed[27] reported a study of 28 coronary artery bypass graft (CABG) patients that investigated the accuracy of their CABG critical pathway and determined how variance from the pathway affected postoperative length of stay. They found that 57% of patients were discharged according to the critical pathway. A significant positive correlation was found between adherence to the pathway and postoperative length of stay. Significant predictors of length of stay were found to be telemetry use and activity level.

PRACTICE APPLICATIONS
Virginia Mason Cardiothoracic Surgery Model

Virginia Mason Medical Center is a private, nonprofit teaching medical center in Seattle, Washington. The medical center includes a 277-bed acute care hospital, an outpatient clinic, and a research center. CNSs are employed in both the clinic and the hospital.

The section of cardiothoracic surgery performs an average of 300 open heart surgeries annually, and the cardiothoracic surgery team consists of three cardiothoracic surgeons, a CNS, a physician's assistant, and a section manager. Typically, three surgical resident physicians are part of the cardiothoracic surgery team caring for hospitalized patients.

The role of the CNS in cardiothoracic surgery originated in 1985. This population-based CNS (PB-CNS) role is based in the clinic but is responsible for patients and their families throughout the whole continuum of care, from preoperative workup and preparation, through the acute hospital stay, including postoperative care in the outpatient setting. This responsibility includes education, emotional support, assessment, troubleshooting problems, initiation of referrals, coordination of care within and outside the medical center, and discharge planning. The CNS makes rounds on all cardiothoracic surgery patients twice daily and is available as a consultant to the nursing staff during the day. The morning rounds include consulting with each patient's nurse on patient progress, problems, or educational needs. Rounds with the patient and family at the bedside include addressing their concerns, assessment of their coping ability, and discussing the patient's progress, anticipated discharge date, and educational information. In the afternoon the CNS does rounds on patients with the surgical residents, attending cardiothoracic physician, and the physician's assistant. Other responsibilities include patient outcome tracking and analysis, coordination and management of ongoing research projects, and education material development.

Problem: Costs of Care

In 1988, in response to increasing costs and competition, an analysis of the cardiothoracic surgery practice was done by section members. The analysis revealed the following deficiencies: charges above the local average, no standardized care management, overutilization of ancillary services, and no expectation for length of stay.

Plan: Creation of a Case Management System

To correct the deficiencies, a plan was developed to determine resource inputs and create a collaborative case management system that coordinated care of the CABG patient across all settings of the medical center. A collaborative case management group was brought together consisting of a surgeon and the CNS from cardiothoracic surgery, the two CC-CNSs in the hospital, the nursing clinical coordinator for intensive care and telemetry, and members of other disciplines on an as-needed basis. The case management group set the following goals for CABG case management: (1) contain costs; (2) prevent fragmentation; and (3) enhance quality of care.

Other objectives included designating an accountable person to monitor and facilitate critical pathway progression and to coordinate care and services received; reducing the incidence of unplanned variance in CABG patient care resulting from unanticipated or avoidable patient complications; strengthening collaborative patient care through mutually agreed on outcomes, time lines, and processes; and improving professional development and satisfaction of nursing staff.

Tools for Case Management

CABG Critical Pathway. The pathway (Figs. 6–1 and 6–2) is a series of stepwise increases in physical activity and education and decreases in physiologic support. Each step is termed a "pathway" and contains elements that analysis have shown the average patient could satisfy on successive days after operation. The pathway is constructed with the above listed items on the left-hand side and pathdays across the top. Areas of physician difference, or items requiring judgment calls, are listed with a question mark preceding. Arrows across the pathway indicate that an item is ongoing. The discharge plan section is incorporated to ensure early planning for discharge from the hospital.

Development. To coordinate, streamline, and ensure continued quality of care, the case management groups decided to develop a critical pathway for the CABG patient. The first step was to analyze data from the cardiothoracic surgery section data base to determine the postoperative length of stay for the pathway. Postoperative length of stay data were analyzed for the previous 3 years. Data from patients who died were not included in the analysis, because these data would skew results. The length of stay during this period varied from 5 to 178 days. The mean length of stay was calculated after excluding patient outliers with a length of stay greater than 30 days. This was computed to get a more representative mean, and 30 days is the Medicare cutoff. The recalculated mean length of stay was 9 days with the mode at 7 days. Since the mode is the measure of central tendency that occurs most frequently, 7 days was chosen as the target postoperative length of stay to analyze.

The next step was to complete a prospective and retrospective chart review of patients with a 7-day postoperative length of stay. Retrospective review was done on 15 charts from patients operated on in the past year. Prospective review was done on 10 charts. The following information for each patient was listed every day of their hospital stay:

- Location in the medical center
- Consultations or visits by _____
- Tests
- Treatments, both medical and nursing
- Medications
- Diet
- Activity
- Education or support

This information was shared with the members of the cardiothoracic surgery section. Each item was evaluated to discern its necessity and therapeutic value. Less expensive alternatives were decided on when applicable, such as pulse oximetry instead of an arterial blood gas to wean patients from mechanical ventilator. Admission laboratory tests were evaluated and consensus reached by the surgeons. A representative from the case management group then negotiated with the laboratory to develop a cardiothoracic battery for preoperative laboratory tests at a reduced rate over requesting each test individually.

The case management group used information from this review meeting to develop the CABG interdisciplinary critical pathway. Since patient care was to be more coordinated, it was decided to set the target length of stay for the pathway at 6 days. A draft of the CABG pathway was taken back to the cardiothoracic surgery section for re-

CABG CRITICAL PATHWAY

	PREOP	SURGERY	PATHDAY 1
LOCATION:	ADMIT TO 8E Preop clinic if AM admit	OR/ICU POD 0	ICU/8E POD 1
VISITS BY:	Cardiologist, CT surgeon, Anesthesia, CT CNS, PT, RT	Cardiologist, CT surgeon, Anesthesia, CT CNS, PT, RT	Cardiologist, CT surgeon Anesthesia, CT CNS, PT, RT
TESTS:	Check if done - CT PRE battery, ABG, T&C 2 units, CXR, ECG, UA, Bleeding time if ASA intake within 7 days	Ebatt, Hct, ABG, CXR,-STAT TT, PTT, PT, PLT count- STAT RBATT & ABG @ 4h then qAM k+ q6H X 48h	ECG CXR-post CT removal RBATT & ABG in AM K+ p6h, CPK (MB if high)
TREATMENTS:	Enema, shave/prep, HT/WT, betadine shower	Foley, I/O, WT O2 vent SG-SVO2/AL Cardiac monitor Chest tubes IV x 2 Pacer wires/pacer ?NG if gastric dil.	D/C foley O2 vent to mask/NP D/C SG-SVO2/AL Telemetry D/C Chest tubes when <10cc/hr ?D/C NG if improved
MEDICATIONS:	Continue pts own except ASA	IV antibiotic MS, Valium ASA supp. ?antiarrhythmic, ?digoxin ?diuretic, ?KCL	
DIET:	Regular - NPO @ 2400	NPO	Clear liquids-advance as tolerated
ACTIVITY:	Up ad lib. Self care	Level I. Bedrest Total care Passive ROM	Level II Self feed, partial self care, OOB/chair
EDUCATION/ SUPPORT:	Preop (CNS, PT, RT) Family visit ICU (8E staff) ICU video, ?CTS video		
DISCHARGE PLAN:	DISPOSITION AFTER D/C		

Figure 6–1 CABG critical pathway, part 1. (Courtesy Virginia Mason Medical Center, Seattle, Washington.)

CABG CRITICAL PATHWAY

	PATHDAY 2	PATHDAY 3	PATHDAY 4	PATHDAY 5	PATHDAY 6
LOCATION:	8E POD 2	8E POD 3	8E POD 4	8E POD 5	8E Discharge
VISITS BY:	Cardiologist, CT surgeon, CT CNS, PT, RT	Cardiologist, CT surgeon, Anesthesia, CT CNS, PT, RT	Cardiologist, CT surgeon CT CNS, PT, RT	Cardiologist, CT surgeon, CT CNS,PT, RT	CT CNS
TESTS:	CXR, post chest tube D/C, K+ in AM CPK-MB (if 1st value high) →	ECG K+ in AM (if diuretics) → CPK-MB (if...........)	CXR PA/LAT w/wire D/C		
TREATMENTS:	I/O, WT, D/C foley ————————		D/C - I/O, WT when @ preop wt.		
	Decrease O2 per protocol until off ————————		D/C - O2		
	Telemetry ————————		D/C tele if stable NSR or Afib with stable rate D/C heparin lock		
	Heparin lock ————————				
	Pacer wires/pacer d/c pacer if stable	→ D/C wires if stable NSR or Afib with stable rate			
MEDICATIONS:	Percocet ————————————————————————→ Dulcolax if no BM			Dulcolax if no BM	
	ASA ————————————————————————→ Order discharge			Order discharge meds	
	?Digoxin				
	DSS, MOM prn ———————————————————→				
	?Diuretic, ?KCL		MOM if no BM		
DIET:	Regular as tolerated, unless diabetic				
ACTIVITY:	Level II-III Amb 1-5 min self care	Level III Amb room prn Amb 3-5 min.	Level IV Amb hall prn Amb 5-7 min. Shower if wires out	Level V Amb 7-10 min. 1/2 to 1 flight stairs	?Referral Phase II
EDUCATION/ SUPPORT:	Begin classes: Heart Surgery ———————————————————→ Heart smart ———————————————————→				Med teaching Appt. given D/C teaching
DISCHARGE PLAN:	DISPOSITION AFTER D/C				

Figure 6–2 CABG critical pathway, part 2. (Courtesy Virginia Mason Medical Center, Seattle, Washington.)

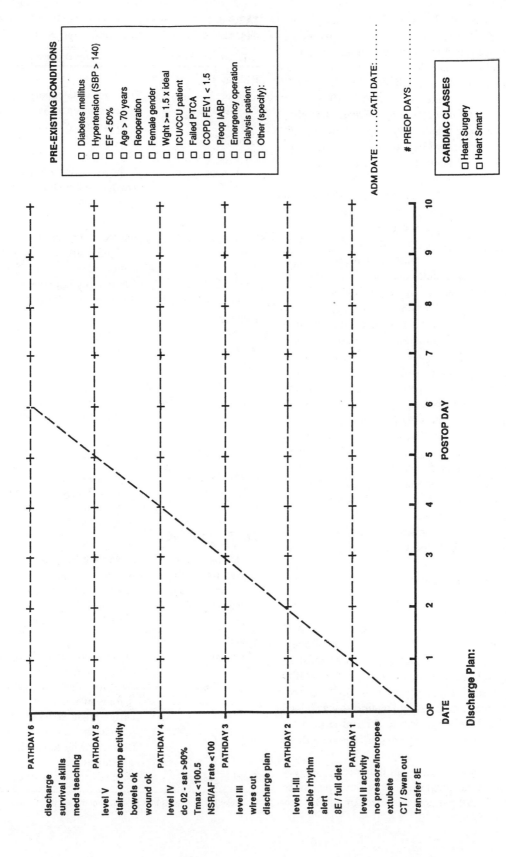

Figure 6–3 CABG clinical tracking form. (Courtesy Virginia Mason Medical Center, Seattle, Washington.)

view and approval. The case management group decided that the cardiothoracic CC-CNS would be the person accountable for daily tracking of patient progress and outcome analysis. The cardiothoracic surgery case management system for the CABG patient was implemented in August 1989.

The CABG Clinical Tracking Form. The clinical tracking form graphically displays an individual patient's progress (Fig. 6–3). The critical indicators are listed under their corresponding pathday on the Y-axis and postoperative days are on the X-axis. The dotted angular line, the line of identity, respresents the course that a patient would take if he or she progressed one pathday for each successive postoperative day. Below the graph is a space to write in the discharge plan for the patient. To the right of the graph is the box containing the list of preexisting conditions. A section is included to check off the cardiac classes that a patient or family attends. Space is also given to list admission date, heart catheterization date, and number of preoperative days. This space allows for monitoring of length of stay before surgery.

Development. The CABG clinical tracking form was developed to facilitate tracking individual patient progress on the CABG critical pathway in an easy to use, highly visual format. This format allows for ongoing analysis of individual patient progress to highlight deviations from the pathway as they occur so additional therapeutic measures can be implemented. Data generated from the clinical tracking form enable group analysis for practice and outcome assessment. Evaluation of these data is used to revise the CABG critical pathway as needed.

To develop the clinical tracking form, information from each pathday on the CABG critical pathway was condensed into four or five main objectives, termed "critical indicators." Table 6–2 describes these critical indicators for each pathday. Studies have been done that document preexisting patient conditions that increase risk of mortality following CABG surgery (Table 6–3).[28-31] A section listing these preexisting conditions was added to the clinical tracking form to determine their relationship to pathway progression and length of stay.

Implementation. The cardiothoracic surgery case management program has been in effect since August 1989. All patients admitted for CABG sur-

TABLE 6–2 Descriptions of Critical Indicators Listed on CABG Clinical Tracking Form (Figs. 6–3 to 6–5)

Critical Indicators	Descriptions
Pathday 1	
Transfer 8E	Transfer to telemetry unit
CT/Swan out	Chest tubes and Swan-Ganz line removed
Extubate	Extubated
No pressors/ inotropes	No longer requiring IV pressors or inotropes
Level II	Dangle to ambulating 1–3 min
Pathday 2	
8E/full diet	On telemetry unit eating regular diet
Alert	Patient alert
Stable rhythm	Cardiac rhythm stable
Level II–III	Ambulating 1–5 min
Pathday 3	
Discharge plan	Discharge plan made
Wires out	Temporary pacing wires out
Level III	Ambulating 3–5 min
Pathday 4	
NSR/AF rate <100	Normal sinus rhythm or atrial fibrillation with rate <100
T_{max} <100.5	Maximum temperature <100.5
dc O_2—sat >90%	Supplemental oxygen removed; oxygen saturation >90%
Level IV	Ambulating 5–7 min
Pathday 5	
Wound ok	Incisions healing well
Bowels ok	Bowels moved since surgery
Stairs or comparable activity	Stairs climbed or comparable activity done
Level V	Ambulating 7–10 min
Pathday 6	
Meds teaching	Medication instruction given to patient/family
Survival skills	Describe signs and symptoms of infection
	Differentiate between sore chest and angina
	Describe who to call if problems
Discharge	Discharge from hospital

Courtesy Virginia Mason Medical Center, Seattle, Washington.

TABLE 6–3 Definitions of Preexisting Conditions on CABG Clinical Pathway Form (Figs. 6–3 to 6–5)

Diabetes mellitus: any type
Hypertension: any documented history
EF <50%: cardiac ejection fraction <50%
Age >70 years: at time of surgery
Reoperation: history of CABG in the past
Female gender
Wght > = 1.5 × ideal: preoperative weight
  ≥1.5 × ideal weight
ICU/CCU patient: in ICU or CCU preoperatively
Failed PTCA: failed percutaneous coronary angioplasty at this admission
COPD FEV$_1$ <1.5: chronic obstructive pulmonary disease with forced expiratory volume in 1 second
Preop IABP: intraaortic balloon pump inserted preoperatively
Emergency operation: CABG an emergency
Dialysis patient: patient on dialysis preoperatively

Courtesy Virginia Mason Medical Center, Seattle, Washington.

gery are case managed. Copies of both the CABG critical pathway and the CABG clinical tracking form are placed in a patient's chart on admission for use by all disciplines involved in the care of the patient. The clinical tracking form is stamped with the patient's name and hospital number. The CNS in cardiothoracic surgery checks the applicable preexisting conditions during preoperative or early postoperative rounds.

Patient progress is recorded on the clincial tracking form daily during rounds with the cardiothoracic surgery team. Failure to achieve all of the critical indicators for a given pathday results in a horizontal line of deviation to the right of the line of identity with notation as to the cause (Fig. 6–4). This results in focused attention on the whole team to correct the problem and implement therapeutic measures as needed. Three types of deviations are noted and tracked to evaluate their effect on patient progress and outcome:

1. Patient condition (e.g., atrial fibrillation)
2. System in the medical center (e.g., no beds available on the telemetry unit so patient remains an extra day in the ICU)
3. Provider of any service to the patient (e.g., physical therapist not in to see a patient when requested)

A coding system has been recently developed to assist in data analysis of the variances (Table 6–4).

Evaluation. Virginia Mason Medical Center embarked on a system-wide project of cardiovascular cost containment 6 months after initiation of the cardiothoracic surgery case management system. An outside consulting group was hired to evaluate the medical center's status on the major cardiovascular and DRGs, including those for CABG. This process was beneficial to the cardiothoracic case management system in that a cardiovascular cost containment task force was formed to evaluate and develop further opportunities for reducing charges while maintaining quality. This task force aided in the development of several policies and protocols that enhanced the CABG case management project.

Individual patient progress is evaluated daily, as mentioned above. The clinical tracking form is removed from the patient's chart on discharge (Fig. 6–5) and taken to the cardiothoracic section of the clinic. The cardiothoracic surgery CNS routinely does the postoperative follow-up examination in the outpatient clinic and documents any changes since discharge. It is at this time that hospital and early postdischarge complications are noted. This information along with information from the clinical tracking form information is entered into a computerized data base. To improve patient care, data analysis is done to examine trends in deviations from the normal pathway and reasons for deviation. The grouped patient data are analyzed annually, and revisions to the CABG critical pathway are made.

Results. The reduction in postoperative length of stay since implementation of the CABG critical pathway is demonstrated in Figure 6–6. The postoperative length of stay in 1989, before implementation of the pathway, was 8.5 days, represented by the bar on the graph labeled B-89. This was reduced to 7.3 days for the first 6 months after implementation. The postoperative length of stay continued to decrease to 6.5 days in 1990 and held at that level for 1991.

Initial analysis of the length of stay by preexisting condition demonstrated interesting results. The mean length of stay for a patient with none of the tracked preexisting conditions was 6.6 days (Fig. 6–7). The four preexisting conditions with

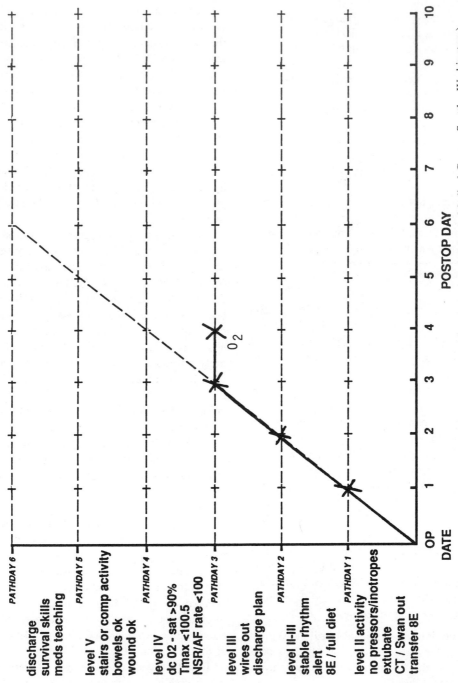

Figure 6–4 Clinical tracking form, example of deviation. (Courtesy Virginia Mason Medical Center, Seattle, Washington.)

TABLE 6–4 Pathway Deviation Codes

Patient
  A1: atrial fibrillation/flutter
  A2: ventricular arrhythmias
  A3: need for supplemental O_2
  A4: activity reduced because of fatigue
  A5: activity reduced because of nausea
  A6: activity refused by patient
  A7: confusion/disorientation
  A8: constipation
  A9: patient anxiety
  A10: other

System
  B1: bed not available in telemetry unit
  B2: order not processed
  B3: other

Provider
  C1: order not written
  C2: order not responded to
  C3: other

Courtesy Virginia Mason Medical Center, Seattle, Washington.

the longest mean length of stay were redo operation (8.5 days), diabetes (8 days), hypertension (7.5 days), and ejection fraction (7.3 days). The results over the next 2 years demonstrate a drop in mean length of stay in the diabetes and hypertension preexisting condition groups, a slight drop in the mean length of stay in the no preexisting condition group, and small increases in the mean length of stay for both the redo and ejection fraction groups (Fig. 6–8).

Mean length of stay by number of deviations was analyzed on the first full year of data (Fig. 6–9). The mean length of stay for those patients with no deviations to the right of the line of identity was 5.2 days. The mean length of stay increased with the number of deviations from one deviation with a length of stay of 6.2 days to greater than two deviations, demonstrating a mean length of stay at 11.9 days. The two most frequent reasons for deviation were atrial fibrillation with a mean length of stay at 7.4 days and prolonged need for supplemental oxygen with a corresponding mean length of stay of 7.4 days. In response to these results a research study, which will be discussed later, was developed to investigate prophylactic use of a beta

blocker to prevent atrial fibrillation. The respiratory therapy department is consulted for additional pulmonary care in patients at risk for prolonged use of supplemental oxygen.

A 6-month analysis of patient charges revealed a drop for both DRG 106 (heart catheterization and CABG surgery) and DRG 107 (CABG only). These were 24% and 29% reduction, respectively. Further analysis over the next year revealed the consistency of these reductions.

Operative mortality and morbidity results for the years 1989 and 1990 are listed in Table 6–5. Following implementation of case management, no clinically significant differences in mortality or in major or minor complication rates occurred.

Discussion. Initiation of the cardiothoracic surgery case management system has accomplished both length of stay and charge reduction while maintaining and even improving some patient outcomes. Unlike other systems of monitoring patient deviation, the clinical tracking form, with its graphic, visual documentation of patient progress, allowed for rapid, easy recognition of patient deviation. This was found to be useful to both nursing and house staff, especially in orienting new staff. The clinical tracking form not only aids in reducing variance by early intervention, but also documents the reason for prolonged length of stay for further analysis.

The clinical tracking form has been a valuable tool for the CNS to analyze trends and group variance for revision of patient care planning. Originally, the CABG critical pathway had patient transfer from the intensive care unit to the telemetry unit on pathday 2. Analysis of patient trends 1 year following implementation revealed that 80% of patients were able to be transferred from the intensive care unit on pathday 1. The CABG critical pathway and the clinical tracking form were then revised.

Use of the clinical tracking form has led to several research studies directed at improving patient care. Analysis of the types of patient variance revealed a 30% incidence of atrial fibrillation, which prolonged postoperative length of stay by 2 days. Investigation was done by literature review into methods to prevent the occurrence of postoperative atrial fibrillation. Some studies demonstrated good results using beta-blocker medication postoperatively. A multidisciplinary research group was

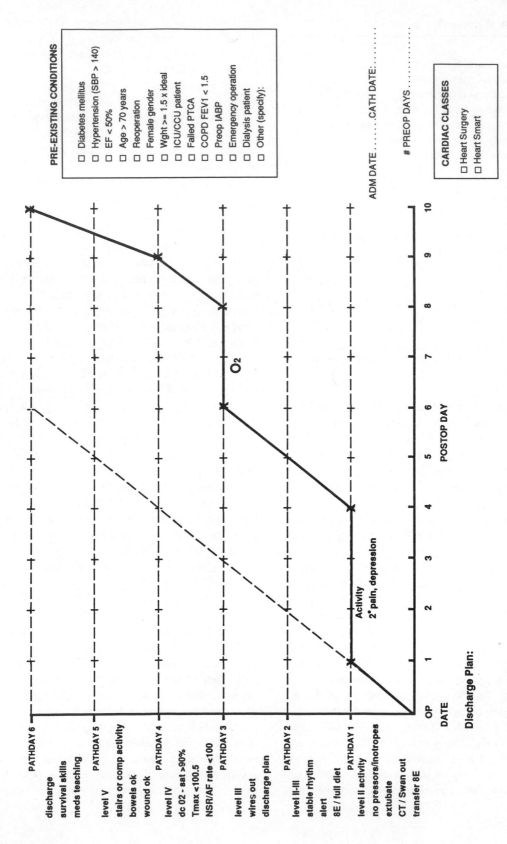

Figure 6–5 Clinical tracking form, Case study. (Courtesy Virginia Mason Medical Center, Seattle, Washington.)

74

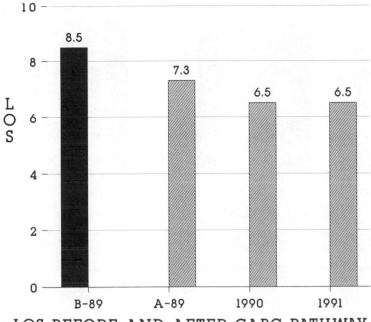

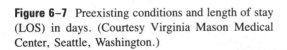

LOS BEFORE AND AFTER CABG PATHWAY

Figure 6–6 CABG pathway and length of stay (LOS) in days. (Courtesy Virginia Mason Medical Center, Seattle, Washington.)

Figure 6–7 Preexisting conditions and length of stay (LOS) in days. (Courtesy Virginia Mason Medical Center, Seattle, Washington.)

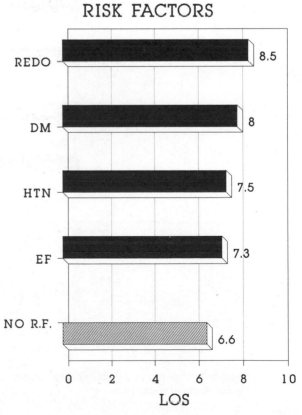

RISK FACTORS

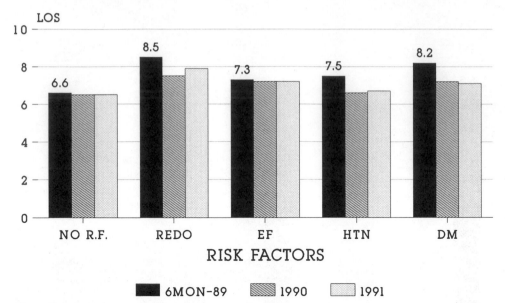

Figure 6–8 Preexisting conditions and results after 2+ years. (Courtesy Virginia Mason Medical Center, Seattle, Washington.)

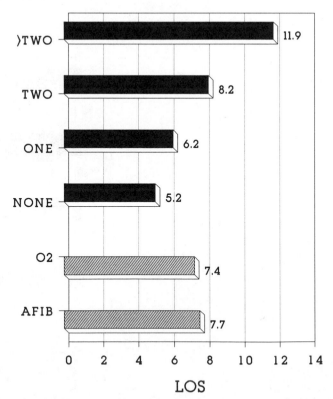

Figure 6–9 Pathway deviations and length of stay (LOS) in days. (Courtesy Virginia Mason Medical Center, Seattle, Washington.)

TABLE 6–5 Result Comparison (1989 vs. 1990)

	1989	1990
Mortality (%)	2.2	1.2
Major complications (%)		
Reoperation	1.2	1.2
Myocardial infarction	4.0	3.2
Other	9.4	6.4
Minor complications (%)		
Atrial fibrillation	29	31
Other	12	9

Courtesy Virginia Mason Medical Center, Seattle, Washington.

brought together to discuss the issue. A single-blind, randomized study was designed and is ongoing to examine the effects of beta-adrenergic blockade to prevent supraventricular arrhythmias following CABG.

The clinical tracking form was a useful tool to document patient progress in a study done comparing CABG patients admitted the day before surgery with those admitted the same day as surgery.[32] Future nursing studies are planned to investigate types of deviation leading to increased length of stay in patients with diabetes and patients undergoing reoperation.

This case management model has proven its value in improving the quality and cost effectiveness of cardiac surgery patient care. I recognize that this model may not be as easily adopted in other critically ill patients, particularly those patients with multiorgan failure. Management of the more complex critically ill patient using a case management approach has yet to be defined. The complex critically ill patient requires the collaboration of even greater numbers of health care personnel. Coordinating these individuals to manage one patient's care is the future challenge for the CC-CNS case manager. The following case study demonstrates the role of the CNS as case manager for a cardiac surgery patient.

CASE STUDY

Mr. H., a 42-year-old man, was admitted to the hospital with increasing angina at rest. In the 8 weeks before admission he had undergone two angioplasties with eventual restenosis of his involved coronary artery. A coronary angiogram and subsequent angio-plasty were performed on the restenosis. The angioplasty failed to dilate the lesion and resulted in a stable, small dissection. Mr. H. was referred to the cardiothoracic surgery department and taken to surgery the following day for CABG surgery. Before these events the patient had no history of coronary disease. Hypercholesterolemia and a positive family history were his only cardiac risk factors. Figure 6–5 shows his progress on the clinical tracking form.

Psychosocial History Mr. H. was the sole income for a household that included his common-law wife, her 17-year-old son, and two children of his own who lived elsewhere. He had a fifth-grade education, was functionally illiterate, and had been employed for 20 years an an auto mechanic. He was very apprehensive, refusing surgery initially.

Day of Surgery Mr. H. underwent a triple coronary artery bypass without any major difficulties. Following arrival in the intensive care unit he was on an esmolol drip for 2 hours. He stabilized over the night without need for pressors or inotropic support.

Postoperative Day 1 Mr. H. was extubated, his Swan-Ganz line and chest tubes were discontinued early in the day, and he was transferred to the telemetry unit in the afternoon. He achieved pathday 1; however, he was noted to have a flat affect and to be depressed.

Postoperative Days 2 to 4 Mr. H. remained at pathday 1 for the next 3 days, because he refused increased activity secondary to pain. He was noted to be very angry and depressed. He stated he was "too tired to answer questions" and remained unreceptive and withdrawn. He was also unwilling to use his incentive spirometer or participate in pulmonary toilet exercises. Mr. H. verbalized anger and concern over finances during his recovery and suicidal ideations. The CNS and his primary nurse developed a plan to address his various needs. The CNS and his nurses continued to encourage Mr. H. to verbalize his concerns. A referral to social services for financial aid application and emotional support was made. A consultation was made to the psychiatrist for assessment of his depression and suicidal ideation. Pain medication regimens were adjusted. The physical therapist continued to encourage Mr. H. to engage in physical activity. The need for pulmonary toilet was emphasized.

Postoperative Day 5 Mr. H. stated his pain was better and ambulated with his physical therapist for 3 minutes; however, he still appeared depressed and withdrawn. The psychiatrist diagnosed Mr. H. as having an adjustment disorder with depressed mood and suggested medication and supportive listening. The social worker started the process for Mr. H. to obtain public assistance.

Mr. H. developed a fewer of 39.1° C. A chest x-ray was done that revealed moderate atelectasis. Blood and sputum cultures were sent, which showed no growth after 24 hours. Room air pulse oxygen saturation was 74%, so the patient returned to 4 L of supplemental oxygen by nasal cannula. A respiratory therapist was consulted to work with pulmonary toilet. His cardiac rhythm was stable, and he was able to eat small amounts. He progressed to pathday 2.

Postoperative Day 6 Mr. H. was more cooperative and initiated activity and pulmonary toilet. He spent over 2 hours out of bed in a chair and ambulated in the hall twice for 5 minutes each. His temperature dropped to 38° C. His temporary pacing wires had been removed 2 days earlier. The CNS worked with Mr. H. and his wife to formulate his discharge plan. He progressed to pathday 3.

Postoperative Days 7 and 8 Mr. H. continued to increase his activity to 7 minutes on day 7 and 8 minutes on day 8. He still showed signs of depression but denied any suicidal thoughts. He remained at pathday 3 for the next 2 days because of hypoxia. His pulse oximetry oxygen saturation was checked and on room air was 77%. He was returned to 2 L of oxygen by nasal cannula. An arterial blood gas on this setting was pH 7.45, PCO_2 41, and PaO_2 69, with an oxygen saturation of 93%. A repeat chest x-ray was done and revealed a moderate right lower lobe pleural effusion. A chest tube was placed that drained 1150 ml of clear pink fluid over the next 24 hours.

His hematocrit was 21, which was down from 24 on postoperative day 2. No source of bleeding was found. He received 2 units of packed red blood cells, which brought his hematocrit up to 25.

Postoperative Day 9 Mr. H. was able to remove his supplemental oxygen, because his room air pulse oxygen saturation was 89%. He was afebrile and continued in a normal sinus rhythm. He ambulated 8 minutes and had met all the indicators for pathday 4.

Postoperative Day 10 Mr. H. climbed a flight of stairs and ambulated 9 minutes. He stated he was ready to go home. Discharge instructions were given to him and his wife. They verbalized a good understanding of them. Mr. H. was discharged to his home with an appointment to return to the cardiothoracic surgeon's office for a checkup in 2 days.

SUMMARY

The challenge in today's health care environment is how to maintain and even improve quality in a cost-effective environment. Case management is a system that has demonstrated results in meeting this challenge. Case management differs in how it is designed and implemented in every institution. After assessing the institution's needs as well as human and fiscal resources, nursing leaders must design their own specific program. Involvement of the CC-CNS in case management has demonstrated numerous benefits. The CC-CNS has the educational background and clinical expertise to be a valuable resource well suited to play a leading role in case management.

References

1. Cronin CJ, Maklebust J: Case-managed care: capitalizing on the CNS, *Nurs Management* 20(3):38-47, 1989.
2. Coile RC: Managed care: 10 leading trends for the 1990's. I, *Aspen's Advisor* 5(6), 1990.
3. Coile RC: Managed care: 10 leading trends for the 1990's. II, *Aspen's Advisor* 5(7), 1990.
4. Evans SA, Carlson R: Nurse/physician collaboration: solving the nursing shortage crisis, *Am J Crit Care* 1(1):25-32, 1992.
5. Zander K: Managed care within acute care settings: design and implementation via nursing case management, *Health Care Supervisor* 6(2):27-43, 1988.

6. Del Tongo Armanasco V, Olivas GS, Harter S: Developing an integrated nursing case management model, *Nurs Management* 20(10):26-29, 1989.

7. Zander K: Nursing case management: resolving the DRG paradox, *Nurs Clin North Am* 23(3):503-519, 1988.

8. Olivas GS et al: Case management—a bottom-line care delivery model. II. Adaptation of the model, *J Nurs Admin* 19(12):12-17, 1989.

9. Howard JC et al: Cost-related variables: a pilot study, *Clin Nurs Specialist* 3(1):37-40, 1989.

10. Mckenzie CB, Torkelson NG, Holt MA: Care and cost: nursing case management improves both, *Nurs Management* 20(10):30-33, 1989.

11. Zander K: Nursing case management: strategic management of cost and quality outcomes, *J Nurs Admin* 18(5):23-30, 1988.

12. Zander K: Differentiating managed care and case management, *Definition* 5(2), 1990.

13. American Nurses' Association: *Nursing case management*, Kansas City, Mo, 1988, The Association.

14. Strong AG: Case management and the CNS, *Clin Nurse Specialist* 6(2):64, 1992.

15. Maklebust J et al: Results of collaboration between case managers and staff nurses, *Mich Nurse*, p 11, May 1990.

16. Gawlinski A, Boggs R, Quinn A: CNS leadership opportunities in case management, *AACN News* p. 7, Oct, 1989.

17. Walthall S: An enhancement of the role of the clinical nurse specialist, *Mich Nurse*, pp 6-8, May 1990.

18. Convey-Svec C: The clinical nurse specialist and PPS reimbursement, *Nurs Management* 22(5):90, 1991.

19. Schroer K: Case management: clinical nurse specialist and nurse practitioner, coverging roles, *Clin Nurse Specialist* 5(4):189-194, 1991.

20. Schull DE, Tosch P, Wood M: Clinical nurse specialists as collaborative care managers, *Nurs Management* 23(3):30-33, 1992.

21. Gaedeke Norris MK, Hill C: The clinical nurse specialist: developing the case manager role, *Dimen Crit Care Nurs* 10(6):346-353, 1991.

22. Green S: The impact of case management, *Mich Nurse,* p 4, May 1990.

23. Rudy EB, Grenvik A: The future of critical care, *Am J Crit Care* 1(1):33-37, 1992.

24. Garder D: The CNS as cost manager, *Clin Nurse Specialist* 6(2):112-116, 1992.

25. Green S: The impact of case management, *Mich Nurse,* p 4, May 1990.

26. Papenhausen JL: Case management. a model of advanced practice? *Clin Nurse Specialist* 4(4):169-170, 1990.

27. Strong AG, Sneed NV: Clinical evaluation of a critical path for coronary artery bypass surgery patients, *Prog Cardiovasc Nurs* 6(1):30-37, 1991.

28. Kennedy JW et al: Multivariate discriminate analysis of the angiographic predictors of operative mortality from the collaborative study in coronary artery surgery (CASS), *J Thorac Cardiovasc Surg* 80:876-887, 1980.

29. Parsonnet V, Dean D, Bernstein AD: A method of uniform stratification of risk for evaluating the results of surgery in acquired adult heart disease, *Circulation* 79 (suppl I):I-3–I-12, 1989.

30. Kennedy JW et al: Clinical and angiographic predictors of operative mortality from the collaborative study in coronary artery surgery (CASS), *Circulation* 63(4):793-801, 1981.

31. Hannan EL et al: Adult open heart surgery in New York state: an analysis of risk factors and hospital mortality rates, *JAMA* 264(21):2768-2774, 1990.

32. Anderson RP et al: Selection of patients for same-day coronary bypass operations, *J Thorac Cardiovasc Surg,* 105(3):444-452, 1993.

The Critical Care Clinical Nurse Specialist in Continuous Quality Improvement

Leslie S. Kern, RN, MN
Linda Faber, RN, PhD

The current health care system is undergoing sweeping reforms brought on by reduced economic and employment resources, public demands for greater accountability, and political forces that are striving to manage and define health care. Rigorous efforts to control costs of health care (i.e., the prospective payment system) have been accompanied by concerns about the quality of care received. Paralleling these concerns about our health care system have been observations of the success of Japanese industry in producing quality products. It became clear to industries in the United States that to be competitive a new approach to quality was needed. Industries began incorporating the new philosophy of continuous quality improvement (CQI) as the way of doing business. In the service sector the Joint Commission for Accreditation of Health Care Organizations (JCAHO) began to chart a new direction for the health care industry. The JCAHO asserted that quality could not be *assured* but that it could be *improved* by using CQI. "The transition from quality assurance to quality improvement is an inevitable step in the evolution of approaches to managing health care quality."[1]

The critical care clinical nurse specialist (CC-CNS) has provided leadership for quality in the past and will continue to provide leadership for this transition. As an expert practitioner the CC-CNS identifies priority nursing activities to be addressed and determines minimal standards for excellence in practice. As educator the CC-CNS teaches nursing staff CQI concepts by role modeling the process in daily practice and by facilitating CQI team processes. As consultant the CC-CNS coordinates CQI activities with the multidisciplinary team and provides expert guidance in the management of complex patients. As researcher the CC-CNS provides direction for tool development and assists staff to define and measure outcomes of nursing care. In addition, the CC-CNS brings research-based findings to the bedside to resolve nursing care issues identified by the CQI process. As manager or leader the CC-CNS generates motivation about CQI and actively participates in nursing practice change. The CC-CNS fosters an environment of innovative nursing care where the CQI process provides direction and a framework for action.

This chapter focuses on the CC-CNS's unique contribution to quality processes. The history of quality issues in health care is reviewed within the context of current changes in health care. Literature on the CNS role in quality improvement is reviewed. Practice implications for the CC-CNS present a multifaceted approach for CC-CNS leadership in CQI. The 10-step monitoring and evaluation process is described with special emphasis on the CC-CNS role. Finally, case examples from CC-CNS practice are presented for further thought and discussion.

THEORETIC FRAMEWORK
Historical Notes

The beginning of quality improvements in health care can be traced to Florence Nightingale in the 1850s. She tracked various health conditions and outcomes to identify ways to improve health and sanitary conditions for British soldiers. Her meticulous *Notes on Hospitals*[2] and *Notes on Nursing*[3] served for decades as standards for caring for sick persons and as the standard text for nursing.

It was not until the 1950s that the study of quality care became rigorous. In 1951 the American College of Surgeons, American College of Physicians, American Hospital Association, American Medical Association, and Canadian Medical Association established the Joint Commission on Accreditation of Hospitals. (The American Dental Association became a corporate member in 1979, and the Canadian Medical Association withdrew in 1959 to establish its own accreditation program.) In 1980 public members were added, and in 1992 a seat was designated for nursing.

As shown in Table 7–1, quality assurance began with implicit reviews, followed by medical audits, and then by systematic monitoring and evaluation activities.[1] Although JCAHO standards are considered the gold standard for health care providers, standards and quality of care have been addressed within other organizations. The American Nurses' Association (ANA), American Operating Room Nurses' Association (AORN), and American Association of Critical Care Nurses (AACN) are three examples of nursing organizations that have developed nursing practice standards. At the federal level is an agency of the Public Health Service, the Agency for Health Care Policy and Research (AHCPR). AHCPR's mission is "to enhance the

TABLE 7–1 Evolution of Quality Measures

Measure	Example
Implicit review	Morbidity and mortality review
Time-limited studies	Retrospective audits
Ongoing monitoring and evaluation	Quality assurance
Integrated program of continuous improvement	Quality improvement

quality of patient care services through improved knowledge that can be used in meeting society's health care needs."[4] This agency is achieving its goals through research programs, demonstrations, evaluations, and information dissemination activities.

The evolution of quality monitoring has consistently moved toward specificity in defining, measuring, and improving the actual service delivered in the health care industry. This was accomplished by instituting organization-wide programs with measurable criteria. Systematic monitoring and evaluation by departments led to the idea of continuously improving the process of care similar to the Japanese model. With the JCAHO's *Agenda for Change*, CQI replaced quality assurance.

Definitions of Quality

In 1988 the JCAHO[5] defined quality of care as the degree to which patient care services increase the probability of desired patient or client outcomes and reduce the probability of undesired outcomes, given the current state of knowledge. Contemporary thought[5] on the definition of patient care quality incorporates four additional concepts:

1. The structures and processes of care are the focus of attention when drawing conclusions about patient care quality.
2. The assessment of the structures and processes includes their effect on the outcomes of patient care.
3. The structures and processes of care only affect the probability of the outcomes of care. Alone they do not guarantee those outcomes, since outcomes depend on many other variables (e.g., patient risk, compliance with treatment).
4. Because the probability of positive outcomes can be improved (e.g., with new knowledge), patient care quality is not viewed as a static "acceptable level of care"; rather it is subject to continuous improvement.[5]

Hospital Corporation of America (HCA) defined quality within the context of total quality management. For HCA hospitals, quality is defined as the continuous improvement of services to meet and/or exceed the needs and expectations of patients, the physicians, the payers, the employees, and the communities served.[6]

In the health care setting, quality care includes

five components: (1) efficient use of resources, (2) minimal risk to the patient of injury or illness associated with care, (3) competence in performance by health care professionals, (4) patient satisfaction, and (5) compassionate care. For the critical care areas, appropriateness of services rendered to patients is especially crucial, given the high cost of intensive care.

Quality Assurance vs. Quality Improvement

Although current thought focuses on quality improvement, the framework of traditional quality assurance has provided a solid base on which to build continuous quality improvement. *Quality improvement* is an organizational and leadership philosophy that guides organizational operations for the purpose of improving the quality of services provided and to improved customer satisfaction. Quality improvement capitalizes on the strengths of quality assurance while broadening its scope and methodologies and eliminating the negative connotations. Table 7–2 identifies the strengths and weaknesses of quality assurance in transitioning to CQI.

The JCAHO in its 1992 standards began the transition to CQI. The focus of these changes has been on interdepartmental communications and the roles of hospital leaders in CQI. The 1994 standards continue the transition with emphasis on education and training, communications and collaboration, and evaluation of effectiveness of CQI activities.[1]

Agenda for Change

The JCAHO initiated their renewed quest for quality improvement with the launching of their agenda for change. The goals of the agenda are to establish an interactive data system based on established valid and reliable national indicators and to refocus the standards on those important governance, managerial, clinical, and support functions that most affect the quality of care.

National clinical indicator sets (the data base for the agenda for change) have been developed by professional organizations, national leaders, and JCAHO officials. This data base will allow organizations across the United States to communicate with similar institutions regarding outcomes and processes of care.[7] It is planned that data will be entered regularly electronically so that feedback

TABLE 7–2 Strengths and Weaknesses of Quality Assurance and Quality Improvement

Traditional Quality Assurance	Continuous Quality Improvement
Externally driven	Internally driven
Follows organizational structure	Follows patient flow
Problem solving	Continuous improvement
Short-term goals and commitment	Never-ending process
Performed in clinical departments	Hospital-wide
Emphasis on special causes	Emphasis on both special and common causes
Focused on people (peer review)	Focused on process improvement
Actions directed toward people	Actions directed toward process improvement
Can create defensiveness	Promotes team spirit and can break down turf lines
Evaluation based on inspection and documentation	Evaluation based on customer satisfaction
Clinical care	Service quality
Divided analysis of effectiveness and efficiency	Integrated analysis

and comparisons are ongoing. Each of the indicator sets has been rigorously tested and refined.

Leadership and CQI

The assumptions underlying CQI are (1) processes are customer focused; (2) improvement in key processes results in improved outcomes; (3) processes are rigorously studied through measurement, control of variations in processes, and tracking of effectiveness and efficiency; (4) people who are closest to the work (i.e., those who do the work) are involved in the study and redesign; (5) continually improving processes is the driving focus of the measurements systems in the organization; and (6) leadership is involved and committed to quality as an organizational focus.

Successful application of CQI in health care is

contingent on leaders who exercise prudent selection and application of valid indicators. Within the cadre of clinical team members, the CC-CNS is in a unique position to cut across functional departmental boundaries to improve outcomes of patient care. The CC-CNS is considered the clinical expert, the clinical care administrator, the clinical program researcher, the clinical performance evaluator, and the staff development coordinator. Thus the CC-CNS has the vantage point of leading the way for continuous improvement in patient care.

REVIEW OF LITERATURE

Although many CNS publications expound quality improvement as an important role function,[7] little has been published on the topic for CNSs in general or critical care practice. This section will therefore provide a framework for the CC-CNS role in quality processes.

CC-CNS Role: Transitioning from Quality Assurance to CQI

As quality assurance activities make the transition to CQI, the CC-CNS can assist in translating the indicator assessments of quality of care into more rigorous, systematic studies, including more precise methodologies and more valid criteria and indicators. For example, the CC-CNS could suggest using one of the AHCPR guidelines for pain to develop indicators for postoperative patients.[8] Use of the scientific process and statistical process control is key to continuous quality improvements.

The CC-CNS is already accepted by members of the health care team as a translator of patient care among disciplines for the welfare of the patient. The CC-CNS has always been in a position to facilitate communication among practitioners by presenting the clinical situation in easily understood terms. This role has a natural extension into the CQI process, which studies important cross functions believed to have the greatest impact on quality patient outcomes. During daily clinical rounds with a team of physicians, discharge planning rounds, case presentations, or morbidity and mortality reviews, the CC-CNS can play an important role in identifying opportunities for care improvements. The CC-CNS is also an excellent choice as quality improvement team leader or facilitator.

The CC-CNS working with the physician has played a pivotal position in outlining critical paths of care (see Chapter 6). The continued monitoring and evaluation of patient progress and the aggregation of data for recovery patterns lend themselves well for future scientific study of processes of care. These studies have implications for resource utilization and costs of health care. In this manner the CC-CNS has the potential for influencing national health care policy, specifically regarding financing and allocation of health care resources.

A knowledgeable and informed CC-CNS guided by continuous improvement data can play a critical part in the survival of a health care organization. The CC-CNS can assist administrators to identify market niches and garner the organization's share of reimbursement allocations. Third-party payers and patients (the ultimate customer) are asking for data to support care decisions and choices of preferred providers. Program evaluation and CQI data with valid and reliable indicators of important processes can be marketing points.

CC-CNS Role in Linking Standards with CQI
Defining Standards

A standard is a statement of quality that serves as a model to facilitate and evaluate the delivery of optimal nursing care.[9] Three types of standards have been identified as being essential to the quality improvement process: structure, process, and outcome. Structure refers to the environment and resources (both equipment and staffing resources) required for the delivery of patient care. An example of a structure standard is the requirement that every intensive care unit (ICU) be equipped with a defibrillator. Process standards refer to nursing process activities and the steps included in the process. An example of a process standard is the requirement that ICU nurses know of the advanced cardiac life support (ACLS) algorithms and are prepared to apply them in an arrest situation. Structure and process standards for critical care nursing are described in the 1989 text *Standards for Nursing Care of the Critically Ill* published by AACN.[10]

Outcome standards refer to the results of a treatment or intervention.[11] Outcome measures are considered by some to be the most valid indicators of quality of care.[12] Outcome monitoring is the preferred quality assurance approach, since the information gained from measuring outcomes has potentially the greatest impact on the quality of care.

Although outcome measures are key to quality monitoring, they are useless without structure and process measures. For example, a patient admitted with an active variceal bleed may be treated aggressively and receive the best possible care but still die. In this case, process is good, but the outcome is bad. Conversely, another patient with massive gastrointestinal bleeding may be inappropriately admitted to a non–intensive care setting, allowed unnecessarily to deteriorate, but ultimately survive. In this case the process was bad, but the outcome was good. Quality indicators should therefore reflect structure, process, and outcome measures of care. The CC-CNS can assist the quality of care committee in identifying structure, process, and outcome indicators so that the continuum of patient care activities can be comprehensively evaluated.

Measuring Outcomes of Nursing Care

Under the guiding principles of CQI, indicators must have the scientific rigor of validity and reliability. The CC-CNS has the knowledge and expertise to identify valid and reliable indicators that impact meaningful processes of care and patient outcomes. The CC-CNS is able to interpret physiologic as well as psychologic and sociologic information as it relates to patient care outcomes.

In AACN's book *Outcome Standards for Nursing Care of the Critically Ill*[9] nursing diagnoses are used as the framework for defining outcomes of nursing. This text was recently cited as one of the rare examples of an outcome framework specific to nursing.[11] Table 7–3 gives examples of outcome criteria from this text. The criteria described here are measurable and adapt easily for use in CQI studies.

At this time in nursing, outcome indicators remain broad in scope, such as "absence of infection" or "patient hemodynamically stable." Although these outcomes reflect nursing phenomena, they also depend on the action of other disciplines and are influenced by multiple physiologic variables not controlled by nursing and therefore do not accurately reflect nursing's particular effect on the patient. The question then becomes "What are outcomes of *nursing* care? How do we measure the results of nursing? What is the most accurate framework for nursing outcomes: a nursing diagnosis framework, a functional status framework?" These and other questions related to measuring patient

TABLE 7–3 AACN Outcome Indicators and Criteria for Critically Ill Patients

Nausea is absent or controlled
"Sick to stomach" complaints absent
Adverse reaction to food or food odors absent
Salivation normal

Pain is absent or controlled
States pain relieved or manageable
Manifestations of pain absent
Respiratory rate, heart rate, and blood pressure normal
Body relaxed

Communication is effective
Acknowledges affirmatively when caregiver correctly repeats content of message sent
Banging on side rails absent or reduced
Uses interpreter, communication tool
Parent indicates preverbal child's needs
Stuttering absent or reduced
Slurred speech absent or reduced
Level of frustration, anger, anxiety, helplessness, fear decreased

Family coping is effective
Family available
Intrafamily cooperation with decision making
Expresses realistic understanding of health status

Coping is effective
Participates in decisions regarding health
Support from social network garnered
Physical limitations acknowledged
Sleep/wake pattern normal for person, activity in unit
Decrease in fear, anger, withdrawal

Dyspnea is absent or reduced
Indicates unpleasant sensation with breathing absent or reduced
Completes sentence without stopping for breath
Accessory respiratory muscle use appropriate to activity level
Respiratory rate normal or reduced

From American Association of Critical Care Nurses: *Outcome standards for nursing care of the critically ill,* Laguna Niguel, Calif, 1990, The Association.

outcomes are the focus of current research and dialogue in nursing.[11] For the CC-CNS involved in the CQI process, the definition of outcomes becomes challenging. The general nursing research literature[13-19] and critical care nursing research literature[20-27] can assist the CC-CNS in identification of valid nursing outcome criteria. As described above, the AACN's *Outcomes for Nursing Care of the Critically Ill* is also an excellent reference.

Research Case Study: Use of Mortality Statistics as an Outcome Indicator for Nursing Care. One recent example in the nursing literature examined the effects of monitoring activities on patient mortality. Since much of the critical care nurse's time is spent in monitoring activities, this study is presented here.

Rubenstein et al.[28] studied the effects of implementation of Medicare's prospective payment system on patient outcomes. This study was conducted in a national sample of 14,012 patients, representing 297 hospitals. To do this a scale, called the RN Assessment Scale, was developed to monitor the process of nursing surveillance. Nursing surveillance consisted of key signs and symptoms for each disease. The scale was specific for five patient diagnoses studied: congestive heart failure (CHF), myocardial infarction (MI), pneumonia, cerebrovascular accident (CVA), and hip fractures. For each scale, criteria were identified for selected activities that a nurse performs to monitor the clinical status of a patient. These criteria included physical examination activities and the process of gathering historical data. In the development of the tool, the researchers tested its predictive ability; that is, if the nurses scored lower on this assessment scale, did this predict a negative outcome for the patient? They found that the quality of nursing surveillance was strongly linked to patient outcomes when controlling for sickness at admission. The 30-day postadmission mortality among patients with CHF with good nursing surveillance was 11% vs. 17% for patients with poor surveillance. Acute MI patients with good nursing surveillance had a 24% mortality compared with a 27% mortality for patients with poor surveillance. This study is a good example of how mortality statistics can be used as indicators of outcomes of nursing care. In addition, correlation among scales (nurse and physician) indicated that improved nursing surveillance was accompanied by improvements in physician assessment, diagnosis, and treatment.

These findings have important implications for the critical care practitioner. This study lends validity to an emphasis on monitoring activities as an important nursing process activity. In addition, it validates the importance of collaborative partnerships with physicians, a concept that is not new in critical care. Nursing assessment may be linked to other critical aspects of the nurse's role. As Rubenstein and colleagues[28] observe:

> For example, nurses who monitor shortness of breath to assess the clinical condition of a patient with CHF also may be attentive to other aspects of the patient's condition, whereas nurses who fail to perform the critical initial step of assessing the patient may be likely to fail in other aspects of nursing process as well.

With the physician relying on the nursing assessment to make critical treatment decisions, an inattentive nurse could start a series of inappropriate treatment decisions, resulting in increased patient mortality.

This study points to the importance of monitoring nursing processes, such as surveillance, when developing CQI study indicators for critically ill patients. It also demonstrates the value of patient mortality as an outcome measure for nursing. Improvements in the structures and processes surrounding patient care can result in improved outcomes.

CC-CNS Role in Linking Quality Assurance, CQI, and Research

One of the five roles of a CC-CNS is researcher. This researcher role is conceptualized in the broadest sense of the research continuum. The research continuum begins with everyday problem solving for immediacy of resolving clinical problems in patient care and culminates in conducting rigorous study on researchable topics in the quest for knowledge and building the scientific base of nursing practice.

Research Continuum

Problem Solving	Quality Assurance	Program Evaluation	Scientific Research

On this continuum traditional quality assurance is considered to be less rigorous than program evaluation, which is less rigorous than pure research science. The similarity in all positions on the continuum is that each is with solving patient care problems using a very similar process with varying degrees of scientific rigor. Table 7–4 provides a parallel between the steps involved in the quality assurance monitoring and evaluation process and the scientific research process.

The CC-CNS is well versed in problem-solving skills for resolving complex care issues as well as

TABLE 7–4 Comparison of Nursing Process, 10-Step Monitoring and Evaluation, and Nursing Research

Nursing Process	10-Step Monitoring and Evaluation	Nursing Research
Problem identification through assessment	Assign responsibility	Formulate and limit research problem
	Delineate scope of care	
	Identify important aspects of care or function	Review related literature
	Identify indicators: structures, process, outcomes	Develop theoretic or conceptual framework
	Establish thresholds for evaluation	Identify variables
		Formulate hypotheses
		Select research design
Develop care plan	Specify methodology and population	Specify population and sample
		Operationalize variables
Implement plan and collect information	Collect and aggregate data	Conduct pilot study
		Collect data
Evaluate information	Interpret information for evaluation of care	Analyze data
Revise plan	Take actions to solve problems	Interpret results of study
	Assess actions and document improvement	
	Communicate relevant information	Communicate study findings

equally versed in the rigors of science. The CC-CNS is in a pivotal position to begin tracking or graphing quality assurance results that begin the process of amassing patterns or trends to be subjected to more scientific study. Often quality assurance data provide the baseline for scientific study.

Research utilization leads to refinements of guidelines and protocol and institutionalization of practice changes. The CC-CNS is often the resource for bringing research findings to the attention of clinical staff for critique. The topic could be based on findings of quality assurance or differential practice patterns observed through continuous quality improvements. The CC-CNS working with a nurse researcher could conduct meta-analyses of relevant literature and evaluate the resulting practice protocol. Some practice changes addressed through research utilization are saline flushes for peripheral lines, temperature measurement, failure to thrive practice guidelines, urinary incontinence practice guidelines, pressure ulcer protocols, and pain management protocols.

The role of the CC-CNS in quality assurance or CQI brings with it unique opportunities for application of research principles and identification of researchable questions. For example, in studying the practice protocols for care of CVC lines, quality assurance data revealed wide variation in practices within a hospital, among employees, and across communities. A national survey conducted by one of the authors (L.F.) revealed that there is little agreement on types or rotations of cleansing agents, the procedure for cleaning and changing lines, or the procedure for dressing changes. A search of the literature did not clarify the process, because published findings were inconsistent and were not amenable to metaanalyses for development and testing of a practice protocol. Through quality assurance activities a very important clinical problem for study was identified.

In summary, there are distinct advantages in linking quality assurance, CQI, and the research process. The outcomes of quality assurance and CQI are the developmental seeds for research programs, assist in establishing the scientific, empiric basis of standards, and assist in building the scientific knowledge base for practice. The follow-up actions to improve the quality of care can include managerial, behavioral, educational, and equipment/supply changes. These corrective strategies could be researched to determine which has a greater impact on quality of patient care. Although the goals of CQI and research may differ, their processes are complementary and the CC-CNS is in a key position to affect the links for quality patient care.

PRACTICE IMPLICATIONS

As hospitals restructure their quality of care program, the CC-CNS's special skills can foster restructuring within the organization at the unit level. Initially the CC-CNS's role may be one of mentor, until staff members develop expertise and comfort with the process. The mentoring role of the CC-CNS may extend beyond nursing, with the CC-CNS providing leadership for other disciplines as well. As others develop confidence with the CQI process, the CC-CNS role becomes one of facilitator. The CC-CNS role, however, is not limited to formal monitoring and evaluation activities. During multidisciplinary rounds and case conferences, the CC-CNS has an opportunity to practice the CQI process and focus discussion on what can be done to improve the quality of care. The CC-CNS draws from the expertise of peers in other disciplines to assist in the CQI process and to identify appropriate patient interventions. Finally, the CC-CNS oversees the evaluation phase of the monitoring process, implementing and maintaining innovations in practice. The CC-CNS role in CQI is therefore one of mentor, facilitator, catalyst, and maintainer of changes in practice.

Empowering Staff

The CC-CNS and nurse manager are ultimately accountable for the CQI process on a nursing unit, but the process alone cannot affect patient care without the acceptance and support of nursing staff. The CQI process is truly a change process, because the identification of important aspects of care that are below threshold indicates an action is needed to resolve the problem. As with any change process, the involvement of those individuals most affected by the change is key to success. Therefore responsibility for CQI needs to be shared with nursing staff.

In the past, quality assurance evoked negative feelings, because this process focused on identification of problems and often ended in searching for the "bad apple." Staff members were uncomfortable with the process and avoided membership on quality assurance committees. Thus quality assurance was often left to the CC-CNS and nurse manager to either impose on staff or complete themselves. Although the CQI process also looks at problems, the focus is not on individual behavior, nor is the focus on problems. The focus is on outcomes and all of the individuals and processes that contribute to an optimal outcome. Because the opportunity is to fix system problems, staff can more readily see the relevance of the topics for study and how the results could affect patient care and practice standards. Data collection is expected to occur concurrently rather than retroactively so that actual care being delivered may be improved.

Although these changes from quality assurance to CQI may help alter some of the negative response to CQI, the CC-CNS must continually role model this important process and demonstrate its applicability to daily practice. The CC-CNS strives to empower staff with this process (Table 7–5) so that they are comfortable with it and value it.

The challenge for the CC-CNS is to familiarize staff with this process. Nursing literature reveals

TABLE 7–5 Strategies for Empowering Staff with CQI

Introduce staff to CQI process early in orientation
Provide formal education about process
Share past successful CQI projects with new staff
Reward staff for participation in process
Reward staff for achieving outcomes of care
Appoint a staff nurse to represent unit at a divisional CQI meeting
Consult with nurse manager to provide paid time for staff to work on CQI projects
Promote staff accountability for CQI results by having staff members report results to unit director and divisional CQI committee
Reward creative solutions to problems identified in CQI process
Have CQI committee members provide formal report on activities at all staff meetings
Develop staff nurse leadership to assume committee chairperson responsibilities (unit and divisional)
Include CQI activities in evaluation process
Have staff identify important aspects of care to be studied from problems that they face in their clinical practice
Have staff involve patients or significant others in examining delivery of care

that an individual's level of commitment and involvement in quality processes is related to the individual's valuation of the program[29]; that is, the higher the value placed on this process, the greater the nurse's involvement. The most effective way for a CC-CNS to ensure quality is to work closely with the people who deliver patient care and to influence their valuing of the CQI process. Through daily observations in clinical rounds and in working directly with staff, the CC-CNS has the opportunity to role model the CQI process.

Moving into a Multidisciplinary CQI Program

Most institutions are transitioning from quality assurance to CQI. This time of transition is an opportunity for the CC-CNS to act and take a leadership role in CQI. One of the major changes of this transition is the emphasis on a multidisciplinary approach. The CC-CNS can initiate movement toward CQI by talking with staff from nursing and other disciplines on her or his unit to begin looking at how each discipline contributes to the goals of patient care. CQI focuses on the patient as a whole and therefore promotes the monitoring and evaluation process as a team process. Although individual quality assurance activities continue at the department level, CQI activities demand a shared approach with all disciplines accountable for desired outcomes.

The CC-CNS has an opportunity to support physician colleagues in transitioning to CQI. The CC-CNS can schedule time with the unit director and other active physicians to review the CQI committee's annual plan. The CC-CNS can enlist physician support by providing information on how the process will benefit their patients. The CC-CNS can clarify the goals of the CQI process by providing information on the differences between quality assurance and CQI. CQI's focus is on the customer and meeting the needs of the customer. The physician is a customer in the health care system. The CQI process gives physicians the tools they need to do what they are trained to do as scientists, namely, to examine outcomes and use the information to improve treatment. Most physicians, once exposed to the CQI process, welcome it because it helps them to provide better care for patients.

CQI in Action: 10-Step Monitoring and Evaluation Process

Central to CQI is the problem-solving process. In this section, the 10-step monitoring and evaluation process is described and examples from critical care practice are presented.

Step 1: Assign Responsibility. This first step in the monitoring and evaluation process is to ensure an organized approach to quality monitoring. Usually this information is part of a unit quality improvement policy. Health care personnel are assigned roles in the monitoring and evaluation process (Table 7–6). It is important that the CC-CNS identify her or his role in this process. The JCAHO manual for accreditation has indicated for critical care areas that the unit director has overall responsibility for quality of care.[5]

Step 2: Delineate Scope of Care and Service. Annually the quality care committee should identify its scope of care and services. This statement includes clinical care activities such as treatments, procedures, modalities used, and types of services provided. Key concepts to be covered are types of conditions treated, managed, and prevented; and what treatments are rendered to whom, when, where, and by whom. Appendix 7–1 provides an example of a scope of care and service for an intensive care nursery.

Step 3: Identify Important Aspects of Care. From all the activities listed in the scope of services and care, the CQI team identifies those activities or processes that contribute the most to patient outcomes. The committee focuses on what patient groups are high volume, are high risk, or have recurring problems related to outcomes of care.

Important aspects of care include functions, procedures, treatments, processes, or other activities that direct patient care. They are the aspects of care that are most important for increasing the probability of a desired patient care outcome and decreasing the probability of undesired outcomes of care. These important aspects of care constitute the priorities for the CQI process. Table 7–7 gives important aspects of care for a medical-surgical intensive care unit.

Step 4: Identify Indicators. Indicators are measurable variables relating to the structure, process, or outcomes of care[5] (Table 7–8). Indicators should be measurable and well defined for ease and reli-

TABLE 7-6 Assigning Responsibility for CQI

Staff	Hospital Governing Body	Section on Critical Care	Medical Director of ICU	ICU Quality Assurance Committee	CNS	ICU Staff	Quality Assurance Staff
Steps							
1. Establish overall responsibility	X	X	X	X			
2. Delineate scope of care		X	X	X	X		
3. Identify important aspects of care		X	X	X	X	X	
4. Identify indicators		X		X	X	X	
5. Establish thresholds		X		X	X	X	
6. Collect and organize data						X	X
7. Evaluate care		X	X	X	X	X	
8. Take action		X	X	X	X		
9. Assess actions		X	X	X	X		
10. Report relevant information		X	X	X	X	X	
Comments:							

TABLE 7-7 Important Aspects of Care for an Intensive Care Nursery

1. Medication delivery
2. Management of suspected sepsis
3. Ventilator management of patients with acute respiratory failure
4. Nutritional support
5. Patient and family education
6. Interhospital transfer
7. Intravenous (IV) therapy management
8. Thermoregulation
9. Measuring and documenting bilirubin light irradiance
10. Inspired gas temperature
11. Mechanical ventilation
12. Oxygen therapy
13. Aerosol therapy treatments
14. Artificial airway management and maintenance
15. Drug orders

From Joint Commission on Accreditation of Health Care Organizations: *Quality improvements in special care units*, Oakbrook Terrace, Ill, 1990, The Commission.

TABLE 7-8 Indicators of Structure, Process, and Outcomes of Care for Critically Ill Patients

Type	Indicators
Structure	Patients receiving intraaortic balloon pump therapy will receive 1:1 nursing care.
	Emergency cart will be restocked within 30 minutes after use.
	Patients with infectious illnesses will not be admitted to transplant intensive care unit.
Process	Lidocaine is administered according to unit protocol.
	Pulmonary artery pressure measures are taken from paper printout.
	Elevated v waves on a pulmonary wedge tracing are read as the mean value from paper printout.
	Sepsis site is identified within 8 hours of admission.
Outcome	Patient has normal breath sounds.
	Patient is without dysrhythmias for 24 hours.
	No reintubation is done within 48 hours of elective extubation.

ability of data collection. Sources of indicators include hospital and unit standards, professional society guidelines (AACN, ANA), clinical literature, laws and regulations (JCAHO), government guidelines (AHCPR guidelines), and staff expertise or experience.

Step 5: Establish Thresholds for Evaluation. "The threshold is the pre-established level or point in the cumulative data analysis that will trigger an intensive evaluation. When the pre-established level (threshold) is exceeded, an in-depth evaluation of that aspect of care is conducted to determine why."[30] Thresholds are usually expressed as a percent but can also be listed as a ratio or number. They should be realistic and not too high or too low. Table 7–9 illustrates a data collection instrument with indicators and thresholds for a medical intensive care unit.

Step 6: Collect and Organize Data. Data collection tools are developed and the data collection

TABLE 7–9 Sample Indicators and Thresholds for Evaluating an ICU*

INTENSIVE CARE UNIT: MANAGEMENT OF PATIENTS WITH SEPTIC SHOCK

Indicator 1: Identification of sepsis site within 8 hours of admission
  Threshold 1: 90% of cases (i.e., cases with septic shock)

Indicator 2: Use of antibiotic therapy timely and appropriate
  Indicator 2a: Antibiotic therapy started within 2 hours of the septic episode or of admission (prescribed on the basis of clinical assessment, smears, and/or available culture results)
    Threshold 2a: 90% of cases
  Indicator 2b: Antibiotic therapy confirmed, adjusted, or changed within 72 hours of septic episode or of admission on basis of culture results
    Threshold 2b: 90% of cases

Indicator 3: Patient oriented to time/place/person by 48 hours of septic episode or admission
  Threshold 3: 90% of cases

Indicator 4: Respiratory failure:
  • Mechanical ventilation required because of impaired gas exchange (hypoxemia, hypercarbia) as follows:
    —Acute respiratory acidosis (pH of less than 7.30 with a corresponding elevated P_{CO_2}), or
    —Severe hypoxemia (failure to maintain arterial blood oxygen of 60 mm Hg with inspired oxygen concentrations of more than 40%)

• Endotracheal intubation without mechanical ventilation required if performed for airway protection, delivery of continuous positive airway pressure, or frequent suctioning†
Threshold 4: 10% of cases

Indicator 5: Stabilization of vital signs by 48 hours after septic episode or admission:
  • Blood pressure, pulse, respiratory rate
  • Body temperature
  Threshold 5: 85% of cases
Indicator 6: Oliguria recognized and efforts made to prevent acute renal failure
  Indicator 6a: Physician notified for urine output less than 30 ml/hr for 2 consecutive hours
    Threshold 6a: 10% of cases
  Indicator 6b: Blood urea nitrogen and creatinine measured if urine output unstable
    Threshold 6b: 100% of applicable cases
  Indicator 6c: In face of oliguria, if hemodynamic analysis reveals hypovolemia (low central venous pressure or pulmonary wedge pressure), fluid challenge given
    Threshold 6c: 100% of applicable cases
  Indicator 6d: Acute renal failure
    Threshold 6d: 5% of cases

Indicator 7: Draining or debridement of pus or necrotic tissue from sepsis site when appropriate
  Threshold 7: 98% of cases

From Joint Commission on Accreditation of Health Care Organizations: *Quality improvements in special care units,* Oakbrook Terrace, Ill, 1990, The Commission.
*These indicators are not definitive or comprehensive; neither are they intended to be standards of care. To be developed into definitive indicators, many would require further refinement for greater specificity and objectivity and to reflect concerns in the individual health care organization.
†Spath PL: Expand occurrence screening into appropriate peer review program, *Hospital Peer Review* 12(5):62, 1987.

methodology defined. Some of the decisions to be made in this phase include sources of data to be used, who is responsible for data collection, sample selection criteria, sample size, who will organize data, how data will be displayed, and available computer resources. When deciding on what size sample to collect data on, a sampling table (Table 7–10) can be used. Examples of data collection instruments are shown to right and on page 92.

The CC-CNS may choose to be involved in data collection or may serve as a coordinator of the process. Staff members should participate in the data collection process for several reasons: (1) it heightens their awareness of the discrepancies in practice; (2) it allows them to evaluate their own practice against their peers; and (3) it serves as a means of educating staff regarding accurate procedures and processes.

Data organization and presentation can take many forms. Graphs, tables, and diagrams (Fig. 7–1) bring visual impact and interest to presentations of results.

Step 7: Evaluate Care. When cumulative data reach the threshold for evaluation, quality committee members should evaluate the care provided to determine if a problem is present.[5] This evaluation may include an analysis of patterns or trends in the care suggested by the cumulative data. If the results of the evaluation point to care provided by an individual practitioner, then peer review is undertaken. The CC-CNS can work with the nurse manager to counsel the staff member. Out of the evaluation come opportunities to improve care.

Pattern and trend information is shared with all health care providers. Information sharing can be done through many media: staff meetings, posted results, daily rounds, or incorporation into edu-

TABLE 7–10 Appropriate Sampling According to Patient Volume

4-week Inspection Unit Population	Sample Size
91-150	20
151-280	32
281-500	50
501-1200	80
1201-3200	125
3201-10,000	200

From *Sampling procedure and tables for inspection by attribution,* U.S. Government Printing Office.

SAMPLE MONITORING AND EVALUATION DATA COLLECTION FORM

IMPORTANT ASPECT OF CARE:

INDICATOR:

THRESHOLD FOR EVALUATION:

DATA SOURCE:

SAMPLE SIZE:

FREQUENCY OF DATA COLLECTION:

RESPONSIBILITIES:
   Who will collect data?
   Who will aggregate data?
   Who will analyze data?
   Who will take action (if necessary)?
   Who will communicate findings?

TRENDS:

SUSPECTED PROBLEMS:

ACTION TO BE TAKEN:

FOLLOW-UP ACTIVITIES:

RESULTS:

From Joint Commission on Accreditation of Health Care Organizations: *Quality improvements in special care units,* Oakbrook Terrace, Ill, 1990, The Commission.

NURSING QUALITY ASSURANCE MONITORING AND EVALUATION DATA RETRIEVAL FORM

MR #: _____

Date: _____

Diagnosis: _____

Instructions

1. Identify patients with the nursing diagnosis "skin integrity impairment, potential or actual, related to pressure."
2. Review is to be conducted twice each month.
3. Complete the data retrieval form utilizing review of the medical record, patient care plan, and patient inspection.
4. Return completed forms to nurse manager.

Important Aspect of Care

Patient safety

Nursing diagnosis: skin integrity impairment, potential or actual, related to pressure

<u>Characteristics of wound</u>:   Length _____ Width _____ Depth _____

Indicator

Compliance with the patient care standard for nursing diagnosis of skin integrity impairment, potential or actual, related to pressure, as evidenced by:

Process	Met	Not Met	N/A	Threshold for Evaluation
1. Patient's skin integrity is assessed every 8 hours	___	___	___	_____
2. Patient's response to nursing interventions documented q 8 hours in nurse's notes	___	___	___	_____
3. Patient repositioned q 2 hours if immobile	___	___	___	_____
4. Use of appropriate assistive device (alternating pressure mattress, sheepskin, therapeutic bed)	___	___	___	_____
5. Mobilization of patient (if not contraindicated)	___	___	___	_____
6. Daily dressing change unless contraindicated	___	___	___	_____
7. Plan of care documented on patient care plan	___	___	___	_____

Outcome

Pressure sores are minimized/healed. _____

Comments: _____

_____

Reviewer: _____

Courtesy R.E. Thomason Hospital, El Paso, Texas.

---

cational programs. Colorful graphs posted in the unit (out of view of patients and families) can attract attention and enable the CC-CNS to review the results with staff members.

When quality indicators review an individual nurse's care, the nurse can be assigned a number that only she or he knows. Data involving an individual nurse's practices can then be posted, with each nurse identified by number. This allows nurses to evaluate how their own practice compares with that of their peers.

Step 8: Take Actions to Solve Problems. In this phase, areas for improvement and the actions to be taken are identified. Possible actions outlined by JCAHO[1] include the following:

• For system problems: improved communications, changes in organizational structure, ad-

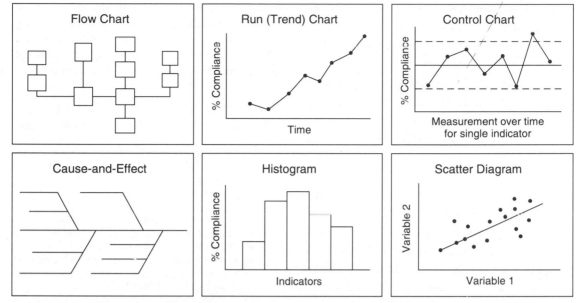

Figure 7-1 Seven helpful charts for presentation of results. (Adapted with permission from GOAL/ QPC, 13 Branch Street, Methuen, MA 01844-1953. Tel: 508-685-3900. Source: Seven Tools of Quality Control © 1985 GOAL/QPC.)

justments in staffing, changes in equipment or chart forms
- For knowledge problems: in-service education, continuing education, making data or scientific reports accessible, and circulating informational material
- For individual skill problems: changes in assignments, informal or formal counseling, and disciplinary action

The CC-CNS makes a significant contribution at this step. The CC-CNS can identify a plan of corrective action and assist in implementing such a plan. For example, a CQI study in a trauma ICU revealed that nurses used a variety of reference points for abdominal pressure monitoring. Some nurses used the symphysis pubis, some the sternal angle, and others the phlebostatic axis. The CC-CNS discussed this finding with the nursing staff and found that career staff members were well informed on the proper location for transducer placement and that the problem was with float and registry nurses who were not properly oriented to the procedure. The CC-CNS discussed this finding with the nurse manager, who was concerned about the current system of orientation for float and registry personnel. They received a general critical care orientation but were not oriented to a specific unit's needs. With this and other data, the CC-CNS and nurse manager were able to convince the critical care division nursing director to make funding available for unit-specific orientation time for float and registry personnel.

Step 9: Assess the Effectiveness of Actions and Assure Improvement is Maintained. This step evaluates the effectiveness of actions. Continued monitoring and evaluation should provide the information necessary to determine if the problem has been successfully solved. Even when a problem is solved, monitoring should be repeated at a later date to ensure long-term success.

Step 10: Communicate Results to Relevant Individuals and Groups. Quality committees are required by JCAHO to maintain records of monitoring and evaluation processes. These records should reflect trend data and be readily retrievable should this be required.

CASE STUDY

The indicator for this case was the unanticipated return of a patient to the special care unit within 72 hours. The important function being monitored and evaluated by the clinical team was the appropriateness of triage decisions. The threshold was set at 0%. This quality improvement topic evolved from two sources: (1) regulatory agency recommendations for refinement of transfer criteria and (2) trend data from incident report records presented during morbidity and mortality rounds. In addition, the floor staff has registered complaints to the special care unit staff that "they were tired of receiving patients who were sent too soon."

The nursing staff, with assistance from the CC-CNS, conducted an intensive review of all patients who returned to the ICU within 72 hours of transfer. Precipitating events and supporting clinical data leading to the unanticipated return to the ICU were reviewed. The CC-CNS and physician staff, in addition to the respiratory therapist, reviewed the clinical course of the patient within 36 hours before the transfer in an attempt to identify trends or patterns that may have predicted or indicated that the patient was not stable enough to be transferred to a less intense care unit. Their review included various clinical parameters such as hemodynamic monitoring patterns; clinical laboratory trends; specific treatments, procedures, and outcomes; and medication dosage patterns.

The quality of care assessment results for these cases showed that a respiratory crisis (code) was usually the precipitating event for the return to the ICU. The CC-CNS identified that these paients had been extubated less than 12 hours before transfer.

Based on these data, the transfer criteria were reviewed and revised, using the Society of Critical Care Medicine (SCCM)-AACN intrahospital transfer standards as a resource. The quality improvement study continued to monitor and evaluate improvement in patient outcome following transfer decisions.

SUMMARY

The CC-CNS has the content expertise and process expertise to facilitate quality activities within critical care settings. Working within a collaborative practice model, the CC-CNS is the ideal person to lead the transition from unit-specific quality assurance to an interdepartmental program of CQI. In the past the CC-CNS's role has been concerned with the quality of patient care delivered. The CC-CNS will continue to make significant contributions to quality during this evolution in health care.

References

1. Joint Commission on Accreditation of Health Care Organizations: *An introduction to quality improvement in health care,* Oakbrook Terrace, Ill, 1991, The Commission.
2. Nightingale F: *Notes on hospitals,* London, 1859, John Parker & Sons.
3. Nightingale F: *Notes on nursing: what it is and what it is not,* London, 1860, Harrison & Sons.
4. U.S. Department of Health and Human Services: Agency for health care policy and research. In *AHCPR program notes,* Rockville, Md, 1989, The Department.
5. Joint Commission on Accreditation of Health Care Organizations: *Quality improvements in special care units,* Oakbrook Terrace, Ill, 1990, The Commission.
6. Nadzam DM: The agenda for change: update on indicator development and possible implications for the nursing profession, *J Nurs Qual Assur* 5(2):18-22, 1991.
7. Martin JP: From implication to reality through a unit-based QA program, *Clin Nurse Specialist* 3(4):192-196, 1989.
8. U.S. Department of Health and Human Services: *Clinical practice guideline: acute pain management: operative or medical procedures and trauma,* Rockville, Md, 1992, The Department.
9. American Association of Critical Care Nurses: *Outcome standards for nursing care of the critically ill,* Laguna Niguel, Calif, 1990, The Association.
10. American Association of Critical Care Nurses: *Standards for nursing care of the critically ill,* Laguna Niguel, Calif, 1989, The Association.
11. Lang NM, Marek KD: Outcomes that reflect clinical practice. In U.S. Department of Health and Human Services: *Patient outcome research: examining the effectiveness of nursing practice. Proceedings of the State of the Science Conference, 1991,* NIH pub. no. 93-3411, Rockville, Md, 1992, The Department.
12. Naylor MD, Munro BH, Brooten DA: Measuring the effectiveness of nursing practice, *Clin Nurse Specialist* 5(4):201-215, 1991.
13. Bloch D: Evaluation of nursing care in terms of process and outcome: issues in research and quality assurance, *Nurs Res* 24(3):256-253, 1975.
14. Blom MF: Dramatic decrease in decubitus ulcers: VA quality assurance program stimulated changes, *Geriatr Nurs* 6(2):84-87, 1985.
15. Bulechek GM, McCloskey JC: Nursing intervention taxonomy development. In McCloskey JC, Grace HK, editors: *Current issues in nursing,* St Louis, 1990, Mosby–Year Book, Inc.
16. La Monica EL et al: Development of a patient satisfaction scale, *Res Nurs Health* 9(1):43-50, 1986.
17. Marchette L, Holloman F: Length of stay: significant variables, *J Nurs Admin* 16(3):12-20, 1986.

18. Marek MD: Outcome measurement in nursing, *J Nurs Qual Assur* 4(1):1-9, 1989.

19. Olson RK, Heater BS, Becker AM: A meta-analysis of the effects of nursing interventions on children and parents, *Matern Child Nurs* 15(2):104-108, 1990.

20. Brooten D et al: A randomized clinical trial of early hospital discharge and home follow-up of very-low-birth-weight infants, *N Engl J Med* 315(13):934-939, 1986.

21. Hartz AJ et al: Hospital characteristics and mortality rates, *N Engl J Med* 321(25):1720-1725, 1989.

22. Hazlett DE: A study of pediatric home ventilator management: medical, psychological, and financial aspects, *J Pediatr Nurs* 4(4):284-294, 1989.

23. Heater BS, Becker AM, Olson RK: Nursing interventions and patient outcomes: a meta-analysis of studies, *Nurs Res* 37(5):303-307, 1988.

24. Kerr ME, Rudy EB, Daly BJ: Human response patterns to outcomes in the critically ill patient, *J Nurs Qual Assur* 5(2):32-40, 1991.

25. Knaus WA et al: An evaluation of outcome from intensive care in major medical centers, *Ann Intern Med* 104(3):410-418, 1986.

26. Mitchell PH et al: American Association of Critical-Care Nurses demonstration project: profile of excellence in critical-care nursing, *Heart Lung* 18(3):219-237, 1989.

27. Toth JC: Measuring the stressful experience of hospital discharge following acute myocardial infarction. In Waltz C, Strickland O, editors: *Measurement of nursing outcomes,* vol 1. *Measuring client outcomes,* New York, 1988, Springer.

28. Rubenstein LV et al: Measuring the quality of nursing surveillance activities for five diseases before and after implementation of the DRG-based prospective payment system. In U.S. Department of Health and Human Services: *Patient outcome research: examining the effectiveness of nursing practice. Proceedings of the State of the Science Conference, 1991,* NIH pub. no. 93-3411, Rockville, Md, 1992, The Department.

29. Leuze MS: Correlation of nurse's knowledge and valuation of the qualtiy assurance process, *J Nurs Qual Assur* 4(2):37-50, 1990.

30. Stevens B: Implementing a quality assurance program at the unit level in intensive care: essential elements for successful implementation, *AACN Clin Issues* 2(1):69-76, 1991.

Chapter Seven Appendix

SCOPE OF CARE AND SERVICES FOR AN INTENSIVE CARE NURSERY

In this hospital, the Intensive Care Nursery accepts any patient who is a neonate with a presently or potentially life-threatening medical or surgical condition. The 25-bed unit is jointly managed by the medical and nursing staff. The Neonatology staff of the Department of Pediatrics provides the unit with physician coverage 24 hours a day. The program also includes ICN fellows and residents.

The ICN Medical Director is responsible for implementing the policies established by the Chiefs of Professional Services of North Carolina Baptist Hospital as they pertain to the operation of the Intensive Care Nursery. The Director, along with the other members of the Neonatology staff, is responsible for making decisions regarding triage of patients from the unit when necessary. The Medical Director is responsible for assuring the quality, safety, and appropriateness of patient care in the ICN. These measures will be accomplished by monitoring and evaluating these services in the manner described by the Quality Assurance Plan of the Intensive Care Nursery. Other qualified designees from the Neonatology staff will be readily available for administrative and consultative decisions when the Medical Director is not available. The Medical Director also serves as Chairman of the Multidisciplinary ICN Committee and another member of the Neonatology staff serves as Chairman of the Quality Assurance Subcommittee.

Nursing staff includes a nurse supervisor, head nurses, assistant head nurses, staff nurses (RN's and LPN's, [physician's assistants], PA's) and unit secretaries. Patients are provided nursing care by an RN and LPN supervised by RN staff through a modified primary care process, with the unit staffed in RN, LPN-to-patient ratios of 1:1, 1:2, or 1:3.

Respiratory care is provided continuously within the ICN. The Respiratory Care staff includes a supervisor, assistant supervisors, and both registered and certified therapists.

Pharmacy support is provided by a dedi-

From Joint Commission on Accreditation of Health Care Organizations: Quality improvement in special care units; Oakbrook Terrace, Ill, 1990, The Commission.

cated satellite pharmacy staffed by licensed pharmacists and pharmacy technicians.

Nutritional support is provided by registered dieticians who provide consultative services for patients receiving enteral and parenteral nutrition.

Patients are triaged to one of two levels of care: Intensive or Intermediate. All beds have bedside monitors and recording capabilities. Each monitor provides at least electrocardiography, two channels of pressure monitoring and pulse oximetry. Each patient head-wall has at least three oxygen and air outlets and three vacuum outlets. All beds are equipped with both Servo-controlled and manual overhead heating elements to maintain a neutral-thermal environment. All beds have emergency backup power. Other available equipment includes ventilators, phototherapy lights, and volume pumps to control IV fluids.

Therapies provided by the ICN include:

1. Airway care and management, including:
   a. Mechanical ventilation
   b. Oxygen therapy
   c. Continuous positive airway pressure
   d. Inhaled bronchodilators
2. Parenteral nutrition
3. Enteral nutrition
4. Neutral-thermal environment
5. Antibiotic therapy
6. Phototherapy

Monitoring includes:

1. Electrocardiography
2. Pulse Oximetry
3. Continuous temperature monitoring
4. Hemodynamic Monitoring
5. Ventilatory mechanics
6. Arterial blood gas analysis

It is the responsibility of the ICN medical director, or a designated member of the Neonatology staff, to insure proper administration of the ICN, to oversee the admission and discharge of patients from the ICN, and for the continued education of the nursing and respiratory care staff. In addition they are responsible for the education of house staff on the ICN rotation and Neonatology Fellows.

The attending neonatologist assigned to the patient is directly responsible for supervising and directing the patient's care. The physician makes daily rounds, visiting and examining the patient, and reviewing and altering the care plan. Since the hospital is a teaching institution, the attending physicians are assigned residents who are responsible for administering routine medical care to the patients. The residents do pertinent physical exams several times each day and assess the patients' status.

It is the responsibility of the ICN medical director or a designated member of the Neonatology staff to decide if a patient meets requirements for admission to the ICN. Final decision on the admission or discharge of a patient is made by the ICN attending physician based on the admission and discharge criteria for the ICN.

A patient may be admitted to the ICN if he/she weighs less than 10 kg and is 3 cm shorter in length than the longest internal bed length measurement, and meets the following criteria:

A. Respiratory compromise
   1. Imminent intubation or acutely intubated patient
   2. Respiratory condition that requires oxygen therapy
   3. Intubated post-op patient
B. Hemodynamically unstable
   1. Unable to maintain BP without vasoactive drugs and other invasive cardiovascular monitoring devices
   2. Required arterial line for blood pressure monitoring
C. Multiple organ system failure
   1. Compromise of more than one body system which is unstable either in conjunction with A, B, or C, or alone
D. Congenital anomalies
E. Immaturity: gestational age less than 38 wks.

A patient may be discharged from the intensive care nursing if he/she meets the following criteria:

A. Respiratory stability
   Respiratory stability is defined as:
   1. Does not require mechanical ventilation or endotracheal intubation
   2. Respiratory status stable for 24 hours after extubation

Part III

The Critical Care Clinical Nurse Specialist as Educator

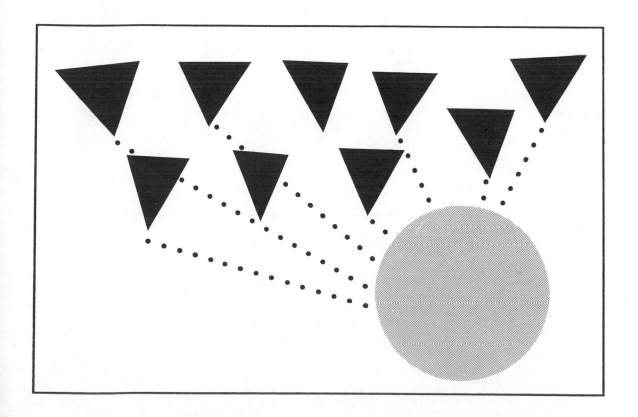

The Critical Care Clinical Nurse Specialist in Critical Care Staff Education

Maureen Keckeisen, RN, MN, CCRN

Over the past 20 years, critical care has evolved into a highly technical and sophisticated specialty requiring extensive theoretic knowledge and clinical practice skills. As a result of the increasing number of specialty units (e.g., cardiac, transplant, neuroscience, and trauma units), the need for unit-based, hospital-wide, and community critical care education specific to a particular patient population of specialty has become increasingly apparent.

Economic constraints within hospital organizations have also impacted the nursing education process. Education departments have been down scaled, and fewer resources are available to support educational programming. Alternative forms of patient care delivery systems implemented within critical care settings have required the CC-CNS to extend the traditional scope of staff education to include responsibility for a diverse group of health care workers including registered nurses (RNs), licensed vocational nurses (LVNs), licensed practical nurses (LPNs), and nurse assistants or technicians. Considerable flexibility is required of the critical care clinical nurse specialist (CC-CNS) educator. The educator role of the CC-CNS has evolved and adapted to meet specialized educational needs in an economically unstable environment.

As educator the CC-CNS may assume teaching responsibilities for many groups, including patients and families, nursing students (graduate and un-dergraduate faculty), peers, and interdisciplinary members of the health care team.[1,2] From 22.9% to 56.3% of the CNS's time is spent in the role of educator, depending on the CNS's particular phase of role development.[3]

To meet the educational and developmental needs of the staff, the CC-CNS participates in a number of activities including orientation of new staff, role modeling while in direct patient care, assessing and identifying learning needs of both new and experienced staff, developing and implementing in-service workshops, conducting informal and formal programs, and evaluating effectiveness of teaching in the clinical setting. Staff education encompasses not only clinical education topics such as assessment, pathophysiology, and related nursing interventions, but also topics related to advanced practice and professional issues such as leadership, nursing care delivery systems, and research utilization.

The essence of the CC-CNS educator role is the sharing of theoretic knowledge and advanced practice skills with staff at the bedside. The CC-CNS stimulates staff to enhance the quality and delivery of care to critically ill patients through one-on-one clinical education and problem solving of actual patient situations.[4,5] Key to successful implementation in the role of educator is good communication and collaboration with the nurse manager, medical director, members of the health care team, and the staff development department.

THEORETIC PERSPECTIVES

Adult learning theory encompasses a body of literature by theorists such as Kidd,[6] Miller,[7] and Knowles.[8-11] Knowledge of the principles of adult learning enables the CC-CNS to more effectively meet the educational needs of critical care staff. Table 8–1 summarizes the main principles of adult education adapted from leading adult learning theorists[6-8] and related nursing literature[12-14] with practice implications for the CC-CNS educator.

Novice to Expert

An understanding of skills acquisition as conceptualized by Benner[15] provides the CC-CNS with the framework to meet the educational needs of nursing staff at the various levels of clinical experience along the continuum of novice to expert. Table 8–2 provides an overview of Benner's Novice to Expert Paradigm as well as implications for the CC-CNS as educator. Incorporating content and

skills acquisition into preceptor training programs enables the preceptor to better understand the progression from novice to expert. Sharing with a novice nurse the normal progression in which skills are acquired may assist in "reality basing" the nurse on completion of preceptorship and orientation. A frame of reference for normal development and progression in the acquisition of skills may lessen the novice nurse's perception of anxiety and reality shock often experienced within the first 3 to 6 months following orientation.

Competency-based Education

Competency-based education (CBE) was initially conceptualized by Del Bueno[16] in 1977 as a philosophy of education that could be utilized in orientation of nurses. CBE focuses on the development of critical performance skills or competencies based on specific performance expectations.[17] CBE is a cost-effective alternative to traditional

TABLE 8–1 Principles of Adult Learning

Principles	CC-CNS Implications
1. Adult learners are self-directed. They generally like to direct their own learning and make decisions regarding program content.	When assessing learning needs of experienced critical care nurses, encourage staff to take part in program planning and in decisions regarding content and type of educational offerings best suited to their needs.
2. Adult learners are motivated if they perceive that the learning experience will help them solve a problem. Learning must be relevant to a perceived need.	Take advantage of a readiness to learn and opportunities for impromptu teaching when staff members perceive a need for an educational offering to solve a clinical problem.
3. Adult learning is enhanced when the learners are able to actively participate in the learning process by sharing and building on past experience.	Encourage active participation, sharing, and discussion of experiences in the classroom setting.
4. Adult learners value time. The learning experience must be worth while or relevant to practice or time is considered not well spent.	Ensure that the content of the educational program is relevant, practical, and readily applicable to clinical practice. The CNS provides the critical link between nursing theory and practical application.
5. Learning is enhanced when the content is presented over time instead of at one session.	Program planning should be critically reviewed to ensure that content is presented in time frames that allow frequent opportunities for breaks over the day, particularly when material is highly technical or complex.
6. Adult learners differ in learning styles and rate of learning based on previous experience. Current learning is influenced by the nurse's self-concept and past life experiences.	Maintain an informal, nonthreatening atmosphere conducive to learning. Consider alternative forms of learning.

TABLE 8–2 Novice to Expert Paradigm: Implications for the CC-CNS Educator

Stage	CC-CNS Implications
1. Novice: possesses principles and theory related to critical care nurses but *not* the contexts in which to apply theory; judgment may be acquired only through context of real situation	Must be given "rules" to guide performance (could be in form of standards and protocols)
2. Advanced beginner: has begun to identify cues in context of patient situation but is unable to differentiate cues as being more or less important than others	Provide guidelines for recognizing cues in patient context; advanced beginner needs more experience before becoming proficient at recognizing and differentiating cues; needs help prioritizing in clinical setting
3. Competent: develops in a 2- to 3-year period; is able to differentiate and prioritize; nursing care is conscious and deliberate but lacking speed and flexibility of a more proficient nurse	Teaching strategies like decision-making games and simulation enable nurse to practice, plan, and coordinate care of multiple, complex patient care needs
4. Proficient: is able to perceive situations and patient as a whole as a result of experience; able to anticipate long-term goals; perceives "nuances" in situations that are not clear-cut; able to recognize deterioration and early warning signals before overt changes occur in vital signs	Education should include case studies, group discussion, and sharing of clinical experiences; rules and guidelines may frustrate proficient nurse; for every rule, nurse will find an exception; case studies should contain extraneous material and insufficient information and be ambiguous and complex to challenge proficient nurse
5. Expert: has an "intuitive" grasp of situations and can zero in on exact problem without need to consider all possible alternatives; does not rely on rules, guidelines, or nuances; will respond with "it felt right" or "it was a gut level feeling" when asked to explain rationale	Performance difficult to capture using usual criteria for performance evaluation; encourage expert staff to systematically describe expert performance, their decision-making process, and effect on patient outcomes, and then share experiences with others

orientation within the classroom, because less time is often required to orient new nurses when existing competencies can be validated and learning is focused on critical performance skills within the practice setting.

Del Bueno and Altano[17] have identified three dimensions of performance in the determination of competence: (1) technical skills, (2) interpersonal relations skills and (3) critical thinking components. Evaluation of competencies requires criterion checklists, which are used to evaluate psychomotor and technical competencies; a skills laboratory to evaluate high-risk and high-frequency psychomotor technical skills such as defibrillation; and video simulation to evaluate critical thinking and interpersonal skills. Development of competency is seen as a responsibility shared by CC-CNS, educators, managers, and employees.

One currently available program to assess the baseline competencies of critical care nurses is the

Performance Based Development System (Baxter Healthcare), which is theoretically based on Del Bueno's constructs of CBE.[16,18] The system can be used during initial orientation to assess entry-level competencies of an individual's clinical judgment, technical skills, and interpersonal relationships. The system validates existing competencies and identifies areas where performance development is needed, using a variety of assessment tools, including video simulation and priority-setting exercises. Preceptors are able to use the assessment data to streamline and individualize orientation based on identified learning needs. Key to implementation of this system within the institution is financial and philosophic support from nursing administrators and a commitment from administrators, nurse managers, clinical specialists, and preceptors in collaboration with nurse educators within the nursing education department. The system also supports documentation requirements and expectations held by licensing agencies that orientation of new personnel be grounded in validation of competencies before administration of patient care.

The literature supports the use of two methods to facilitate development of competencies in critical care nurses[19,20]: simulations and debriefing. Simulations support active participation instead of passive observation.[20] They represent a "rehearsal" in which nurses are able to practice setting priorities, making decisions, and developing hands-on psychomotor skills without the consequences of actual patient emergencies. Examples of simulated activities include laboratory simulation (i.e., use of manikins, monitoring equipment), role-playing, video simulation of patient situations, and simulation games.[18,19,21-24] All forms of simulation allow a nurse to enhance competencies in a nonthreatening setting without compromising the patient. The use of simulation helps staff to integrate complex patient situations and stimulate critical thinking while enhancing the development of competencies.

Debriefing sessions would follow simulated activities or real-life situations in the critical care setting. With the CC-CNS as a facilitator to assist with group process, significant learning may take place when participants are able to summarize their thoughts, share feelings about the experience, and discuss possible alternatives, the reason for their decisions, and how that experience might be applied to future clinical scenarios.[19,23] Debriefing also serves as a mechanism to assess the effectiveness of the learning experience.

Alspach[25] has conceptualized CBE in the context of critical care education along a continuum of entry level to experienced staff. CBE ensures the initial acquisition of competencies at entry level, in-service education ensures that the competency is maintained over time, and continuing education provides a means for further development of critical care nursing competencies. An understanding of CBE provides the CNS with an excellent theoretic base with which to plan, implement, and evaluate educational offerings in staff education.

ANA Standards for Educator Role of CNS

The CNS in the role of educator is described in the American Nurses' Association (ANA's) *The Role of the Clinical Nurse Specialist*[26] as providing "information when there is a knowledge deficit and when new information is needed to resolve a health problem or improve the quality of care. The document also describes the many functional components or subroles of CNS educator, which encompass teaching nurses, patients, and families within the community and across different health care disciplines.

AACN Position Statement and Competency Statements on CC-CNS as Educator

The American Association of Critical Care Nurses' (AACN's) *Role Definition Position Statement*[27] initially identified the role of the critical care CNS as an educator. In 1989 AACN published *Competency Statements for Critical Care Clinical Nurse Specialists*[28] in which the role and competencies of the CNS as educator were further defined. This document provides the framework for development in the role of educator. Mastery of advanced knowledge and skills as an educator is demonstrated by (1) facilitating the acquisition and application of clinical knowledge, theoretic knowledge, and decision-making skills by nurses, nursing students, and other health care providers; (2) contributing to nursing knowledge through scholarly publications and presentations on clinical topics and issues in critical care nursing; and (3) assessing learning needs and designing, implementing, and evaluating comprehensive teaching programs for specific patient populations, health care providers, and community groups to improve patient outcomes.

Clearly delineated in the AACN position statement and competency statements is the importance of incorporating research-based practice in the role of CC-CNS as educator. The role of educator lends itself to sharing the most current research during educational offerings. By consistently integrating theory and recent research findings into presentations and contributing to the literature, the CC-CNS not only encourages research-based practice but also stimulates scientific inquiry among critical care nurses.

Standards in Critical Care Education

The development of *AACN Education Standards for Critical Care Nursing*[29] has helped to standardize the educational process for critical care nurses. The AACN standards serve as guidelines for development of institutional-specific standards.

An additional resource for the CC-CNS is an AACN publication entitled *Critical Care Orientation: a Guide to the Process*.[13] It is a comprehensive guide to critical care orientation and also includes theoretic and practical aspects related to staff education. A working knowledge of the practice standards for critical care education will enable the CC-CNS to more effectively implement the role of educator.

RELATED LITERATURE AND RESEARCH

Within the literature the CNS is described as an educator and role model, unique and potentially influential in integrating theory and advanced practice skills at the bedside.[30-32] Much of the literature related to the CNS as educator, however, focuses on a global description of the CNS educator as patient educator, staff educator, or nursing faculty member. There is a paucity of research or related literature that specifically addresses operationalization of the CNS role in staff education and implementation of specific strategies into practice.

Robichaud and Hamric[33] have described various educational activities in their operational definition of the CNS educational role component. Their definition of the role was described within the framework of a time documentation instrument used to evaluate CNS practice. Ryan-Merritt et al.[34] operationalized the CNS educator role by identifying behaviors and developing competency statements. The competencies, however, were identified primarily for use for teaching and curriculum development in the academic setting.

Definition of the role and time spent by the CNS as educator has been well documented within the literature.[2,3,35-38] Holt[37] initially described the educator role within developmental stages of the clinical nurse specialist role. The model outlined various activities that the CNS as educator might expect to engage in within a set time frame (stage 1 [PreCNS] through stage 6 [7+ years as CNS]). Baker[35] expanded Holt's model and identified specific educational role activities based on personal experience. In the first 2 years the CNS may initiate education on "need to know" topics and focuses on maximizing teaching at the bedside. In the third and fourth years, educational activities may include implementation of educational programs based on identified needs and problem areas, the development of alternative forms of learning such as self-

instructional modules or videos, and participation in educational programs as a lecturer outside the institution. Educational activities for years 5 and 6 include continual refinement of previously stated activities and development of state and regional recognition in areas of expertise. Sparacino and Cooper[2] expanded on the educational activities cited in previous studies and proposed teaching at the national level in the fifth year of role implementation.

Cooper and Sparacino[36] cited a study by the University of California, San Francisco,[3] which reported the amount of time spent in various stages of educational role development. Whereas it was estimated that the CNS at UCSF spends 10% to 25% of time in the education role, the actual time spent ranged from 22.9% to 56.3% during different phases of role development (years 1 to 4 in CNS role). Robichaud and Hamric[33] found that 27% of the CNS's time was spent in education; however, their study did not control for variations in time spent at the various stages of role development. No data addressed time spent specifically on staff education; however, one can interpret the results of these studies as guidelines for allocating time in the role of educator as opposed to time in the other CNS role components.

Buchanan and Glanville[39] described a model that provides the CNS with a process for implementation of the educator role in clinical practice. Four components of the model include (1) assessment and diagnosis of learning needs, (2) instructional planning, (3) implementation, and (4) evaluation of the teaching-learning process. These authors used a framework describing the CNS role and responsibilities as educator in terms of a process, method, and competencies needed for effective implementation of the educator role.

Ways in which the CNS might facilitate the development of critical thinking and clinical reasoning skills in staff have been addressed in the literature.[40,41] Toliver[41] describes the use of inductive reasoning to enhance critical thinking skills and foster competence in the clinical setting. Three critical steps in inductive reasoning were described, including (1) gathering all information available and elaborating on it; (2) differentiating relevant information from irrelevant; and (3) identifying the consequences of the relevant data. Implications for the CNS include frequent practice and exposure to clinical situations with feedback to enhance pattern recognition and ability to differentiate what is relevant vs. not relevant. Farrell and Bramadat[40] discussed the use of paradigm case analysis and simulated recall as educational strategies that can be used by the CNS to develop clinical reasoning skills. Both strategies encourage verbalization and documentation of excellence in practice. Sharing this knowledge with other nurses enhances learning potential. Although these strategies may have educational and practice implications for the CC-CNS educator, more documentation is needed about implementation of the CC-CNS educator role.

PRACTICE IMPLICATIONS

Critical care nursing education is defined by Alspach[25] as "education that is directed at facilitating the acquisition and application of the knowledge, skills, and attitudes that are required for competent critical care nursing practice." The four major components of critical care education address the acquisition of (1) knowledge or cognitive skills, (2) psychomotor or technical skills, (3) interpersonal or attitudinal skills, and (4) critical thinking ability.[12,13]

In many institutions the CC-CNS has centralized as well as decentralized educational responsibilities including mandatory cardiopulmonary resuscitation (CPR) or advanced cardiac life support (ACLS) courses and critical care orientation programs, as well as unit-specific educational offerings and in-service workshops. The CC-CNS frequently interfaces with the staff development educator in the planning, marketing, implementation, and evaluation of these programs. In some institutions the CC-CNS will collaborate with a unit-based clinical educator. Development of collaborative relationships with nurse educators will assist the CC-CNS in accomplishing the many tasks associated with program implementation and broaden the perspective of educational needs within the hospital and community.[42]

This section addresses implementation of the CC-CNS educator role. Formal and informal program development, marketing, and evaluation are covered, along with the CC-CNS role in assessment of staff educational needs and organization of an orientation program.

Learning Needs Assessment

For an educational program to be meaningful and effective, educational planning should begin with a needs assessment. This needs assessment should include the four components discussed above.[9,12,43-46]

Learning style is defined as the way in which an individual conceptualizes, processes, and organizes information.[47] The importance of assessing learning style in a needs assessment is well documented within the literature.[13,37,48,49]

A needs assessment may be formal or informal. There are various types, kinds, and advantages of formal and informal methods. A formal approach to needs assessment includes a survey, an open-ended questionnaire, or a checklist.[44,46,50,51] The advantages of a formal assessment (Fig. 8–1) are that it is systematic and quantifiable; the disadvantage is that it is time consuming. Figure 8–1 asks the critical care nurse to rank various topics relative to critical care practice (i.e., chest x-ray interpretation, defibrillation, blood gas interpretation). The nurse is asked to indicate level of need (no need, moderate need, or great need) as well as level of content needed (basic, intermediate, or advanced). Assessment tools of this kind enable the CC-CNS to plan specific educational programs for the calendar year.

Incorporating open-ended questions in the needs assessment encourages staff to identify "perceived" learning needs. Examples of open-ended questions include asking staff to identify areas of interest and potential topics for educational programs. Figure 8–2 gives a needs assessment that incorporates open-ended questions into the assessment format.

Informal approaches to needs assessment include discussions or interviews with staff, identification of learning needs through rounds, and continuous quality improvement activities. Informal discussion with staff is a very effective means of determining both learning need and learning style of participants. The CC-CNS can learn a great deal about individual or group preferences regarding use of case studies, role-playing, video or computer simulation, self-instructional learning packets, or scheduling of abbreviated vs. full-day programs. Data obtained informally are far less time consuming but require validation of identified need.[46] Given the many options available to the CNS,

EDUCATION NEEDS ASSESSMENT

Instructions: Please read each item and circle the number corresponding to your *need for information* about the subject.

If you have circled a letter indicating a need for information, please indicate the *level of content* by circling the appropriate number.

	Level of Need			Level of Content		
Clinical Knowledge/Skills	**No Need**	**Moderate Need**	**Great Need**	**Basic New**	**Intermediate**	**Advanced**
1. Chest X-ray Interpretation for the Critical Care Nurse	1	2	3	1	2	3
2. Thermodilution Cardiac Output	1	2	3	1	2	3
3. Taking a 12 Lead EKG	1	2	3	1	2	3
4. Defibrillation/Cardioversion	1	2	3	1	2	3
5. Chest Tube Management	1	2	3	1	2	3
6. Continuous Arterio-Venous Ultrafiltration	1	2	3	1	2	3
7. Nutritional Assessment	1	2	3	1	2	3
8. Parenteral Nutrition	1	2	3	1	2	3
9. Interpretation of Blood Chemistries	1	2	3	1	2	3
10. Mock Code	1	2	3	1	2	3
11. Blood Gas Assessment	1	2	3	1	2	3

Figure 8–1 Formal learning needs assessment tool. (Courtesy University of California, Los Angeles, Medical Center.)

methods that support cost-effective use of time and resources should be considered.

Assessment of learning needs and styles is a critical component of educational program planning. Although the nurse manager may collaborate in this process, I believe that the CC-CNS has primary responsibility for this activity. Many units have staff nurse committees (or individuals) responsible for planning 1 year of in-service programs, including the needs assessment. In this instance the CC-CNS serves as a resource and facilitator of this process. Encouraging staff participation in the identification of their own learning needs not only recognizes their role in planning an educational program but also is consistent with the principles of adult education. The CC-CNS should also consider learning needs of staff in the context of current changes in the hospital environment and implementation of various models of health care delivery. Collaboration with the unit director will enhance the needs assessment process

by providing the CC-CNS with valuable information and insight into the learning needs and competencies of the staff.

In performing a needs assessment, it is important to solicit information from a majority of staff, including night staff. A less than 50% return rate on this assessment is not acceptable. The CC-CNS may need to use creative means of ensuring staff cooperation, such as giving forms out at report and collecting them 3 hours later, watching the nurse's patients while the form is being completed, and provision of incentives (e.g., food) for completion of the form during the shift. Once completed, the needs assessment form can be placed in the individual staff member's educational file.

Formal vs. Informal Educational Programs

Critical care education may take the form of formal or informal programs, which include alternative methods of education. Formal educational programs may take the form of an extensive critical

---

UCLA DEPARTMENT OF NURSING MEDICAL ICU LEARNING NEEDS ASSESSMENT

NAME: _____

Certifications: _____ BCLS   Exp. Date: _____

                   _____ ACLS   Exp. Date: _____

                   _____ CCRN   Exp. Date: _____

1. Are you interested in ACLS _____ and/or CCRN _____ certification or re-certification?

2. Are you currently enrolled in a nursing program? _____ If yes, what type of program and when do you plan to graduate?

    _____

3. What type of educational programs do you prefer? (check as many as apply)

    _____ Unit based inservices (e.g., at staff meetings)

    _____ Bedside teaching

    _____ All day seminars at UCLA

    _____ Outside programs

    _____ Self study (video, computerized learning)

    _____ Other (list) _____

4. What types of patients do you currently feel *most* comfortable caring for? (examples: chronic obstructive pulmonary disease, weaning patients, bone marrow transplants, diabetics, liver patients, gastrointestinal bleeders)

    _____

    _____

    _____

5. What types of patients do you feel *least* comfortable caring for?

    _____

    _____

    _____

6. List three topics you would like to learn more about this year:

    _____

    _____

    _____

Figure 8–2 Learning needs assessment tool incorporating open-ended questions. (Courtesy E. Henneman, UCLA Department of Nursing.)

7. On a scale of 1 to 4 with 1 being not at all comfortable and 4 very comfortable, please rate yourself in the following areas:

_____ Caring for a patient with a Swan Ganz catheter

_____ Caring for a patient who is dying

_____ Caring for a patient with SVO_2 monitoring

_____ Caring for a patient with a Hickman catheter

_____ Caring for a patient with a distressed family

_____ Caring for a patient in septic shock

_____ Caring for a patient who is immunosuppressed

_____ Caring for a myocardial infarction patient

_____ Caring for a weaning patient

_____ Caring for a patient with disseminated intravascular coagulation

8. Would you be interested in participating in nursing rounds on the unit?

yes _____   no _____

9. How can I as the clinical specialist assist you in meeting your educational needs in the MICU? (Check as many as apply)

_____ By offering continuing education classes in the unit.

_____ By keeping you up to date on classes in the community.

_____ By sharing nursing research findings.

_____ By holding educational seminars (all day)

_____ By assisting with patient care

_____ Other (list) _____

_____

10. Comments/Suggestions: _____

_____

_____

Figure 8–2 *Continued*

care orientation program or a 1-day seminar. Informal educational programs on topics such as skin care or wound management, arrhythmias, coping, or alterations in hemodynamic values or waveforms may take the form of brief in-service programs for staff or impromptu staff education at the bedside during clinical rounds. Alternative forms of education may include self-study, skills laboratories, videotapes, educational newsletters, or use of computer-assisted instruction. Depending on the developmental phase (i.e., novice or experienced CNS), the CC-CNS may implement the role quite differently. For example, a novice CC-CNS may want to focus on developing a needs assessment, identifying the learning needs of the staff, participating in informal teaching at the bedside, conducting in-service workshops, and developing a core of lectures and classes. Experienced CC-CNSs may implement the role differently and focus on maintaining staff competence, developing the role of educator in senior staff nurses, and serving as an educational consultant to these nurses. Incorporating recent research and literature into educational programs will enable both the novice and experienced CNS to more effectively operationalize the educator role and respond to the continuing educational needs of critical care nurses.

Formal Educational Programs: Planning and Implementation

Formal programs may require considerable time in planning, development, and implementation. The CC-CNS will need to allocate sufficient time for the development of learning objectives, program outline, lecture material (content/outline), audiovisual (AV) materials, and program evaluation.

Program planning and implementation also require the CC-CNS to consider the (1) cost for duplication of a syllabus or outlines, brochures, fliers, mailings, and refreshments; (2) procurement of speakers, their availability and fees, if any; (3) room availability and reservation; (4) arrangements for AV equipment such as slide or overhead projectors, video cassette player, and adjunct equipment. One strategy to defray some of the costs associated with program implementation is to seek sponsorship from vendors or drug company representatives. Many companies maintain funds to make endowments for educational programs or pro-

vide sponsorship for an educational speaker. In return for sponsorship, companies may require a brief presentation time for a sales representative or at the very least an acknowledgment to appear on the syllabus or be given verbally during the program.

Planning a formal educational program needs to begin at least 4 to 6 months in advance. It may be helpful for the CC-CNS to develop a timetable (Table 8–3) for completion of the tasks associated with program planning and implementation.[52] Allocation of time may be a real challenge for the CC-CNS educator, and the CC-CNS may consider consulting with resources such as the education department. Many education departments support various aspects of program planning, marketing, implementation, and evaluation. Support staff from the education department may also assist the CC-CNS with registration and distribution of contact hours certificates to participants. The expertise of other CNSs, nurse educators, physicians, pharmacists, respiratory therapists, and other health care team members may be helpful in program planning as well as implementation.

Strategies for Marketing Within Hospital or Community. Advertising and marketing an educational program are key to reaching potentially interested staff in the institution or persons within the community. Fliers are the most cost-effective way to advertise within the hospital setting. Brochures that are mailed to the community need to include a program description, objectives, faculty, continuing education hours offered, cost of program, and a brief schedule of the day. The marketing expense associated with mailing brochures and using journals to advertise an educational program must be considered.

Successful implementation of an educational program is the result of careful planning, development of AV aids that facilitate learning, and effective presentation of educational material. AV aids include slides, overhead transparencies, audiotapes, or videotapes. AV aids can greatly enhance presentation of lecture material if used effectively. Whereas slides are an excellent way to highlight key concepts during a presentation to larger groups, overhead transparencies are very effective in small group presentations and offer much flexibility in that the lecturer can return to a transparency to reinforce a previously discussed concept

TABLE 8–3 Timetable for Formal Program Planning

Time Frame	Tasks
4-6 months before program	Secure date(s) without competing programs (e.g., check with nurse manager for potential conflicts)
	Develop program objectives, outline, evaluation, budget
	Determine audience (local, regional, national)
	Determine availability of speakers
	Reserve classroom and AV equipment
	Apply for continuing education credit
2 months before program	Market program to critical care staff; target audience (send brochures, post fliers)
	Seek local support for program marketing to boost attendance
	Develop lecture content and outline
1 month before program	Complete lecture content, program evaluation
	Develop AV materials to supplement lecture
1-2 weeks before program	Complete course syllabus
	Order refreshments
Day of program	Check that AV equipment is in good working condition
	Distribute program syllabus with lecture outlines, handouts
	Completion of posttest and program evaluations by participants
	Distribute continuing education certificates
1 week following program	Complete program paperwork
	Send thank-you notes to speakers

without having to flip back through a series of slides.

Before program implementation, the CC-CNS must allow adequate time to prepare for the actual lecture presentation. Rehearsing the lecture and reviewing slides and transparencies are key to being prepared and organized. Additional strategies for preparing for presentation include reviewing an audiotape recording, videotaping oneself, or presenting to a small group of friends and asking for feedback, followed by practice, practice, and more practice! Table 8–4 gives some general guidelines with suggested time frames for lecture presentation.

Formal Program Evaluation. In the context of the CNS as educator, evaluation of an educational program should communicate the quality and effectiveness of the program in terms of learner outcomes, serve as documentation of the effect of the CC-CNS on nursing practice in a clinical setting,[39,53-55] and contribute to decisions regarding ways in which future programming may be improved.[52-56]

Figure 8–3 shows a program evaluation form developed at the UCLA Medical Center Department of Nursing Research and Education Department. This instrument includes several components: (1) the speaker in terms of teaching style and effectiveness; (2) the course in terms of objectives met, relevance to practice, use of AV materials, and overall rating; (3) suggestions for improvement and future program planning; and (4)

TABLE 8–4 General Guidelines for Lecture Presentation

Time Frame	Tasks
1 week before presentation	Complete final lecture outlines, slides, overhead transparencies
1-2 days before presentation	Review relevant literature related to topic to refresh your memory and update most recent facts and figures
1 day before presentation	Rehearse your lecture (including slide presentation)
	Rehearse mentally, both progression and flow of presentation
	Preview slides and overhead transparencies beforehand while rehearsing your lecture
Day of lecture	Arrive early to check room, lighting, presence and functioning of appropriate AV equipment
	Position podium in location that does not block view of audience

---

UCLA DEPARTMENT OF NURSING RESEARCH AND EDUCATION
PROGRAM EVALUATION

PROGRAM TITLE _____   _____
                                                                                      DATE(S)

_____

SPEAKER EVALUATION:
Use the following scale: 4/Excellent   3/good   2/fair   1/poor

We would appreciate your comments with regard to the organization, clarity, style, and effectiveness of the speaker.

TOPIC	INSTRUCTOR	RATING	COMMENTS

COURSE EVALUATION:

1. The program objectives were met:

   Yes_____   No _____   Comments:

2. The program content was relevant to my practice:

   Yes _____   No _____   Comments:

3. The outlines & handouts were well written and useful:

   Yes _____   No _____   Comments:

4. The AVs helped to reinforce my learning:

   Yes _____   No _____   Comments:

5. Overall rating of the program: 5   4   3   2   1
                                            Excellent   Poor

6. Suggestions for improving the classes:

7. Suggestions for future classes:

8. How did you hear about this program? _____ Flyer; _____ Brochure; _____ Friend;

   _____ Professional Organization; _____ Outreach Program; _____ Other:

9. Would you come to another UCLA Program?

   Yes _____   No _____   Comments:

10. Overall Comments:

Figure 8–3 Program evaluation tool. (Courtesy UCLA Department of Nursing.)

program marketing. Numerous authors provide examples of formal course examinations.[13,57-60]

Informal Educational Programs: Planning and Implementation

The essence of informal program planning and implementation is to make each moment count. In comparison to formal programs, informal programs require far less time in planning, preparation, and implementation. Informal programs are less structured and offer more flexibility, enabling the CC-CNS to share information in a time-efficient and cost-effective way. Examples of informal education are in-service workshops and impromptu teaching.

Strategies for Implementing In-Service Workshops on Unit Level. Several strategies are available to the CC-CNS to meet the educational needs of staff on the various shifts without the use of formal program planning. For example, the CC-CNS could make rounds on all shifts to initially identify the learning needs of day, evening, and night shift staff. Having monthly night shift "midnight chats" might also enable the CNS to assess other clinical issues, problems, or educational needs that differ from those identified on the day shift. The absence of interruptions on the evening and night shifts provides an excellent opportunity for impromptu teaching at the bedside or discussion about a particular patient whose diagnosis and medical therapy are unusual. The presence of the CC-CNS on the different shifts may also motivate the staff to become interested in communicating their educational needs, particularly if staff members perceive the CC-CNS as available and taking a personal interest in reaching all shifts.

Scheduling an in-service lecture for both day and night shifts does not mean automatic attendance. Unless an in-service lecture is adequately marketed and there is adequate coverage, staff may not be motivated or able to attend. The CC-CNS can help maximize attendance. If the CC-CNS is not doing the actual in-service lecture, offering to provide patient coverage will enable more staff to attend. Timing the in-service lecture to coincide with the time immediately following change of shift report might enable staff from both shifts to attend if staff members cover for each other for 1 hour after their shift. Often the staff with the great-

est need for the lecture are unable to attend because it is scheduled on their day off. Consulting the schedule and working with the nurse manager before scheduling an in-service lecture in addition to coordinating adequate coverage are ways to reach those staff. Learning will always be more meaningful and effective if the CC-CNS uses the principles of adult learning by making the educational offerings convenient, relevant, and individualized to the needs of the staff.

Alternative Forms of Staff Education

In addition to in-service workshops the CC-CNS may use various alternative forms of staff education such as self-study packets, use of learning or skills laboratories, computer-assisted instruction, or audiotapes and videotapes that offer many options for the adult learner in critical care.

Self-study packets enable the learner to learn at her or his own pace at a convenient time and place. Programmed instruction self-study offers immediate feedback and reinforcement as the individual progresses through the program. Although preparing self-study packets is very time consuming for the CC-CNS, it may be well worth it for topics such as basic dysrhythmia or learning how to calculate drips when staff members need to review and practice their theory and skills following a more formal classroom program.

A learning skills laboratory offers staff an opportunity to practice and refine skills in an environment that is less threatening than the clinical setting. A skills laboratory enables staff to practice skills such as defibrillation/synchronized cardioversion, blood gas drawing, phlebotomy, tracheotomy care, or hemodynamic line setups without time constraints or chancing patient safety. The CC-CNS may need to negotiate for space as well as a commitment from administration for appropriate funds for skills laboratory equipment that is not used in direct patient care.

Computer-assisted instruction is an excellent means of teaching critical thinking skills, decision making, and priority setting in an interactive yet individualized format. One research study found no significant differences in knowledge, retention, or attitudes between a computer-assisted instruction group and a (traditional) lecture group.[61] An example of a computer-assisted instruction program is the AACN self-learning module used to prepare for the certified clinical care nurse (CCRN) examination. A complete list of critical care computer-assisted instruction programs is available through AACN.

Another alternative form of staff education is an educational newsletter to communicate clinical updates, clarify misconceptions, and reinforce standards of care. A newsletter format enables nursing staff to be updated at a convenient time. Each subject heading is followed by a brief summary of the topic in three or four sentences. It is a way in which the CC-CNS might "clinically connect" with each staff person on a monthly or bimonthly basis. It is also a means of sharing information with all staff members consistently and systematically. One subject heading might be clinical trivia. In a few sentences the staff might learn about the presence of "extra" P waves on the electrocardiogram (ECG) of a cardiac transplant patient, reinforced with a strip of a transplanted patient's ECG tracing. Figure 8–4 gives an example of a clinical trivia segment of a clinical newsletter. Development of a unit-based library provides another alternative for learning by making references and resources more accessible when the need for information arises. An article file could be placed in such a library.

Videotaped lectures, audiotapes, and models could be stored here. A staff library allows accessibility during breaks to peruse educational materials in a relaxed setting.

Educational bulletin boards may also be situated within the unit or within the employee break area. Postings on these bulletin boards might include upcoming in-service workshops, educational programs, CCRN information, or clinical updates and reminders. The 10-minute learning break was one strategy used by a nurse educator who posted weekly and monthly fliers with various themes on clinical updates, stress management, team building, or side effects of certain drugs.[62]

A clinical update notebook containing recent literature and articles to update staff on the latest technology, new procedures, new drugs, or any clinically relevant topic is another strategy. Placing the update notebook on the unit or in the break room will make it readily available to staff when the need or interest arises.

The CC-CNS can creatively impart information to staff in an atmosphere that is conducive to learning in numerous ways. Providing alternatives to the traditional method of learning in the classroom setting encourages self-directed learning and is consistent with principles of adult learning.

7. JUST FOR FUN...Clinical Trivia - Did you know that a Cardiac Transplant patient's EKG strip may often show 2 "p" waves per cardiac cycle? The reason for this is that the patient's old Sinus Node is left in place when his/her heart is surgically removed, and the new transplanted heart has it **own** Sinus Node. Therefore "P" waves can be seen on EKG for both sinus nodes, but only one (the newly transplanted heart) is able to initiate conduction through the electrical system!

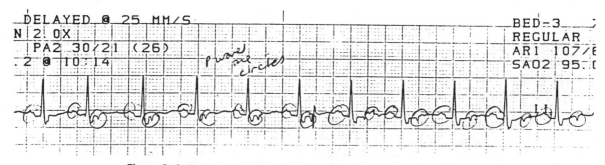

Figure 8–4 Example of clinical trivia segment in a clinical newsletter.

Orientation

New Staff in Critical Care

Trends in the current economic climate indicate that great challenges are in store for the CC-CNS in orientation of new staff, which may be a diverse group of health care personnel. The CC-CNS will need to adjust orientation according to the level of experience (new graduates vs. experienced), length of employment (temporary agency staff, registry staff, or float team personnel), and scope of practice (RN vs. LVN vs. nurse's assistant). The CC-CNS along with the nurse manager has a tremendous responsibility for ensuring that patient care personnel are appropriately prepared for their responsibilities.

A detailed discussion of the orientation of new staff members to critical care is beyond the scope of this chapter. There are, however, excellent resources available to assist the CC-CNS in staff orientation, including *Critical Care Orientation: a Guide to the Process*.[13] Both theoretic concepts and practical implications are provided for the CC-CNS assuming responsibility for orienting new staff into critical care.

New Graduates into Critical Care

AACN's position statement on integration of new graduates into critical care[63] provides the CC-CNS with a perspective of the advantages, concerns, and strategies for the successful integration of new graduates into the critical care setting. New graduates are generally very eager to learn, possess great enthusiasm in their practice, and are willing to take on the challenges of new learning experiences.[63] New graduates, however, have greater learning needs and require a more extensive and lengthy orientation.[64-66] In a study of 50 nurses new to critical care, Houser[65] found that predictors of job performance included prior clinical experience, postorientation test scores (used to measure knowledge level), and educational background. Preceptorships,[67-69] internship programs,[70] and nurse advocate projects[71] have been cited within the literature as programs that facilitate the transition of new graduates into critical care. The AACN document has outlined specific strategies and guidelines that may be utilized by the CC-CNS in the orientation of new graduates.[63]

Preceptorship

Preceptorship as a means of integrating new nurses into the critical care unit is well documented.[67-69] Using a preceptor is a viable and effective method of orientation for new graduates as well as experienced staff in critical care.[72-74] Compelling advantages include increased job satisfaction and decreased turnover among new staff. The CC-CNS plays an important role in the development and training of persons within the unit via role modeling and formal educational programs. Alspach's *From Staff Nurse to Preceptor: A Preceptor Training Program*[75] is an excellent resource and offers theoretic as well as practical guidelines to assist the CC-CNS in the development of a preceptor program. A preceptor/orientation committee may also facilitate orientation of a new nurse into the intensive care unit (ICU). The committee, composed of experienced staff members who serve as preceptors within the unit, may help structure the new staff's orientation, provide support and guidance for both the new nurse and preceptor, and provide continuity for the new nurse in terms of tracking learning needs. It is imperative that the CC-CNS work closely with the preceptor/new nurse team, providing structure, support, and encouragement to both new and experienced staff.

Orientation Manual

Developing an orientation manual often helps to streamline the orientation process. The manual might contain a welcome letter and a brief description of the unit and its various patient populations. The manual should also include the unit-specific care standards and protocols as well as the various skills checklists that must be completed before the end of orientation. An orientation manual will ensure that all new nurses receive the same information and will serve as a resource long after the completion of orientation.

Skills Competence

Various strategies ensure the competency of staff in the critical care setting. One strategy is to develop a clinical competency skills checklist by identifying common unit procedures that are considered high frequency and high risk or problem-prone critical care skills.[17] Examples of critical care skills include assisting with insertion of a pulmonary artery catheter, setting up hemodynamic lines, assisting with intubation and extubation, or suctioning patients on a ventilator.

Offering a critical care skills laboratory to practice high-risk or problem-prone procedures at regular intervals during the year and routinely scheduling mock codes on the unit will help to ensure entry competencies as well as continuing critical care competencies of experienced staff members. Using clinical scenarios frequently encountered on the unit in the mock codes will ensure population-specific competencies (i.e., assisting with opening chest and setting up for internal defibrillation).

Documentation of initial competencies and continued maintenance of competencies in staff is a critical component of the CC-CNS educator role. Maintaining an educational file on each staff nurse will assist the CC-CNS in tracking staff competencies and continuing education in accordance with Joint Commission on Accreditation of Health Care Organizations (JCAHO) standards and documentation requirements.

Performance Problems

A performance problem is defined as a discrepancy between actual performance and desired performance.[76] Performance problems may be readily identified early in the orientation process or later in the process when the preceptor voices concerns about the new nurse. The nurse manager must be kept apprised whenever a performance problem is identified, and together the CC-CNS and nurse manager should formulate the plan of action. It is important for the CC-CNS to gather information in order to intervene in the most effective manner. Determining if it is a knowledge or skills deficit is the first step. If it is simply a knowledge or skill deficiency, correcting the deficit through additional training or retraining may easily alleviate the performance problem.[76] However, in the absence of a skill deficiency, the manager with input from the CC-CNS will need to determine if the new staff member has the potential to benefit from an extended orientation. Individuals who demonstrate poor clinical judgment or who lack a sense of urgency when caring for critically ill patients are examples of performance problems that may not be the result of a knowledge or skill deficiency. Although the literature supports the idea that clinical judgment and decision making develop over time, developing a sense of urgency may not be

time related. It is important for the new staff member to receive oral and written feedback about performance. The individual must participate in the development of goals and objectives to correct any deficiencies and understand what is expected as well as the consequences of being unable to meet the expectations of improved performance. When all obstacles to performance have been addressed and the new nurse is still unable to perform at entry-level competence, the individual may need assistance seeking employment in a more appropriate clinical setting.

Tracking Progress of New Nurses

One of the important roles of the CC-CNS as educator includes tracking the progress of new nurses who have entered the unit. Although preceptors have played a major role in the initial socialization and clinical orientation at the bedside, it is imperative that the CC-CNS maintain contact with the preceptor/new nurse team. Continual monitoring of progress throughout the orientation period ensures continuity of the learning process. Weekly meetings throughout the orientation process with the preceptor/new nurse team together with the nurse manager will enable the CC-CNS to assess orientation and help to guide the process. Informal meetings individually with the preceptor and new nurse will also enable the CC-CNS to adequately monitor the orientation process. Encouraging constructive feedback between the preceptor and new nurse will enhance the learning experience for both staff members.

On completion of orientation, a formal or informal debriefing session is encouraged to assess current competencies and identify learning needs to be addressed in the future. It is often helpful for the new nurse to have written feedback summarizing the orientation process, identification of learning needs that still need to be addressed, and future clinical or educational goals (both short and long term). A goal might be "to continue to seek resources to assist the new staff in meeting future learning needs" or "to successfully complete an ACLS course within the first 6 months following orientation."

In addition to written feedback, a letter from the CC-CNS and preceptor committee welcoming the staff members and congratulating the individual on successful completion of orientation is key to the socialization process.

In the weeks immediately following preceptorship and orientation, the new nurse will need additional support from the CC-CNS. Without the preceptor present, the new nurse will experience some degree of culture or reality shock. Expectations from the staff are generally quite high. Staff members may forget that the new staff person possesses only entry-level competencies. The CC-CNS must help to structure a supportive environment for the new staff member. Assigning the new staff member a resource person for each shift after formal orientation can further facilitate a smooth orientation.

Consistent with the theory of novice to expert, integration of a new staff member into a critical care unit will initially proceed very slowly. The first 6 months may be a very turbulent time for the new critical care nurse. Caruthers et al.[64] stated that a new nurse may require 6 to 18 months of experience in critical care before being able to function at a high level of productivity. Follow-up sessions with new staff at 3, 6, and again at 12 months will ensure that the learning and developmental needs of new staff continue to be met. Continual reassessment of learning needs and revalidation of competencies are critical to the integration of the new nurse into critical care.

Evaluating an Orientation Program

Evaluation of the effectiveness of an orientation program is multifaceted. Only through evaluation is the CC-CNS able to determine if the program was effective in terms of helping the new staff member acquire entry-level practice skills and what changes or improvements need to be made. Orientation is not truly completed until the new staff member is able to perform competently within the clinical setting. Methods of evaluating competency of staff on conclusion of an orientation program may include (1) course examination at the conclusion of a formal critical care program; (2) clinical evaluation through observation by preceptor via competency (criterion) checklists; (3) direct observation on the part of the CC-CNS; and (4) formal and informal feedback from the new nurse with regard to the preceptor experience and suggestions for program improvement. Each component is valuable to the CC-CNS because the data serve as a basis for future program development and refinement.

The CC-CNS as educator truly has an important role in assessment, planning, implementation, and evaluation phases of a unit-based CBE orientation program.

CC-CNS Educator Role Responsibilities in Staff Education

In the *Accreditation Manual for Hospitals for Special Care Units*[77] JCAHO standards address the need to provide a formal training program of sufficient duration and substance to prepare the nurse to be competent in the delivery of nursing care in the special care unit. These standards address the documentation of initial entry-level competencies of staff members as well as maintenance of staff competency through continuing education programs. Documentation includes staff participation in relevant education programs within the institution as well as programs attended outside the institution. This responsibility is often the nurse manager's but may be shared with the CC-CNS. Knowledge of standards set forth by other regulatory agencies (Centers for Disease Control, state entities) may have additional implications for the CC-CNS.

Many units maintain an in-service and continuing education notebook containing the names of the staff and a listing of in-service lectures and programs attended by individual staff. Each staff person is responsible for updating her or his file regularly. This information is then readily available to the nurse manager and JCAHO reviewers. Since documentation can be a very time-consuming process, it is helpful to know that several computer programming options are available to assist in documenting orientation and tracking continuing education of staff.

Working with the Advanced Clinical Nurse

One of the ways that the CC-CNS educator can meet the learning and developmental needs of advanced clinical nurses is to involve them in aspects of staff education. Many advanced staff members teach informally at the bedside as preceptors and role models. Their clinical experience and expertise provide an exceptionally strong knowledge base that lends itself to teaching inexperienced critical care staff members. Ideas for involving advanced staff members in education include (1) encouraging the staff to give 10- to 15-minute in-service talks on topics of interest and areas of expertise, (2) giving entry-level critical care program lectures in

1- or 2-hour blocks (e.g., pacemakers or arterial line monitoring), and eventually (3) lecturing for longer blocks of time in an intermediate or advanced core course (e.g., intraaortic balloon pump [IABP], intermediate hemodynamic classes). These experiences enable the advanced nurse to gain experience teaching in a more formal classroom setting. The CC-CNS is instrumental in guiding the staff in the development of objectives, lecture content, outlines, and audiovisual aids. Additional experiences may include becoming a basic cardiac life support (BCLS) or advanced cardiac life support (ACLS) instructor. As staff members gain more experience and confidence in public speaking, they will be ready to take on additional challenges such as participating in the planning and development of formal educational programs or symposiums. Making arrangements for staff to spend an afternoon with a physician or nurse practitioner in the clinic setting to refine interviewing, assessment, and diagnostic skills offers additional opportunities for learning. Each of these activities offers an excellent opportunity for the advanced nurse to be challenged and remain motivated while developing professionally. By offering encouragement, coaching, and supportive and constructive feedback to enhance teaching skills, the CC-CNS plays an important role in the development of the advanced clinician.

Keeping Abreast of Changes in Nursing, Medicine, and Health Care

To provide up-to-date information in educational offerings the CC-CNS must keep current and make time for self-education. This can be accomplished by subscribing to critical care journals, reading the latest research in critical care literature, and attending local and national critical care seminars and conferences such as the AACN National Teaching Institute or AACN Leadership Institute.

Attending annual meetings of professional organizations such as the Society of Critical Care Medicine or American Heart Association provides another means of keeping updated on changes in the practice of nursing and medicine. The most recent research and papers are presented at these meetings and offer a more global perspective of the latest trends in critical care. These professional meetings also enable the CC-CNS an opportunity to network with physicians, nurses, and other health care professionals on the national and international levels.

It is also important that the CC-CNS schedule time to work at the bedside to maintain clinical practice skills as well as keep updated on new technology, drug therapies, and treatment modalities. Making rounds with the physician teams provides another means of keeping current.

EXAMPLES OF CC-CNS ROLE AS EDUCATOR
Critical Care Quick Reference Manual

One project that was facilitated by a CC-CNS was the development of a unit-specific quick reference manual. The project was envisioned as a way to meet the needs of new nurses as well as float, traveler, and agency personnel who were not familiar with the variety of surgical patients routinely admitted to the ICU. Each senior staff nurse took responsibility for the development of a quick reference for a particular surgical patient population. Included in the reference was an illustration of the surgical procedure and a brief description of the procedure, special protocols, and team preferences, as well as implications for the nurse caring for that patient (care plan format). Each quick reference was reviewed by the CC-CNS for appropriateness of content and format and revised as necessary. Surgical procedures for more than 15 specialty surgeries were indexed according to surgical service (e.g., liver transplant or head and neck) and placed in a brightly colored loose-leaf notebook and kept on the unit as a reference. Since completion of the project and placement of the quick reference manual in the ICU, the manual has been used innumerable times as a quick reference and educational resource by new and experienced staff members. The manual was an excellent learning experience for the staff who participated in its development. The quick reference guide has enhanced professional development, and more importantly, staff members have felt a sense of pride in providing a much needed reference for the unit.

CC-CNS Grand Rounds in Critical Care Units

In a large medical center the CC-CNS have come together as a group to implement a division-wide grand rounds program. Each critical care unit is assigned 1 month to present a patient. The CC-CNS for that unit is responsible for working with a staff nurse to select a patient who is currently in the unit for presentation. The nurse presents the patient's medical history, nursing assessment, and patient problems. Staff representatives from all critical care areas attend and participate in the discussion of the case. During the discussion the CC-CNSs and staff members draw from one another's expertise to devise a care plan for the patient. In this forum staff members have an opportunity to share their expertise while learning new techniques for managing complex patient care problems. In addition, system problems common to all critical care areas have been identified and rectified as a result of these rounds. Finally, staff members have become more aware of the number of CC-CNSs available for consultation.

SUMMARY

The educator role of the CC-CNS requires specific knowledge of educational principles and refined communication and interpersonal skills. Critical care areas are constantly changing, with new technology, sicker and more aged patients, and refinements in knowledge of resuscitation and medical therapy. The CC-CNS will therefore probably spend a significant amount of time in this role component. The CC-CNS assesses educational needs, plans, markets, implements, and evaluates formal educational programs. Using sophisticated interpersonal skills the CC-CNS informally educates staff members in actual clinical situations and guides them in problem solving patient care dilemmas. As computer technology continues to evolve, the CC-CNS educator role will most likely become increasingly one of developer (of new educational methods) and facilitator (of independent educational processes). This chapter has provided a foundation for the educator today and in the future.

References

1. Priest A: The CNS as educator. In Hamric JB, Spross JA, editors: *The clinical nurse specialist in theory and practice,* ed 2, Philadelphia, 1989, WB Saunders Co.
2. Sparacino PSA, Cooper DM: The role components. In Sparacino PSA, Cooper DM, Minarik PA, editors: *The clinical nurse specialist: implementation and impact,* Norwalk, Conn, 1990, Appleton & Lange.
3. University of California at San Francisco, Department of Nursing Services: Proposed developmental role markers, 1986, The University.
4. Dirschel K: The conception, gestation, and delivery of the clinical nurse specialist. In Rotkovich R, editor: *Quality*

patient care and the role of the clinical nurse specialist, New York, 1976, John Wiley & Sons.
5. Everson S: Integration of the role of the clinical nurse specialist, *J Contin Educ Nurs* 12(2):16-19, 1981.
6. Kidd JR: *How adults learn,* New York, 1973, Associated Press.
7. Miller HL: *Teaching and learning in adult education,* New York, 1964, MacMillan.
8. Knowles MS: *The adult learner: a neglected species,* ed 2, Houston, 1979, Gulf Publishing.
9. Knowles MS: *The modern practice of adult education,* Cambridge, Mass, 1980, The Adult Education Co.
10. Knowles MS: *The modern practice of adult education: from androgogy to pedagogy,* Chicago, 1980, Follett.
11. Knowles MS: Applications in continuing education for the health professions, *MOBIUS* 5(2):80-100, 1985.
12. Alspach JG: *The educational process in critical care nursing,* St Louis, 1982, Mosby–Year Book, Inc.
13. Jiricka MK: *Critical care orientation: a guide to the process,* Newport Beach, Calif, 1987, American Association of Critical Care Nurses.
14. Tobin HM, Yoder-Wise PS, Hull PK: *The process of staff development: components of change,* St Louis, 1979, Mosby–Year Book, Inc.
15. Benner P: *From novice to expert: excellence and power in clinical nursing practice,* Menlo Park, Calif, 1984, Addison-Wesley.
16. Del Bueno DJ: Competency based education, *Nurse Educator,* May-June 1978.
17. Del Bueno DJ, Altano R: Competency-based education: no magic feather, *Nurs Management* 15(4):48-53, 1984.
18. Del Bueno DJ: Clinical assessment centers: a cost effective alternative for competency development, *Nurs Econ,* pp 21-26, Jan-Feb 1987.
19. Boss LAS: Teaching for clinical competence, *Nurse Educator* 10(4):8-12, 1985.
20. DeTornay R, Thompson MA: *Strategies for teaching nursing,* New York, 1982, John Wiley & Sons.
21. Corbett NA, Beveride P: *Clinical simulations in nursing practice,* Philadelphia, 1980, WB Saunders Co.
22. Glanville C, Feldman E: A comparison of two types of learning experiences in a second year nursing course, *Nursing Papers,* 1977.
23. Ulione MA: Simulation gaming in nursing education, *J Nurs Educ* 22(8):349-351, 1983.
24. Vehonick PJ et al: I came, I saw, I responded: nursing observations and action survey, *Nurs Res* 17(1):38-44, 1968.
25. Alspach JG: Designing a competency-based orientation for critical care nurses, *Heart Lung* 13(6):655-662, 1984.
26. American Nurses' Association: *The role of the clinical nurse specialist,* Kansas City, Mo, 1986, The Association.
27. American Association of Critical Care Nurses: *The critical care clinical nurse specialist: role definition position statement,* Newport Beach, Calif, 1987, The Association.
28. American Association of Critical Care Nurses: *Competency statements for critical care clinical nurse specialists,* Newport Beach, Calif, 1989, The Association.
29. Alspach JG et al, editors: *AACN education standards for*

critical care nursing, St Louis, 1986, Mosby–Year Book, Inc.

30. Georgopoulous BS, Christman L: The clinical nurse specialist: a role model, *Am J Nurs* 70:1030-1039, 1970.

31. Menard SW: The CNS as teacher. In Menard SW, editor: *The clinical nurse specialist: perspectives on practice,* New York, 1987, John Wiley & Sons.

32. Sills GM: The role and function of the clinical nurse specialist. In Chaska NL, editor: *The nursing profession: a time to speak,* New York, 1983, McGraw-Hill.

33. Robichaud A, Hamric AB: Time documentation of clinical nurse specialist activities, *J Nurs Admin* 16(1):31-36, 1986.

34. Ryan-Merritt MV, Mitchell CA, Pagel I: Clinical nurse specialist: role definition and operationalization, *Clin Nurse Specialist* 2(3):132-137, 1988.

35. Baker PO: Model activities for clinical nurse specialist role development, *Clin Nurse Specialist* 1(3):119-123, 1987.

36. Cooper DM, Sparacino PSA: Acquiring, implementing and evaluating the clinical nurse specialist role. In Sparacino PSA, Cooper DM, Minarik PA, editors: *The clinical nurse specialist: implementation and impact,* Norwalk, Conn, 1990, Appleton & Lange.

37. Holt FM: *Growth and development of the clinical nurse specialist.* Paper presented at the Virginia Council of Clinical Nursing Specialists' Annual Convention Meeting, 1982.

38. Holt FM: Executive practice, *Clin Nurse Specialist* 1(3):116-118, 1987.

39. Buchanan BF, Glanville CI: The clinical nurse specialist as educator: process and method, *Clin Nurse Specialist* 2(2):82-89, 1988.

40. Farrell P, Bramadat IJ: Paradigm case analysis and simulated recall: strategies for developing clinical reasoning skills, *Clin Nurs Specialist* 4(3):153-157, 1990.

41. Toliver JC: Inductive reasoning: critical thinking skills for clinical competence, *Clin Nurse Specialist* 2(4):174-179, 1988.

42. Blount M et al: Extending the influence of the clinical nurse specialist, *Nurs Admin Q* 6:53-63, 1981.

43. Armstrong DG, Denton JJ, Savage TV: *Instructional skills handbook,* Englewood Cliffs, NJ, 1978, Educational Technology Publications.

44. Bell DF: Assessing educational needs: advantages and disadvantages of eighteen techniques, *Nurs Educ,* pp 15-21, Sept-Oct 1978.

45. Bell EA: Needs assessment in continuing education: designing a system that works, *J Contin Educ Nurs* 17(4):112-114, 1986.

46. Jazwiec RM: Learning needs assessment: a complex process, *J Nurs Staff Dev,* pp 91-96, Fall 1985.

47. Jackson BS, Gosnell-Moses D: Cognitive style: a guide for selecting teaching strategies for learners in critical care, *Crit Care Q* 7(3):18-25, 1984.

48. Kolb DA: *Learning style inventory: technical manual,* Boston, 1976, McBer and Co.

49. Garity J: Learning styles: basis for creative teaching and learning, *Nurse Educator,* pp 12-15, March-April 1985.

50. Lorig K: An overview of needs assessment tools for continuing education, *Nurs Educ,* p 12, 1977.

51. Schwab CZ: Assessing learning needs of the experienced critical care nurse, *J Nurs Staff Dev,* pp 133-135, Summer 1988.

52. Farmer ML: " I have to develop a program: Where do I begin?" *J Nurs Staff Dev,* pp 116-139, Summer 1988.

53. Henker R, Hinshaw AS: A program evaluation instrument, *J Nurs Staff Dev,* pp 12-16, Jan-Feb 1990.

54. Poteet G, Pollak C: Increasing accountability through program evaluation, *Nurse Educator* 11(2):41-47, 1986.

55. Tarcinale MA: The role of evaluation in instruction, *J Nurs Staff Dev,* pp 97-103, Summer 1988.

56. Weiss C: *Evaluation research: methods of assessing program effectiveness,* Englewood Cliffs, NJ, 1972, Prentice-Hall, Inc.

57. Farley JK: The multiple choice test: writing the questions, *Nurse Educator* 14(6):10-12, 39, 1989.

58. Farley JK: Item analysis, *Nurse Educator* 15(1):8-9, 1990.

59. Flynn MK, Reese JL: Development and evaluation of classroom tests: a practical application, *J Nurs Educ* 27(2):61-65, 1988.

60. Layton JM: Validity and reliability of teacher-made tests, *J Nurs Staff Dev,* pp 105-109, Summer 1986.

61. Gaston S: Knowledge, retention and attitude: effects of computer assisted instruction, *J Nurs Educ* 27(1):30-34, 1988.

62. Morton PG: Teaching tips: the 10 minute learning break, *J Contin Educ* 22(1), 1991.

63. AACN's Management SIG: Integration of new graduates in critical care units: management perspective, Newport Beach, Calif, 1988, The Association.

64. Caruthers T, Wallace-Barnhill G, Hudson-Civetta J: A method for qualitative analysis of nursing turnover, *Crit Care Med* 9:225, 1981.

65. Houser D: A study of nurses new to special care units, *Super Nurse* 8(15), 1977.

66. Hughs L: Employment of new graduates: implications for critical care nursing practice, *Focus* 14(4):9-15, 1987.

67. Bartz C, Maloney JP: Preceptor-preceptee relationship in critical care nursing, *Crit Care Q* 7(2):33-41, 1984.

68. Begle MS, Willis K: Development of senior staff nurses as preceptors, *Dimen Crit Care Nurs* 3(4):245-251, 1984.

69. Moyer MG, Mann JK: A preceptorship program of orientation within the critical care unit, *Heart Lung* 8(3):530-534, 1979.

70. Mims BC: A critical care internship program, *Dimen Crit Care Nurs* 3(1):53-59, 1984.

71. Anderson SL: The nurse advocate project: a strategy to retain new graduates, *J Nurs Admin* 19(12):22-26, 1989.

72. Giles PF, Moran V: Preceptor program evaluation demonstrates improved orientation, *J Nurs Staff Dev,* pp 17-24, 1987.

73. McLean PH: Reducing staff turnover: the preceptor connection, *J Nurs Staff Dev* (3):20-23, 1987.

74. Shogan JQ, Prior MM, Kokski BJ: A preceptor program:

nurses helping nurses, *J Contin Educ Nurs* 16:139-142, 1985.

75. Alspach JG: *From staff to preceptor: a preceptor training program: instructor manual,* Secaucus, NJ, 1988, Hospital Publications.

76. Mager RF, Pipe P: *Analyzing performance problems or* *'you really oughta wanna,'* Belmont, Calif, 1970, Fearon Pitman Publisher.

77. Joint Commission on Accreditation of Health Care Organizations: *JCAHO scoring guidelines: accreditation manual for hospitals for special care units,* Oakbrook Terrace, Ill, 1992, The Commission.

Chapter 9

The Critical Care Clinical Nurse Specialist Role in Patient Education

Pamela Becker Weilitz, RN, MSN(R)

Educational responsibilities of the critical care clinical nurse specialist (CC-CNS) include both formal and informal patient and community education.[1] The CC-CNS has a unique set of skills, content expertise in an area of clinical practice, and experience in nursing practice as well as working with patients and families. The CC-CNS has a unique perspective in patient education spanning the acute care phase, home care needs, and potential life-style changes. The CC-CNS may teach patients directly or work through others. As an advanced practitioner, the CC-CNS is in a position to anticipate expected needs and respond to unexpected needs and complications during the hospitalization and in preparation for discharge.

The American Association of Critical Care Nurses' (AACN's) competence statements for the CC-CNS define the role responsibilities in critical care patient education, stating, "The CC-CNS assesses learning needs and designs, implements, and evaluates comprehensive teaching programs for specific patient populations, health care providers and community groups to improve patient outcomes."[2] Specifically, the CC-CNS "seeks to improve patient and family outcomes through the application of educational concepts and skills, assists critical care nursing staff in the acquisition of practice skills and knowledge, and acts as a role model of professional critical care nursing practice in the community."[2] Robichaud and Hamric[1] include participation in unit-based patient education activities, development and implementation of patient education programs, and evaluation of the success of programs as part of the CC-CNS's responsibilities.

THEORETIC PERSPECTIVES

Teaching is the ability to impart knowledge to others in order to change behavior or understanding.[3] Knowles[4] identified five reasons for teaching, namely, to change (1) things known (knowledge), (2) things done (tasks, skills), (3) things felt (attitudes), (4) things valued, and (5) things comprehended (understood).

Nursing traditionally defines learning as a change in behavior or outcomes.[5] Kolb[6] has defined learning as knowledge created through the transformation of experience. Kolb's definition includes the components of experience, perception, cognition, and behavior. The learner receives information, filters it, and applies what she or he perceives to be important or having an impact on life.

Individuals have different learning styles. Samples and Hammond[7] define learning style as the way an individual processes information. The particular style of learning is based on previous experiences and social, cultural, and environmental demands.[6] The four styles of learning identified by Kolb[6] are divergent, assimilative, convergent, and accommodative. Divergent learners value people and like to be involved. Convergent learners like applied knowledge. Assimilative learners value facts and knowledge, whereas accommodative learners are futuristic, risk taking, and artistic.[5]

What Makes a Teacher?

The teacher has mastery of content and the skills necessary to teach that content.[8] Ryan-Merritt et al. define the teacher as the facilitator of learning.[9] Behaviors a teacher should possess include (1) the ability to assess learning needs and readiness to learn, (2) collaboration with students to identify learning needs, (3) an ability to formulate teaching and learning objectives, (4) an ability to plan and select appropriate teaching and learning strategies, (5) an ability to select and prepare appropriate teaching materials, and (6) an ability to identify barriers to learning and evaluate attainment of new knowledge.

Theories of Learning

The *pedagogic model* for learning is content directed. The teacher decides what content needs to be taught and develops the time frame and content outlines. The orientation to learning in the pedagogic model is subject centered and usually not directly applicable to daily situations at the time it is taught.

This model is in contrast to how adults learn. The *androgogy model* of learning states that an adult is self-directed in learning, using experiences from life.[4] As individuals mature they become more independent, increasing in self-direction. They are able to identify their readiness to learn and develop their own opportunities for learning. As part of the maturation process, experiences are accumulated as a "data base" on which future learning is built. Much of the motivation for adult learning is related to changes in life situations such as a new role, job, or health problem. The adult learner is more problem centered and quickly applies the learning to the current life situation.[8]

To provide effective patient education certain principles must be considered: (1) learning depends on a desire and readiness to learn; (2) learning is built on a preexisting knowledge base; (3) patient participation enhances learning; (4) repetition strengthens learning; (5) materials must be adjusted to the patient's level; and (6) reduction of distractions will improve the efficiency of teaching and learning.

Teaching and Learning Process

Bille[10] identified six steps in the patient teaching and learning process: (1) assessment, (2) nursing diagnosis, (3) planning, (4) implementation, (5) evaluation, and (6) documentation. The assessment provides baseline data about the health and health beliefs of the patient and family and is used to establish a plan of patient education. The CC-CNS assesses patients' present level of knowledge about their illness, patients' and families' learning needs, and ethical, cultural, religious, or financial concerns that could be barriers to learning.[10] For example, a patient or family who is preoccupied with the financial aspects of the hospitalization because of an absence of health insurance may find it difficult to concentrate on a patient education session. The same patient and family may not be able to follow the medical care plan, because they do not have the necessary resources. The CC-CNS assesses the information and plans interventions to meet the patient's and family's needs.

The second step is formulation of the nursing diagnosis. Two frequently used diagnoses are lack of knowledge related to . . . and alteration in coping related to. . . . These diagnoses are used because they clearly describe what the patient or family needs to learn as a result of either a knowledge deficit or a change in the patient's life-style. For example, lack of knowledge related to inexperience with the surgical procedure or alteration in coping related to first hospitalization provides a clear diagnosis of the patient's or family's education needs.

The written education plan is based on the assessment and identified diagnosis. The plan contains specific behavioral objectives and patient and family outcomes that will occur as a result of the teaching process. Implementation of the plan occurs with each interaction with the patient or family, providing many opportunities to teach.[10]

After the plan has been implemented the CC-CNS evaluates the effectiveness of the teaching. The patient is asked to repeat what was taught such as the details of a modified salt diet for the cardiac patient or the signs and symptoms of an upper respiratory infection for the patient with chronic obstructive pulmonary disease. The patient is asked to return demonstrate skills taught, such as proper suction technique or care of a tracheostomy. Only through evaluation of the patient's skills and understanding will the CC-CNS be able to assess the patient's learning. The CC-CNS documents what teaching has taken place, the patient's response to the teaching, and the evaluation of the patient's understanding and ability to return demonstrate skills taught.

Barriers to Teaching and Learning in the Critical Care Setting

The major barriers to teaching in the critical care setting are time and the nurse's skills in patient teaching. Nurse barriers include lack of preparation in patient education, lack of adequate communication skills, lack of assessment skills, lack of teaching skills, and low priority.[11] The nurse must be knowledgeable in the subject matter to be taught, familiar with the principles of education, and have time to work with the patient and family. A nurse in the cardiac intensive care unit (CICU) possesses many technical skills and knowledge about the care of cardiac patients; however, she or he may not be effective in patient teaching. Additional skill in communication, patient education theory, and experience in teaching is needed.

Other barriers to effective teaching and learning in critical care may be psychologic, physical, physiologic, and environmental (Table 9–1). In the critical care setting, the CC-CNS should be sensitive to patient discomforts such as pain, recent procedures, previous interactions with other caregivers, and sensory deprivation. Patients who are overtired, stressed, and in pain will not be able to concentrate. The age of the patient can be a barrier to learning. Table 9–2 summarizes strategies for teaching elderly patients.

The patient's literacy level may be a barrier to learning. A literate person is someone who can read and write a short statement about everyday life.[12] Redman[13] points out that 23 million people in the United States are functionally illiterate. The median literacy level nationwide is at the tenth grade with 20% of the population reading at a fifth grade or lower level.[13] A patient may be able to read but may not be able to understand what has been read or what actions are expected.[14] Ask the patient to read aloud the patient education information, and determine if the patient can understand the material by asking for repetition in the patient's own words. Poor reading skills impact the patient's ability to organize thoughts, perceptions, vocabulary, understanding, and interpretation.[14] It may be necessary to provide other educational materials for these patients in alternative media; such as pic-

ture poster boards or structural three-dimensional models.

RELATED RESEARCH AND LITERATURE

The role of the CC-CNS as patient educator is a distinct role and one that cannot be separated from every other CC-CNS role. The CC-CNS has the opportunity to demonstrate leadership skills, act as a change agent, and role model clinical practice through the patient educator role.[3] A study by Boyd[15] found that CNSs spent 25% of their time in the educator role.

Robichaud and Hamric[1] define the CC-CNS role in patient education as part of direct patient care activities. When the CC-CNS provides direct patient care, teaching can be demonstrated through role modeling. As the CC-CNS engages in patient education activities, the staff learn the process. During consultations the CC-CNS teaches through discussions and recommendations for patient care.[3] Welch-McCaffery[16] points out that a unique feature of CC-CNSs' health-related teaching is their ability to assess physiologic factors that may impact the learning process. Buchanan and Glanville[17] identified a model for patient education that expands the role of the CC-CNS beyond direct patient education. They point out that the role of educator is as important as the roles of researcher or consultant and represents advanced nursing practice. The components of the model include assessment and diagnosis of learning needs, instructional planning, implementation of instructional plans, and outcome evaluation. The model provides the CC-CNS an overall perspective and sense of direction of what is important in the interactive learning process.[17]

Teaching the critically ill patient and family requires adaptation of basic teaching and learning principles. The information should be brief and concise, with frequent repetition.[18] It may be difficult to determine what information the patient or family wants to know. Studies have shown that during times of high fear and anxiety the nurse should focus on psychologic content and during low levels of anxiety focus on procedural aspects.[19] It is important not to overwhelm with medical jargon and statistical facts. Present the most important information as concisely and completely as possible, allowing time for the patient and family to ask questions. High stress times for critically ill patients are preoperatively, preceding an unfamiliar procedure or therapy, and at the time of transfer

TABLE 9–1 Barriers to Learning in Critical Care Settings

Barrier	Nursing Implications	CC-CNS Strategies
Psychologic		
Readiness to learn	Decreased retention of information taught	Plan education session with input from patient
Emotional	Decreased concentration	Spend time with patient exploring fears, concerns, and other emotions
Loss of control	Lack of cooperation, anger	Allow patient to participate in learning process, e.g., planning when to teach and, when appropriate, the order in which things are to be taught
Information overload	Fatigue may decrease retention or cause confusion	Plan education with other activities in mind, e.g., test procedures, other caregiver interactions
Physical		
Pain	Patient may not be able to focus on the material taught	Plan education around medication schedules; evaluate patient response to pain medications
Vision	Inability to see materials given	Ask family to bring in patient's glasses; if needed, obtain ophthalmology consultation for patient
Hearing	Inability to understand instructions	Ask family to bring in hearing aid if available; speak directly to patient in clear, short sentences; use clipboard to write instructions
Physiologic		
Hypoxemia and carbon dioxide retention	Decreased mental alertness and ability to concentrate	Assess for oxygenation and ventilation
Altered sleep-wake cycle	Fatigue; altered memory, perception, and concentration	Provide periods of uninterrupted sleep
Fluid and electrolyte imbalance, hemodynamics	Impaired understanding and retention	Monitor electrolytes and fluid balance
Environmental		
Lack of privacy, high noise level, unplanned interruptions, bright, sterile environment	Reduces patient concentration; may make patient self-conscious and uncomfortable	Close patient's door or pull curtain; decrease volume of conversation; reduce level of lighting; plan enough time to present the material in an unhurried manner and allow for questions
Cultural		
Language	Patient's ability to read and understand materials taught	Arrange for an interpreter
Health beliefs	Patient may see illness as a weakness or insurmountable crisis	Assess patient's and family's beliefs about health, illness, and wellness. Develop care plan to assist patient in coping

from the ICU to a general patient care area.[18] Studies have shown that including the family in the education process will reduce patient anxiety and improve patient outcomes.[20,21]

The critical care staff nurse is in an excellent position to provide education with each patient interaction. Narrow[22] and Corkadel and McGlashen[23] believe those persons with the closest patient contact should be responsible for health education. The nurse can present small portions of the material

TABLE 9–2 Strategies for Teaching Elderly Patients

Physical Changes	Strategies
Decreased ability to respond to multiple or complex stimuli	Present material in short segments; break up complex tasks into sections, building on each learning session
Difficulty in discriminating high-pitched sounds	Speak in clear, moderate-to low-pitched voice; reduce environmental noise
Decreased visual acuity	Provide glasses as appropriate; use patient education material in larger print for ease of reading
Difficulty with recent memory	Repeat information frequently; ask patient to demonstrate the material taught; provide written information to supplement material taught
Physiologic changes, e.g., electrolyte changes, and hypoxia reducing retention and concentration	Monitor electrolytes and oxygenation; reinforce material taught, using multiple forms of media

during routine care.[24] It is the CC-CNS's role to provide staff with the knowledge and skills for patient education. The critical care nurse at the bedside can more easily plan the education experiences within the context of the patient's care plan. The CC-CNS assists the staff nurse in assessing the patient and family and in developing the plan.

An extensive research base supports preoperative teaching.[25,26] Research supports the benefit of patient education before medical procedures, such as placement of pulmonary artery catheters, surgery, or intubation. Lindeman[27] reports that preoperative teaching has been shown to be effective as a nursing intervention that influences the recovery of surgical patients. The CURN (Conduct and Utilization of Research in Nursing) Project reviewed the use of structured preoperative teaching and developed protocols for patient education that were evaluated clinically.[28] The results indicated that preoperative patient education did have a pos-

itive impact on patient outcomes. Barr[25] reports that outpatient preoperative teaching for the cardiac transplant patient has resulted in a better teaching and learning experience. Factors identified include less pressure of last-minute teaching, less anxiety of the patient, time for the information to be reinforced, and an opportunity for the patient to participate in teaching during periods of remission.[25]

Methods of teaching need additional research. Most of what has been studied is printed materials. With the high level of illiteracy, research in multiple media is needed to establish alternative means of patient education.[29] Additionally, research is needed to identify optimal educational techniques for patients with shortened lengths of stay or with limited education time.

PRACTICE IMPLICATIONS

There are many advantages to the CC-CNS providing all the patient education, including continuity of the patient education, consistency of content taught, and the expertise of the CC-CNS in working with a particular patient population. The disadvantages include decreased staff involvement, the staff nurses' lack of familiarity with the patients, resulting in missed opportunities to develop patient-nurse relationships, and disruption of a primary nurse model.

The role of patient educator can be very satisfying. The CC-CNS develops a close relationship with the patient and feels a sense of accomplishment when the patient succeeds. The CC-CNS is in a position to facilitate communication with patients, physicians, and nurses about patients' needs. Unit- or service-based novice CC-CNSs may find the patient education role is comfortable and helps establish credibility with staff and physicians, increasing their level of self-confidence.

If the CC-CNS is organizationally based, the role of patient educator can be overwhelming. Potentially every unit in the hospital could request the CC-CNS's time. Role conflicts and frustration result when the CC-CNS cannot meet everyone's requests. Because patient education is time consuming, the CC-CNS may find that there is little time left for consultation, research, and clinical practice. Additionally, the nursing staff does not gain skills in assessing, planning, and implementing patient education if the CC-CNS is expected to be the patient educator.

Novice CC-CNSs may find that patient education is a good place to start their work. CC-CNSs provide role modeling for the staff nurses. As CC-CNSs become more experienced in patient education, they should begin to develop staff in this role. By involving the staff in the assessment, planning, and development of the education materials, staff members already will have a vested interest in the project. The CC-CNS slowly develops the staff's ability in teaching by first asking staff members to accompany her or him during teaching sessions and then asking staff to participate in the actual teaching. Over time staff members will see themselves as patient educators and incorporate teaching into their daily practice. It is important to celebrate the staff's success in patient teaching, sharing the experiences in staff meetings and with the patient education committee.

The mature CC-CNS serves as a consultant to the nursing staff, assisting with assessment of patient education needs and development of the patient education plan. The CC-CNS helps nursing staff members develop patient education plans, teaching materials, and tools and assists with development of patient assessment skills, nursing care plans, and implementation of the patient education plan. The CC-CNS functions as a facilitator of patient education, working with the complex and difficult patient. Participation on a unit-based patient education committee provides modeling for the staff nurse. The CC-CNS may institute daily rounds on specific patients to review the patient education plan and evaluate the patient's and nurse's progress toward the expected outcomes. The CC-CNS is also a valuable resource for new staff members. Part of orientation of the new staff nurse might include a patient education checklist the CC-CNS would review with the nurse. Topics could include how to teach, planning patient education, review of specific patient education material, and how to evaluate patient learning. The CC-CNS role models clinical practice, including development of patient education plans, providing the new staff nurse with orientation to good clinical practice.

The patient education plan would include the appropriate nursing diagnosis, the patient education materials to be taught, and the time frame for teaching. For example, with a nursing diagnosis of lack of knowledge related to inexperience with tra-

cheostomy management, the goal is to have the patient independently doing tracheostomy care and suctioning by discharge. Information to be taught includes suctioning and tracheostomy care. The plan might be as follows:

- Day 1: Teach the patient about the purpose of the tracheostomy tube and the importance of keeping the airway clear.
- Day 2: Show the patient how to suction the tracheostomy.
- Day 3: Have the patient suction the tracheostomy tube with supervision. Begin to teach tracheostomy care.

The plan would continue for each day of hospitalization.

The CC-CNS is in the best position to review the research in patient education and share it with the nursing staff, who can implement it into clinical practice as appropriate. This can be done through informal discussions during daily rounds, through formal journal clubs, during staff meetings, or through posting of pertinent articles in the staff lounge. The CC-CNS can also provide research articles on specific patient education problems or topics as they relate to patients in the ICU.

Assessment of Patients' Education Needs

The first step in developing a patient education program is the needs assessment. The CC-CNS can develop the needs assessment tool or use one found in the literature. If you develop your own tool, check the tool to be sure you are getting the type of information you are looking for. Information to be gathered includes assessment of the patient population, educational level, type of illness, what the nurse or physician feels is important to know, how the patient learns best, the most frequently asked questions by patients, and the types of information the patients feel are important to know before they go home. The needs assessment is given to the professional staff, the nurse manager, the medical director of the unit, and patients or families. The critical care patient education committee could interview other staff members for input, as well as the medical director and nurse manager. The first box on page 126 shows a needs assessment questionnaire directed to nursing and physician staff.

Assessing the patient's and family's needs can be accomplished by interviewing patients who are

CARDIOLOGY PATIENT EDUCATION
NEEDS ASSESSMENT

The Cardiology Patient Education Committee is reviewing current patient education materials. We would like your input in determining the education needs of our patients. Please answer the following questions and place the survey in the box in the lounge.

1. What are the three most frequently occurring diagnoses in the coronary care unit (CCU)?
2. Rank order (1 to 5) the following education topics for patients with coronary disease.

_____ Anatomy   _____ Stress man-
_____ Pathophysiology   agement
_____ Medications   _____ Exercise plan
_____ Life-style   _____ Weight control
        changes   _____ Dietary man-
                                   agement
_____ Other _____
_____ Other _____

3. Given the current length of stay in the CCU, what are the three most important things the patient needs to be taught?
4. What are your greatest barriers to teaching, other than time?
5. If you could have anything you needed to teach your patients, what would you choose, other than time?
6. What do you think is the greatest patient education need in this unit?
7. What methods of patient education have you used successfully with the coronary patient?

currently in the ICU or have been recently discharged. If the patient has been discharged from the hospital, a telephone interview can be used. It is important to get a good cross section of the patients seen at your institution, including age, admitting diagnosis, previous admissions, and case mix. If the tool is to be completed by the patient or family, keep it short, with clear questions that only require short answers.

A coronary care unit patient education committee developed a telephone interview in response to the nursing staff's concern about the information given to patients undergoing cardiac catheterization. The staff developed a list of questions the primary nurse used in a telephone interview following the patient's discharge to home. The box

below shows part of the questionnaire used. From the information obtained, staff members were able to revise the patient education materials and information given to the patient.

Collection of the needs assessment data can be accomplished with the help of the critical care staff. This gives them the opportunity to gather information firsthand and assist with tabulation of the information. The more the critical care staff members are involved in the process, the more they will feel tied to the patient education project.

It is important to meet with the ICU medical director and the nurse manager to obtain their input regarding patient and family educational needs and

TELEPHONE INTERVIEW
QUESTIONNAIRE ON POSTCARDIAC
CATHETERIZATION

Patient Information
Name: _____
Date of Hospitalization: _____
Age: _____ Sex: M   F
First cardiac catheterization?   Y   N
Introduction: Hello, Mr./Ms. _____, this is _____, I was your primary nurse when you were in the hospital. I am calling to see how you are doing and to ask you a few questions if I may.

Questions
1. Did the predischarge information you received meet your needs?
2. Did you have questions that were unanswered?
3. When did you start driving again?
4. When are you supposed to return to your physician?
5. Can you recall when you were told you could resume sexual activity?
6. What medications are you currently on?
7. Do you know when can you begin regular exercise?
8. What can we do to improve our care for you?
9. Once you were home, what questions did you have?
10. Did you find the booklet on cardiac catheterization helpful?

their support in keeping the educational program going when the initial newness wears off. They also are in a position to assist and support the program through staffing and budget recommendations.

When the needs assessment has been completed, the CC-CNS along with the staff, nurse manager, and medical director analyzes the results. Important considerations include the frequency of admission to the hospital and previous exposure to patient education information. The needs assessment results may offer insight to the best time of day to provide education and the type of information perceived as essential for the patient and family.

Development of Action Plan

Once the results of the needs assessment have been tabulated, the CC-CNS should arrange for a meeting with the critical care staff to share the information. The meeting and the assessment results will serve as a start for involving staff in developing a plan of action. Ask the critical care staff nurses what ideas they have about meeting the needs expressed by patients, physicians, and critical care nurses. Have the staff brainstorm their ideas, making a list and then systematically eliminating those suggestions that cannot be accomplished.

It will be helpful to staff members to provide them with recent literature and research on patient education for the population of patients selected. You may decide to do this in a journal club setting, asking the staff to read the articles and present the information at a second staff meeting. This not only gets the staff members involved but also helps them to develop their skills in critical reading.

It is helpful to allow the staff time to learn how to teach patients in the critical care setting. This can be accomplished by staff role-playing patient education situations. The role play can be videotaped to allow the staff member teaching the opportunity for self-evaluation. Patient education materials may already be in place that cover the content to be taught. The novice nurse will benefit from mentoring by a nurse experienced and comfortable with patient education. Having materials such as standards of care, teaching aids, teaching plans, documentation guidelines, and sample documentation in place is helpful in getting the critical care staff ready for patient education.

Staff members need time to share their positive and negative experiences with patient education in the critical care setting. Get the staff nurses together to group problem solve concerns they have shared. One problem frequently discussed is enough time to teach the patient. Have the group exchange ideas of how they can plan patient education activities in the care plans. Each interaction with the patient is an opportunity to teach. "This yellow pill is your furosemide [Lasix]. It will cause you to urinate more often." "You are having an echocardiogram today. It will not be painful." The staff may decide to use overlap time during 10-hour shifts or assign a specific time of day or shift for patient education.

Many critical care nurses are expected to carry out patient education as part of their job descriptions. The staff nurse evaluation should include a section about participation in patient education. Feedback of this type is appreciated by staff and further emphasizes the importance of patient education.

Developing a critical care patient education newsletter to share with staff, patients, and families is one way to provide ongoing patient education in a timely manner.[30] The newsletter provides education for discharged patients as well as patients who live out-of-town or are unable to participate in outpatient educational classes.

One method used to share patient education materials and ideas is to hold an annual patient education open house. The critical care nurses in other units are invited to see the types of patient education materials available and methods used to teach patients and share ideas for future development of patient education programming. This is a wonderful way of reinforcing with staff the variety of materials available and is a positive experience for those nurses who have developed patient education materials.

Unit-Based Patient Education Committee

The needs assessment and analysis of data are the beginning of the unit-based patient education committee. When staff members play an integral part in developing programs, implementation is more successful. The agenda for the first meeting of the unit-based patient education committee would include such items as developing a purpose and goals for the group, establishing regular meeting times, group member roles and responsibilities, and the addition of ancillary staff as members of the committee. See box below for an example of a patient education committee's goals. Future committee meetings can be advertised by placing a flier in the ICU. Establishing a regular meeting time and place allows staff to plan in advance for the meetings.

The decision of who will serve as committee chairperson should come from the committee. During the initial months the CC-CNS may serve as chairperson. After several meetings a chairperson is selected by the group to collaborate with the CC-CNS and learn committee chairperson responsibilities. If staff members are experienced in chairing committees, the CC-CNS would function as a consultant.

Once the committee has been established and a chairperson elected, development of the committee

---

4 WEST ICU PATIENT EDUCATION COMMITTEE PURPOSE AND GOALS

Purpose

The purpose of the 4 West ICU Patient Education Committee is to provide the 4 West patients and families with the education necessary to achieve their optimum level of health. To achieve this the committee has set the following goals.

Goals

1. To assess the educational needs of the patients and families of 4 West ICU
2. To identify teaching materials necessary to meet the educational needs of the patients and families of 4 West ICU
3. To develop needed educational materials to meet the educational needs of the patients and families of 4 West ICU
4. To implement and facilitate the use of educational materials in teaching patients and families of 4 West ICU
5. To evaluate the effectiveness of the educational activities for patients and families of 4 West ICU
6. To assess the knowledge level and skill of the 4 West ICU nursing staff regarding patient and family education
7. To increase the knowledge level and skill of the 4 West ICU nursing staff regarding patient and family education

---

as a working team is beneficial. The CC-CNS spends time with the group reviewing group process theories and problem-solving techniques.

Development of Patient Education Materials
Phase 1: The Needs Assessment

Phase 1 in developing patient education materials is an assessment of what is currently available in the market. Table 9–3 lists sources of patient education materials. The unit-based patient education committee can evaluate the materials available and determine suitability for the specific patient type. Things to consider include application to the population of patients, readability of the materials, complexity of the content, completeness of the information, accuracy of the materials, ease of obtaining the materials, and cost of the materials.

If appropriate materials are not available, committee members will need to decide if they should develop their own. Questions to consider include (1) what would be the time and costs involved in developing your own patient education materials, such as illustrations? (2) is there a funding source for developing patient education materials? (3) are there resources within the organization to help with patient education material development? and (4) is there support for developing materials, such as typing, copying, printing, and collating materials?

Phase 2: Development

The committee and the CC-CNS brainstorm about topics and content to be developed. This is a good time to bring in other health care team members if they are not already on the unit-based patient education committee. The multidisciplinary team decides what content is necessary, using the nursing staff's needs assessment, feedback from

---

TABLE 9–3 Sources of Patient Education Materials

Drug companies
Product companies
American Lung Association
American Cancer Society
American Diabetes Association
American Heart Association
Public Health Services
U.S. Department of Health and Human Services
American Journal of Nursing company

the nurse manager, and input from the medical director.

Once the topics have been chosen, the format for presenting the materials is decided. The patient population who will use the information must be considered. It would be impractical to develop patient education materials on video if the majority of the patients have visual or hearing impairments or do not have access to a video player. If possible, the same information should be available on multiple types of media so the CC-CNS and staff nurse can select the appropriate materials for patients with varying learning styles and educational needs. In critical care, since patients and families are in crisis, information needs to be brief, repeated, and slowly delivered.

In the current health care environment, it is difficult to teach the patient everything you would like to because of the short length of stay. The CC-CNS and patient education committee must be able to evaluate what information is critical for the patient to know in an ICU, after leaving the ICU, and by discharge. In addition, home care visits or education in the outpatient setting may be indicated. For example, a CC-CNS may be consulted regarding discharge planning for a patient going home with a dobutamine drip. The CC-CNS could decide to teach the patient about the purpose and side effects of dobutamine, how to turn on and off the cassette, and how to regulate prescribed dosage settings. The Visiting Nurses' Association (VNA) nurse could be asked to reinforce this teaching in the home environment.

Next, committee members begin the process of the literature review and development of the content. The content should be accurate and current. Avoid overloading the patient and family with unessential information. The written materials should concisely discuss the what, why, and when.[15] Be sure the material is easy to read and written in lay terms with as little medical jargon as possible. Table 9–4 lists guidelines for developing written patient education materials.[20] One method of assessing the reading level of patient educational materials is to use the Smog formula[31] (Table 9–5).

Arrange consultation with media experts to assist in determining the best way to present materials. The process of typesetting and printing can take as long as 3 months depending on the length

TABLE 9–4 Guidelines for Developing Written Patient Education Materials

Keep sentences short and to the point.
Express only one idea in each sentence.
Avoid complex grammatical sentence structures.
Write in active rather than passive voice.
Use one- and two-syllable words.
Keep eye span to 60 to 70 characters.
Present most important information first.
Do not use all capital letters; it is harder to read.

From Boyd M: A guide to writing effective patient education materials, *Nurs Management* 18(7):56-57, 1987.

and size of the document developed. Preparing a video presentation requires development of a script, the taping of the educational session, and editing and may be costly. It is important to get a written estimate of the cost involved before submitting a proposal for the project. If the hospital does not have a media department, consult printing or photographic services to determine if they prepare printed materials. The hospital public relations department may be able to suggest a vendor, since they frequently have printed and other media prepared for advertisements for the hospital.

Phase 3: Obtaining Funding

Funding for developing educational materials may be available from the nursing department, hospital auxiliary, the medical staff of hospital society, drug companies, or grants. Nursing or medical

TABLE 9–5 Smog Formula

Step 1: In any printed material, count 30 sentences, that is, any lists of words ending in a period, a question mark, or an exclamation point. Count 10 at the beginning, 10 in the middle, and 10 at the end of the material.
Step 2: Total the number of words of three or more syllables in the 30 sentences selected.
Step 3: Take the square root of the number in step 2.
Step 4: Add 3 to the square root. This is the grade level of the material.
Example: 30 sentences with 49 three-or-more-syllable words
The square root of 49 is 7
$7 + 3 = 10$ (tenth-grade reading level)

school librarians can run a search to locate funding sources. Professional organizations may have scholarships or research monies available for developing and researching patient education materials. Drug or product manufacturers will often support publication of patient education materials. The CC-CNS should discuss this possible funding source with sales representatives.

Phase 4: Implementation

Implementation of patient education materials into clinical practice involves education of the staff and a plan for incorporation into the care plan. Staff members need to decide where the materials will be kept. Storage on the unit will increase the staff's access to the materials and may improve utilization. One way to remind staff about the patient education materials is to prepare notices or fliers to be posted throughout the unit; for example, "Are you caring for a patient with a Swan-Ganz catheter? Don't forget the new patient education booklet. It can be found in the cabinet next to the nursing station." The CC-CNS can encourage use of the materials by asking staff members if they are using the information, helping staff members plan and use the information, and following up with the staff about problems or concerns. After 7 to 10 days of use, get the staff together to evaluate how things are going. Discuss problems with implementation, storage, and patient response to the materials. It is important to continue to get input from the staff about the materials and include patient education discussions in daily rounds.

Phase 5: Evaluation of Materials

After the educational materials have been developed, test them on patients and staff for feedback. Set clear objectives for measuring what learning is planned and use them to assess the effectiveness of the materials. Use the feedback from patients, families, and professional staff to revise and improve the materials. The process of changing and updating educational materials based on the evaluations is connected to the process of continuous quality improvement.

CASE STUDIES

Developing Patient Education Booklet for Patients with Swan-Ganz Pulmonary Artery Catheter The coronary care unit/coronary observa-tion unit (CCU/COU) patient education committee determined that a booklet was needed on the pulmonary artery catheter, since the unit sees a large number of cardiomyopathy patients requiring hemodynamic monitoring. The CC-CNS for the unit approached a company who supplies the catheter, for funding. The CC-CNS wrote a formal letter to the company, outlining the purpose of the booklet, how many would be needed, the estimated printing costs, and the process that would be used to ensure quality of the final product. The booklet was developed by the committee and reviewed by physicians, nurses, and patients. The booklet was printed in-house and the bill sent to the company. The committee then sent a thank-you note to the company with several copies of the final product. The booklet was so successful that physicians in the clinic areas requested copies to distribute to patients who were going to be admitted for hemodynamic monitoring. In addition, one cardiologist was so impressed with the quality of this booklet, he asked the committee to develop a similar booklet on ablation therapy for dysrhythmias. The committee members experienced great personal satisfaction from this successful and valuable project.

Developing Respiratory Patient Education Program in Respiratory Intensive Care Unit The respiratory intensive care unit (RICU) experienced an increase in the number of ventilator-dependent patients. The pulmonary CNS identified that many patients were going home on their mechanical ventilators and needed to be able to care for their ventilators, airway, and basic needs. The skills identified for the ventilator-dependent patient included care of the tracheostomy, pulmonary hygiene, communication, bathing and toileting, medications, and management of the home mechanical ventilator. The skills most easily taught by the ICU staff were pulmonary hygiene and tracheostomy care.

Review of the literature revealed many articles that discussed home discharge of the mechanically ventilated patient.[32-36] It was easy to find nursing procedures that described the correct way to suction, clean, and change a tracheostomy tube; bathing and toileting; and education about medications. Information for teaching the patient about their home mechanical ventilator was available through the home care companies that provided the ventilator.

A multidisciplinary team consisting of the pulmonary CC-CNS, staff nurses, respiratory therapist, dietitian, social worker, and physical therapist was formed. The team determined what the patient needed to know before discharge based on the American College of Chest Physicians' recommendations[37] and the American Lung Association's[38] and American Thoracic Society's[39] standards for the care of patients with chronic obstructive pulmonary disease (COPD). Table 9–6 lists the topics patients and families needed to know before discharge. The team began by dividing the content among the experts and developing 1-2 to 3-page written information. The information was reviewed by all team members and the respiratory and critical care division physicians for their input. The materials were sent to the sixth grade class of a local elementary school for feedback. The materials were typed on a formatted page so each one looked alike and was identified as part of the respiratory patient education series. The topics were not collated. This permitted the staff to select the individual pages and topics a patient needed and did not overwhelm the patient with all the material at once.

Commentary The materials have been used for the past 6 years with great success. The patients find the single-page format easy to use because of its simplicity and easy to understand. Patients wanting more information are given literature from the American Lung Association and other specialty organizations.

SUMMARY

Patient education is an essential component of quality, comprehensive patient care. Although the value of patient education is recognized, there continue to be inadequacies in patient education programs, particularly in the hospital setting. The CC-CNS is equipped to solve some of the problems related to patient teaching. Through role modeling, staff empowerment, and development of educational materials the CC-CNS can positively impact patient education programs.

TABLE 9–6 Knowledge for the Home Ventilator Patient (Respiratory Patient Education Series)

Topic: respiratory medications	**Topic: oxygen therapy**
Actions	Type used
Side effects	Oxygen safety
Administration schedule	Manual resuscitation bag
Administration methods	**Topic: airway care**
Topic: home ventilator	Tracheostomy tube care
Assembly and disassembly of vent circuit	Cuff care
Cleaning circuit	Changing tracheostomy tube
Ventilator settings	Suctioning
Control knobs	Using home suction machine
Alarm systems	Cleaning suction catheters
Troubleshooting the vent	
Topic: chest physiotherapy	**Topic: exercises**
Using chest percussor	Chest mobility exercises
Topic: when to call the physician	**Topic: signs and symptoms of a respiratory infection**

References

1. Robichaud AM, Hamric AB: Time documentation of clinical nurse specialist activities, *Journal of Nursing Administration* 16(1):31–36, 1986.
2. American Association of Critical Care Nurses: *Competence statements for critical care clinical nurse specialists,* Laguna Niguel, Calif, 1989, The Association.
3. Menard SW: *The clinical nurse specialist: perspectives on practice,* New York, 1987, John Wiley & Sons.
4. Knowles M: *The adult learner: a neglected species,* Houston, 1973, Gulf Publishing Co.
5. Arndt MJ: Learning style: theory and patient education, *J Contin Educ Nurs* 21(1):28–31, 1990.
6. Kolb DA: *Experiential learning: experience as the source of learning and development,* Englewood Cliffs, NJ, 1984, Prentice Hall, Inc.
7. Samples B, Hammond B: Holistic learning, *Science Teacher* 29:28–34, 1985.
8. Murdaugh C: The nurses role in education of the cardiac patient. In Kern LS: *Cardiac critical care nursing,* Gaithersburg, Md, 1988, Aspen Publishers, Inc.
9. Ryan-Merritt MV, Mitchell CA, Pagel I: Clinical nurse

specialist role definition and operationalization, *Clin Nurse Specialist* 2(3):132–137, 1988.

10. Bille D: Patient family teaching in critical care. In Kenner CV, Guzzetta CE, Dossey BM: *Critical care nursing: mind-body-spirit,* ed 2, Boston, 1985, Little Brown & Co.

11. Close A: Patient education: a literature review, *J Adv Nurs* 13(2):203–213, 1988.

12. UNESCO: *Illiteracy in America 1986: extent, causes and suggested solutions,* New York, 1981, National Advisory Council on Adult Education.

13. Redman BK: *The process of patient education,* St Louis, 1988, Mosby–Year Book, Inc.

14. Hussey LC, Gilliland K: Compliance, low literacy, and locus of control, *Nurs Clin North Am* 24(3):605–611, 1989.

15. Boyd MD: A guide to writing effective patient education materials, *Nurs Management* 18(7):56–57, 1987.

16. Welch-McCaffery D: Role performance issues for oncology clinical nurse specialist, *Cancer Nurs* 9(6):287–293, 1986.

17. Buchanan BF, Glanville CI: The clinical nurse specialist as educator: process and method, *Clin Nurse Specialist* 2(2):82–89, 1988.

18. Thelan LA, Davie JK, Urden LD: *Textbook of critical care nursing, diagnoses and management,* St Louis, 1990, Mosby–Year Book, Inc.

19. Hathway D: Effect of preoperative instruction on postoperative outcomes: a meta-analysis, *Nurs Res* 35(5):269–275, 1986.

20. Dziurbejko M, Larkin J: Including the family in preoperative teaching, *Am J Nurs* 78:1892–1894, 1979.

21. Doerr C, Jones J: Effect of family preparation on the state of anxiety level of the CCU patient, *Nurs Res* 28:315–316, 1979.

22. Narrow BW: *Patient teaching in nursing practice,* New York, 1979, John Wiley & Sons.

23. Corkadel L, McGlashen R: A practical approach to patient teaching, *J Contin Educ Nurs* 14(1):9–15, 1983.

24. Brannon PHB, Johnson R: The internal cardioverter defibrillator: patient-family teaching, *Focus* 19(1):41–46, 1992.

25. Barr WJ: Teaching patients with life-threatening illness, *Nurs Clin North Am* 24(3):639–644, 1989.

26. Oberst MT: Perspectives on research in patient teaching, *Nurs Clin North Am* 24(3):621–628, 1989.

27. Lindeman C: Nursing research in patient education, *Annu Rev Nurs Res* 6:29–60, 1988.

28. Horsley JA et al: *Using research to improve nursing practice: a guide,* New York, 1983, Grune & Stratton.

29. Smith CE: Overview of patient education, *Nurs Clin North Am* 24(3):583–587, 1989.

30. Ventura MR et al: Patient newsletter: a teaching tool, *Patient educ Counseling* 15:269–274, 1990.

31. McLaughlin H: Smog grading—a new readability formula, *J Reading* pp 639–645, 1969.

32. Frace RM: Home ventilation: an alternative to institutionalization, *Focus* 13(6):28–36, 1986.

33. Gilmartin M, Make B: Home care of the ventilator-dependent person, *Respir Care* 28(11):1490–1497, 1983.

34. Haynes N, Raine SF, Rushing P: Discharging ICU ventilator-dependent patients to home health care, *Crit Care Nurs* 10(7):39–49, 1990.

35. Mularz LA, Simandl-Gerr RA: Caring for ventilator dependent patients, *Nurs Management* 20(6):26–28, 1988.

36. Thompson CL, Richmond M: Teaching home care for ventilator-dependent patients: the patient's perception, *Heart Lung* 19(1):79–83, 1990.

37. O'Donohue WJ, Grovannoni RM, Goldberg AI, Keens TG: Long-term mechanical ventilation: Guidelines for management in the home and at alternative community sites. *Chest* 90(1):1S–37S, 1986.

38. American Lung Association: *Standards for the care of patients with chronic respiratory disease,* New York, 1971, The Association.

39. American Thoracic Society: Standards for nursing care of patients with COPD, *ATS News,* p 31, Summer 1981.

Chapter 10

The Critical Care Clinical Nurse Specialist Role in Student Education

Suzanne S. Prevost, RN, PhD, CCRN

One of the most exciting and challenging aspects of the critical care clinical nurse specialist (CC-CNS) role is its tremendous diversity. At the very least the CC-CNS is expected to function as an advanced practitioner, educator, consultant, and researcher. Depending on the needs of the institution and the strengths of the individual, additional expectations, such as manager or continuous quality management coordinator, may be added to the list. One strategy for fulfilling this rather overwhelming position description is to accomplish two or three of these activities simultaneously. This concept is probably best exemplified in the role of the CC-CNS as educator. In nearly everything the CC-CNS does, from providing direct care to conducting research, opportunities for education arise. The audience is constantly changing from patients to families to staff nurses to physicians to administrators. Perhaps one of the most challenging teaching responsibilities for the CC-CNS is educating students of the health care professions.

Students who are educated or influenced by the CC-CNS include basic and graduate-level nursing students; medical students, interns, and residents; and those persons from other disciplines such as respiratory therapy, physical therapy, and pharmacy. In the interactions with physicians in training and students of other disciplines, the CC-CNS has an obligation to support quality nursing care and to describe the unique contributions of nursing interventions. The CC-CNS also is responsible for modeling active participation and, frequently, lead-

ership of the multidisciplinary team. The CC-CNS demonstrates appropriate and assertive methods of communicating and collaborating among disciplines with the hope of exerting a positive influence on current and future interdisciplinary relationships.

THEORETIC PERSPECTIVES

The role of the CC-CNS in the education of basic nursing students may range from guest lectures to coordinating clinical rotations to being a preceptor for groups or individuals. The CC-CNS must be prepared to clearly define the role and to demonstrate what differentiates the CC-CNS role from that of the staff nurse.

The most common type of student instruction provided by the CC-CNS is the education of graduate nursing students. This type of teaching may occur in a formal classroom setting but more frequently involves the CC-CNS functioning as a preceptor in the clinical setting. The opportunity to observe, participate, and collaborate with a practicing CC-CNS is essential for the CC-CNS student. The CC-CNS can also provide valuable learning opportunities to students in other specialties. Graduate students in medical-surgical nursing or adult health would certainly benefit from clinical exposure to critically ill patients. When a patient on a medical or surgical unit suddenly becomes critical, the CC-CNS must be prepared to assess the patient and intervene. The CNS student who has an interest in serving a specific population, such as patients with diabetes, needs guided clinical exposure to patients in the critical phases of such illnesses. The CC-CNS can also provide valuable instruction to graduate students in nursing administration by helping them to understand and appreciate the CC-CNS role.

In this role as the educator of graduate nursing students, the CC-CNS fulfills two very important responsibilities. First, the CC-CNS is fostering the development of the future generation of CNSs; and second, the CC-CNS is helping to bridge the gap between academia and practice. Several authors[1,2] have suggested that the CNS is the nurse who is best suited to facilitate this collaborative relationship. The CNS demonstrates commitment to both areas with the primary commitment to patient care, supported by the CNS's foundation of advanced knowledge.

CNSs have created a variety of models to fulfill their roles as educators for graduate nursing students. As previously mentioned, the clinical preceptor model is most common. Other options include functioning in formal or informal joint appointments, coordinating graduate-level courses, providing guest lectures, or serving as a consultant for the development and refinement of graduate nursing curricula. From a less formal perspective the CC-CNS also provides valuable insights to graduate students by serving as a role model, both in the clinical setting and in other realms of the professional community; and in some cases by functioning as a mentor.

RELATED RESEARCH AND LITERATURE
CNS Educational Preparation

Considerable controversy exists regarding what content is essential in CNS educational programs. Likewise, vast differences exist in the various graduate programs across the United States.[3] Several authors have made specific recommendations regarding areas that ought to be strengthened, such as content related to leadership and management, fiscal and budgetary concepts, theories and strategies for change, negotiation skills,[4,5] and research utilization.[3] The competence statements for CC-CNSs published by the American Association of Critical Care Nurses (AACN) in 1989[6] should serve as a logical foundation for designing curriculums for the CC-CNS.

One area where consensus does exist, however, is the importance of clinical practice experience within CNS educational programs. Most authors agree that this experience should be directed and modeled by a CNS preceptor or a faculty member in the clinical setting.[3,5]

Role of Preceptor

A preceptor is a teacher who works directly with the student on a one-on-one basis, over a period of time, to guide the student through essential learning experiences.[7,8] The role of the preceptor in relation to undergraduate nursing students and new graduate nurses has been described by several nurse authors. Expectations for these preceptors include assisting the student with technical skills, role modeling and encouraging acceptable behaviors, evaluating progress, providing continuity of care for the student or new nurse, and serving as a liaison between the student and hospital environment.[9,10] Although these same expectations apply for the CC-CNS who is a preceptor for graduate students, considerable differences do exist. The graduate student usually enters the situation with more clinical experience and technical proficiency than the undergraduate or new nurse; therefore the graduate student functions at a higher level of professionalism and has different learning needs.

Hill[8] published a model for the practicing CNS who is a preceptor for CNS students. Hill described the four major learning needs of the CNS student as advanced clinical skills, communication skills, leadership skills, and group skills. The student must understand foundational theoretic content in each of these areas before clinical implementation.

Shah and Prolifroni[7] used a qualitative method in a study to describe the role of the CC-CNS preceptor. They conducted semistructured interviews with 10 CC-CNSs who had functioned as preceptors for CNS graduate students. Their findings included descriptions of a typical day, time commitments, preceptor responsibilities, and rewards. Specific preceptor responsibilities identified in this study were facilitator, teacher, change agent, resource, nurturer, organizer, director, monitor, role model, and socializer.

PRACTICE IMPLICATIONS
Negotiating Preceptorship Responsibilities

A successful CNS student clinical experience requires three-way collaboration. Thoughtful preparation, planning, and negotiation among the practicing CC-CNS, the CNS student, and the faculty member will help to achieve optimal outcomes for everyone involved. The student must honestly assess and communicate strengths, weaknesses, and interests. The CC-CNS needs a thorough understanding of the student's baseline knowledge and personal objectives, as well as the objectives for the course, to facilitate the learning experience. The faculty member needs to be aware of the types of patients cared for and services provided in the clinical agency and on specific units. The student also needs an understanding of the roles and responsibilities of the CC-CNS preceptor.

Sometimes initial negotiations may involve other people, such as the administrator who evaluates the CC-CNS, nursing staff development instructors, medical intensive care unit (ICU) directors, physicians who manage specific patient populations, or the hospital's legal staff. Most teaching hospitals have specific policies governing licensure, malpractice insurance, and practice limitations for visiting students. If these policies are developed primarily to govern the practice of undergraduate students, the CC-CNS graduate student may need to negotiate exceptions.

In the negotiation phase the CC-CNS should clarify how the course will be graded and what type of evaluation is expected to be provided to the student and the faculty member. Evaluations may range from intermittent verbal reports on the student's progress to anecdotal notes to pass/fail ratings or scores for each of the student's objectives. The preceptor rarely assigns the final course grade, but she or he should be given ample opportunity to provide input into the grading process. The CC-CNS should also be given an opportunity to evaluate the structure of the course for faculty members. For example, are the objectives appropriate? Do they accurately reflect the knowledge requirements for the CNS position? Did the precepting responsibilities mesh well with other components of the CNS's position? Did the CNS feel capable of meeting the student's learning needs?

The graduate student should present a draft of personal and course objectives (Table 10–1) to the CC-CNS on or before their initial meeting. At this point the CC-CNS can help the student to evaluate whether the expectations are realistic within the available time frame and whether the facilities, re-

TABLE 10–1 Example of Student Objectives for a Graduate-Level CC-CNS Course

Goal: At the completion of this practicum the student will demonstrate beginning-level competency in the essential roles of the CC-CNS. Competency will be demonstrated through accomplishment of the following objectives:

As a Practitioner
1. Completes and documents comprehensive assessments of at least eight patients and their families
2. Contributes to the care plan, through documentation and consultation with other care providers, for at least six patients
3. Provides basic and advanced interventions to at least four patients or family members
4. Evaluates patient responses to interventions (from no. 3) and adjusts plan accordingly
5. Participates in clinical rounds with the CC-CNS preceptor

As an Educator
1. Collaborates with the CC-CNS or other staff members to provide staff development programs
2. Plans, conducts, and evaluates at least one unit-level in-service program
3. Provides documentation of educational interventions provided to at least two patients

As a Consultant
1. Observes and documents three examples of consultation provided by the CC-CNS preceptor
2. Identifies one area of marketable, personal expertise within which the student could provide consultation to other nurses
3. Demonstrates successful integration with staff as evidenced by three staff members asking the CNS student questions and five nursing staff members knowing the student's name

As a Researcher
1. Reviews the research literature on at least one nursing intervention
2. Demonstrates creativity in sharing the findings from no. 1 with nursing staff

As a Leader or Manager
1. Documents one example of effective management strategies demonstrated by the CC-CNS preceptor
2. Documents one example of cost savings associated with CC-CNS interventions in the clinical facility

sources, and patients are available. Recommendations can be made for the structure of the clinical experience. For example, it may be helpful for the student to come into the unit early in the morning to participate in surgical staff rounds; the student may want to come on particular days to participate in staff or administrative meetings; or it may be interesting to provide continuity of care to a specific patient and family over several consecutive days.

At this time the CC-CNS can also project the degree of interaction that will be needed and evaluate how this will fit with other responsibilities. The CC-CNS should assist the student in identifying opportunities with mutual benefits for both the preceptor and the student. The student can learn a lot about the CC-CNS's role by actually assuming some portion of the CNS's workload, with supervision, of course. Table 10–2 lists examples of such shared activities.

Even though educating and acting as a preceptor of students are beneficial and logical activities for the CC-CNS, there are times when they can become burdensome because the student requires structure and looks for feedback. Graduate students

TABLE 10–2 Examples of Shared Opportunities for the CC-CNS Preceptor and CNS Student

CNS Responsibility	Student Involvement
Write or revise procedures	Review literature; prepare draft
Conduct educational needs survey	Assist with tool development; administer tool; summarize results
Lecture for staff development	Prepare visual aids/handouts; present a specific topic or team teach with CC-CNS
Coordinate preoperative education	Teach individual patients
Conduct patient care conferences	Work up patient assignment; prepare for patient care conference
Report on quality improvement	Collect and/or summarize data
Consult with telemetry staff on dysrhythmia interpretation	Audit records on telemetry unit to identify common dysrhythmias
Conduct clinical research studies	Review literature; obtain consents; collect data

are accustomed to a staff nurse role with a structured day and visible outcomes. As is true with many nursing responsibilities, the CC-CNS who is most comfortable and proficient with teaching will be called on most frequently. In large teaching hospitals, CC-CNSs may be called on by faculty from various courses (i.e., the undergraduate critical care instructor, the graduate level critical care instructor, and the individual teaching CNS role theory) or by faculty from more than one university.

Since clinical practice is the primary commitment for most practicing CC-CNSs, clinical responsibilities may at times preclude one's ability to teach effectively. The CC-CNS must be assertive and honest in communicating limitations to students and faculty members. The CC-CNS should specifically identify the months, days, and times when teaching would fit well with other responsibilities. If the CC-CNS becomes overwhelmed to the point of having to refuse a request to teach students, it is extremely important to explain why. Otherwise, faculty and students tend to become suspicious about why a CC-CNS would refuse the "help" of a graduate student. The CC-CNS can help to educate both the student and faculty by explaining the nature and extent of responsibilities related to the various CC-CNS roles and the amount of time and intervention involved in the clinical teaching of students at various levels.

Integrating Students into Clinical Setting

Regardless of the experience level of the CC-CNS student, the first few days in a new clinical setting will be primarily observational and will require a considerable time commitment from the preceptor. As with any new employee, the student needs a guided tour of the unit and facility if they are unfamiliar. The CC-CNS serves as the liaison between the student and the institution. The graduate student should be introduced to as many of the staff members (nursing and medical) as possible, with specific mention of status as a graduate student with previous nursing experience. The CC-CNS should look for opportunities to facilitate integration and staff acceptance of the student, such as introduction at staff meetings, participation in rounds, posting student objectives on the unit bulletin board, and invitations to informal social events. The student may need to be reminded of the importance of nonverbal behaviors, such as attire appropriate for the clinical setting and providing a helping hand when the unit is busy. Pairing the student with a staff nurse for 3 or 4 hours may help to orient the student to unit practices such as documentation; storage of supplies; and ordering of tests, medications, or equipment.

Orientation to the role of the CC-CNS generally requires detailed explanation followed by several days of observation and participation in various activities. It is unfortunate that the times when the CC-CNS is the most busy are often the best times for the student to learn about the complexity of the CNS role, yet these are the times when the CC-CNS is least available to explain and instruct. The CC-CNS may need to have a "debriefing" session with the student at the end of a busy day. If the student is commited to actively participating in the learning experience and if the CC-CNS is able to share portions of the workload with the student, both will benefit. The CC-CNS should encourage students to expand their understanding of the role by talking with staff nurses or nurse managers about the types of support they have received from the CC-CNS and their expectations of the CNS.

Clinical Activities

The structure of the clinical experience will depend highly on the course objectives. If the primary goal is to learn more about the area of specialization, the experience should be patient-focused clinical practice. However, if the primary goal is to understand the role of the CC-CNS, more diverse activities will be required. Another issue related to structure is the level of involvement. Will the student spend most of the time in observational experiences or actively intervene? Frequently the CC-CNS uses the clinical time to make brief observations of multiple advanced practitioners, specialty units, and unique procedures. Although these opportunities serve to broaden the student's perspective, they do little to extend the student's expert knowledge in an area of specialization. Students should be encouraged to spend concentrated amounts of time with complex patients and their families and to actively participate and contribute to CC-CNS functions.

Expert Practice

The student should be given opportunities to participate to some degree in each of the CC-CNS roles, with the greatest concentration of time in direct and indirect patient care. In some cases, graduate students may avoid spending time in the clinical practice role, because they feel they have already developed their clinical expertise through several years of practice at the staff nurse level. They may feel more challenged by the opportunity to participate in roles such as education or research that are regarded as advanced-level activities. In such situations the preceptor may need to remind the student that advanced clinical practice is the foundation of the CC-CNS role. Students should be challenged to articulate and demonstrate how their advanced patient care differs from that of the experienced staff nurse. For example, they may have the opportunity to spend more time with the family than the staff nurse and develop interventions that can support families during crisis. This activity can help the student to further understand the expert practice role, and it can help the staff to differentiate the role of the graduate student from that of the undergraduate student.

One of the most valuable clinical experiences for students is to observe patients through the course of their hospitalization. The CC-CNS may help the student to identify appropriate patients in the emergency deparment or other admitting areas. Providing care to the patient and family throughout the stay in the operating room, ICU, and general unit and even after discharge offers several benefits. First, the patient receives a greater level of continuity of care than usual. The student has an opportunity to provide more specific assessments and interventions and to develop more intimate relationships with the patient and family. The student gets a much broader understanding of the entire illness experience. This situation also gives individual patients a greater understanding and appreciation for the role of the student and the CC-CNS.

The student should also be encouraged to participate actively in clinical rounds with the CC-CNS and the medical staff. This experience helps the student to understand the type of observations and assessments the CC-CNS makes and the level of interventions provided. The CC-CNS can role model for the student effective communication and collaboration strategies in working with physicians and other members of the multidisciplinary team.

Education

In the area of education the student should again be encouraged to differentiate the educational role of the CC-CNS from the educational role of the experienced staff nurse. Experienced staff nurses are expected to participate in staff education through in-service presentations or being preceptors and to provide individualized patient education. The CC-CNS should explain how her or his educational responsibilities differ. For example, the CC-CNS may be expected to coordinate orientation for a whole group of new nurses rather than acting as a preceptor for one at a time. The CC-CNS may have specific and unique methods for validating staff competency. She or he may be responsible for educating the staff on new equipment or procedures. The CC-CNS may formally or informally educate professionals in other disciplines about issues related to nursing care.

In terms of patient education the CC-CNS may be responsible for educating patients and families with complex educational needs, such as discharge teaching for patients on ventilators (see Chapter 9); or the CC-CNS may need to work with patients who have learning difficulties, such as illiteracy, sensory deficits, or language barriers. By making rounds with the CC-CNS, the student can observe how the CC-CNS identifies specific learning needs, which patients the CNS teaches, and what types of teaching strategies are used.

A common dilemma for the CC-CNS is the tendency of staff nurses to expect the CC-CNS to do all or most of the patient education for specific patients. The CC-CNS can advise the student regarding how to avoid this pitfall by providing resources and strategies to empower staff nurses in their roles as patient educators. An appropriate activity for the CC-CNS student is development of patient education materials related to a particular illness or procedure.

Research

For the CC-CNS student the research role is usually perceived in one of two ways: fascination or intimidation. The CC-CNS's attitude and participation related to research can have a profound effect on these students. If the CC-CNS models value and respect for research by incorporating research into practice, the student will be positively influenced. On the other hand, if research partic-

ipation and utilization are low priorities for the practicing CNS, students who are fascinated will be squelched and students who are intimidated will feel justified.

Many options exist for student participation in research. Whenever possible, activities related to thesis research should be incorporated into clinical experiences. The CC-CNS can assist the student in identifying and refining clinically relevant research questions. If the student is in the early stages of the thesis project, the CC-CNS will probably have a broader knowledge of the existing research literature in various areas related to critical care. The CC-CNS can help to direct the student in terms of what has already been done and what questions remain unanswered in particular areas. On the other hand, the student who has already begun to develop a proposal may have a better command of the recent literature in the area of interest than the CNS. The CC-CNS may benefit from the student's literature review and the student's insights on the topic. The CC-CNS can also be very helpful in designing feasible methodologies for clinical research. And perhaps the most valuable service the CC-CNS can provide is to guide the student through the intricacies of the approval process.

In addition to thesis research activities, the student can actively participate in the research role of the CC-CNS. Students can assist with reviewing literature, obtaining patient consents, collecting data, or entering data into the computer. All of these activities will facilitate the CNS's research productivity and provide valuable learning opportunities for the student. Research utilization activities are particularly appropriate for the CNS student. For example, the student may investigate the research base for specific procedures; the student may lead a journal club and review research articles with the staff; or the student may summarize the research on a particular topic and develop a poster or bulletin board display for the staff.

Consultation

Most CC-CNSs who are well established in clinical facilities spend a large portion of their time providing consultation, particularly in light of the trends toward increasing levels of patient acuity and expanding technology, both in the ICU and on medical-surgical units. CC-CNSs are frequently consulted to assist staff nurses with highly technical procedures, such as insertion of a pulmonary artery catheter or troubleshooting a peritoneal dialysis system. The CC-CNS may be consulted to perform physical assessments or validate assessment findings on patients experiencing a critical change in status. Dysrhythmia analysis and complex wound care are two additional areas where CC-CNSs frequently provide consultation. CNSs are also commonly called to provide psychosocial or family-oriented consultation when there is evidence of ineffective coping or disruptive behaviors.

It is unfortunate that it is usually difficult for the CNS student to actively participate in the consultant role. Recognition, acceptance, and utilization of the CC-CNS as a consultant follow consistent demonstrations of clinical expertise and the display of a helpful attitude. CNS students rarely have the time to develop that level of trust and credibility with the staff. However, the student who has become integrated with the staff may find staff nurses approaching her or him with questions and informal consultation. Therefore the student's experience with consultation in the clinical setting is primarily observational.

The CC-CNS can, however, impart valuable insights to the student related to the processes of consultation. The CC-CNS can suggest strategies for establishing clinical credibility, marketing CC-CNS availability to the staff, and documenting consultations.

Documentation is a critical element of the consultation process to promote adherence to recommendations and to help justify the services the CC-CNS provides. If the consultation is patient focused, documentation in the patient's record should include the reason for consultation, who requested the consultation, who (the CNS) provided the consultation, assessment findings, diagnosis, plan, immediate interventions and recommendations for future interventions, and plans for follow-up evaluation. (See Chapter 11.) A similar process is used to document other types of consultation, such as staff-oriented or system-oriented issues. However, the documentation is provided to the person being consulted, rather than a patient's record. In any case the CC-CNS should retain copies of the documentation for her or his own records to help justify how the CC-CNS is being utilized and the interventions provided. The CC-CNS student should also be encouraged to keep some form of documentation, such as 3×5 cards, related to the patients the CC-CNS has worked with.

Leadership/Management

The management responsibilities of the CC-CNS vary considerably depending on whether the CC-CNS is fulfilling a line or staff position; but, regardless of whether the power base is formal or informal, the CC-CNS must be recognized as a leader to be effective. In addition to actual management of staff, CC-CNSs can use their administrative leadership skills by chairing committees and managing clinical programs or research projects. Another important administrative function for the CC-CNS is fiscal responsibility, which may be demonstrated through documentation of the CC-CNS's own cost effectiveness, development of cost-containment strategies for the unit, and participation in budget proposals and other financial decisions.

Once again, it is unlikely that the CNS student would be able to function as a leader or manager during the clinical experience. Thus the role modeling provided by the CC-CNS preceptor in this area is critical. Specific lessons helpful to the student include how to successfully manage meetings, how to calculate cost savings and revenue generation, and how to document CC-CNS activities or time utilization. Copies of the forms or logs used by the CC-CNS to track activities and outcomes should be shared with the student. Students may be challenged to attempt to use a similar format to document how they spend their own time during their clinical experience.

Other important aspects of the role that should be shared with the student are "after hours" responsibilities and accountability. Few CC-CNSs limit themselves to a 40-hour work week. The CC-CNS's day is often longer than a standard shift, and it may include taking paperwork home, being called during the night for patient or staff problems, providing nursing expertise in community activities, or participating in professional organization functions. The preceptor can help the student to develop realistic workload expectations and to identify strategies for time management and establishing personal limitations.

Legal and Ethical Considerations

Another common area of responsibility for the CC-CNS is dealing with legal issues and ethical dilemmas. Most graduate students will have some degree of exposure to the theoretic perspectives of current legal and ethical issues in their course work. The CC-CNS preceptor can expand the student's understanding of the dynamics of such situations by exposing the student to actual cases in the clinical setting and demonstrating strategies for resolution (see Chapter 12).

The CC-CNS should expose the student to institutional and unit policies related to informed consent, advance directives, "do not resuscitate" orders, and dying patient protocols. Ethical issues relating to resource allocation, such as admission and discharge criteria and unit staffing policies, are also common areas of involvement for the CC-CNS. The student should be reminded of expectations related to confidentiality, particularly if the student is expected to relay clinical experiences in conferences with faculty and student peers.

SUMMARY

The CC-CNS has several educational responsibilities. Among the most challenging is preparation of the future generation of CNSs. Although the CC-CNS may participate in many forms of graduate-level education, from guest lectures to consultation to directing an entire course; the most common method is by acting as a preceptor for students in the clinical setting. Guided clinical experiences are essential for the graduate student to learn and assimilate the role of CNS. These experiences are best facilitated under the supervision of an established CC-CNS who participates in all components of the CC-CNS role, demonstrates a passion for her or his work, and possesses the self-confidence and patience required to generously share time and talents. Like most aspects of the CNS role, clinical preceptorships can be demanding and time consuming, but the outcomes can be productive and mutually rewarding for the graduate student and the CNS.

References

1. Minarik PA: Collaboration between service and education: perils or pleasures for the clinical nurse specialist? *Clin Nurse Specialist* 4(2):109–114, 1990.
2. Kenton LG: The CNS in collaborative relationships between nursing service and nursing education. In Hamric AB, Spross JA, editors: *The clinical nurse specialist in theory and practice,* ed 2, Philadelphia, 1989, WB Saunders.
3. Snyder M: Educational preparation of the CNS. In Hamric AB, Spross JA, editors: *The clinical nurse specialist in theory and practice,* ed 2, Philadelphia, 1989, WB Saunders.
4. Edlund BJ, Hodges LC: Preparing and using the clinical nurse specialist: a shared responsibility, *Nurs Clin North Am* 18:499–507, 1983.
5. Lewis E: The purposes and characteristics of master's education. In *Developing the functional role in master's education in nursing.* NLN no. 15-1840, New York, 1980, National League for Nursing.
6. American Association of Critical Care Nurses: *Competence statements for critical care clinical nurse specialists,* Laguna Niguel, Calif, 1989, The Association.
7. Shah HS, Prolifroni EC: Preceptorship of CNS students: an exploratory study, *Clin Nurse Specialist* 6(1):41–45, 1992.
8. Hill AS: Precepting the clinical nurse specialist student, *Clin Nurse Specialist* 3(2):71–75, 1989.
9. Chickerella BG, Lutz WJ: Professional nurturance: preceptorships for undergraduate students, *Am J Nurs* 81:107–109, 1981.
10. Limon S, Bargagliotti L, Spencer JB: Providing preceptors for nursing students: what questions should you ask? *J Nurs Admin* 12:16–19, 1982.

The Critical Care Clinical Nurse Specialist as Consultant

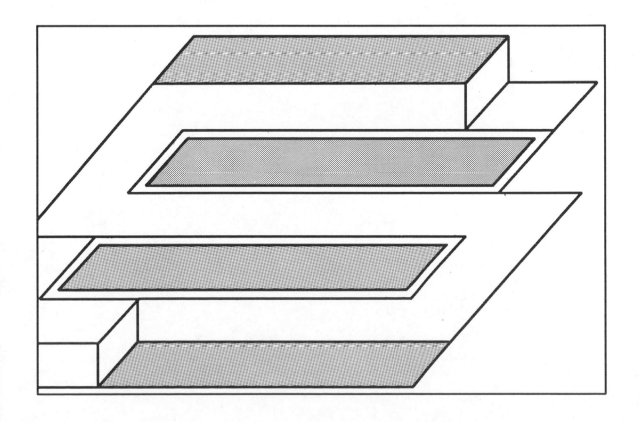

The Critical Care Clinical Nurse Specialist Role in Consultation

Susan M. Walsh, RN, MSN, CS, CCRN

Consultation is an important and essential component of the critical care clinical nurse specialist's (CC-CNS's) practice.[1,2] CC-CNSs are frequently consulted for their content and process expertise in a specific area of clinical nursing. Consultation is defined as a process of communication between professionals.[3] As a process it has clear steps that can guide the CC-CNS in interactions with patients and colleagues. To be effective as a consultant the CC-CNS needs to understand the consultation process and how to apply the process in the critical care environment.

THEORETIC PERSPECTIVES

Descriptions of the CNS include consultation as an important subrole.[2,4-7] Consultation is independent of the other roles of clinician, educator, researcher, and leader/manager and has been described as the foundation for practice of the CNS.[8-10] As a consultant the CNS provides expertise in a variety of ways. Consultation may occur for direct patient care, to guide other nurses in providing care, to provide education, or to guide systems in developing and evaluating health care programs. Whether describing consultation as a subrole of the CNS or the framework for CNS practice it is important to understand and apply consultation process and principles.

Role of Nursing Consultant in Critical Care

The CC-CNS faces a unique challenge in defining and implementing the consultant role. Patients are often in the critical care unit for only a short time, thereby limiting the CC-CNS's time for patient contact. The patient's acute physiologic needs often take precedence over more complex nursing problems that may best be addressed by a CC-CNS. Advanced-practice CC-CNS skills are seen when the CC-CNS interprets complex hemodynamic waveforms, troubleshoots an intraaortic balloon pump (IABP), or counsels families about resuscitation decisions. As the skills of the staff nurse increase, the CNS may do less direct patient care. Nurses generally are comfortable with using other nurses for consultation. When the CC-CNS engages in consultation, staff responsibility for implementation of the consultant's recommendations must be clarified. If not, confusion will hinder the effectiveness and acceptance of the consultant role. Evaluating the outcomes of a CC-CNS consultant is also difficult, since patients who benefit most from consultation are those at risk for complications. It is helpful to keep these characteristics in mind when approaching and evaluating the CC-CNS consultant role.

Consultee-Consultant Relationship

The consultee-consultant relationship is key to the CC-CNS's success as a consultant. The consultant relationship is defined as a collaborative one where the nurse and CC-CNS are equal. Successful consultation requires a certain openness and mutual respect between the CC-CNS and the consultee. Developing this trust depends on understanding the unique aspects of the consultee-consultant relationship and the readiness of the consultee to engage in a collaborative relationship.[11] Factors influencing the readiness of the consultee are the amount of time the consultant has worked in the particular unit, the length of time the consultee has known the CC-CNS, the organizational support for collaborative relationships, the presence of the CC-CNS, and previous experiences of the consultee.

The collaborative relationship differs from a supervisory relationship in that the CC-CNS has no authority over the nurse. The consultant relationship also differs from that of educator.[11] The educator-pupil relationship is one where the teacher possesses information that the student lacks. This places the teacher at a higher level than the pupil. In the consultant relationship both the CC-CNS and the nurse care for the patient. Since the CC-CNS is often educated at a higher level than the staff nurse, the CNS must stress the collaborative nature of the learning experience and the importance of the staff nurse's contribution. Comments such as "the information you shared is essential to helping this patient" aid in recognizing staff expertise and knowledge.

One of the most important aspects of the consultant relationship is clarification of the responsibility and authority of the nurse and the CC-CNS. Authority and responsibility in the consultative relationship flow from a crucial premise: that the nurse who is caring for the patient retains authority and responsibility for the patient. The nurse maintains the right to accept or reject the recommendations of the CC-CNS except when patient safety or continuity of care is an issue.[4,12,13] The CNS who believes the patient's condition is jeopardized has a responsibility to the patient, the nurse, and the organization to resolve the conflict. The CC-CNS should first make every attempt to clarify with the nurse the significance of the CC-CNS's recommendations and why the patient is at risk. If conflict continues, the CC-CNS must discuss the case with the nurse manager responsible for patient care in the unit. The CC-CNS needs to inform the nurse of this action before approaching the manager, again emphasizing the critical nature of the problem and significance to patient care.

Many units do not have a primary nursing care system, and negotiating with multiple nurses to implement the CC-CNS's recommendations may be cumbersome. The CC-CNS needs to identify formal and informal methods of communication in the unit and access these to implement recommendations. Care plans, change of shift reports, and follow-up telephone calls or visits may help to establish consistency among staff. The CC-CNS must

remember, however, that violating the nurse's authority for patient care destroys the essence of the consultant relationship.

Since the nurse maintains authority and responsibility for the patient, the CC-CNS must negotiate and clarify which parts of the nursing process will be assumed by the nurse and which will be assumed by the CC-CNS. The delegation and assumption of each part of the consultation will depend on the availability and expertise of the nurse and the trust relationship that the CC-CNS maintains with the consultee. Since these factors change, the CC-CNS is responsible for clarifying with each consultation who will assume responsibility and accountability for each component of care.

Models for Consultation

Since consultation is a process that can be applied in many different clinical settings, it is helpful to understand several models of consultation for use by the CC-CNS. These models can be used to set boundaries and clarify role expectations for the consultant and consultee. Application of models for consultation can help strengthen the effectiveness and eliminate confusion about the consultant role in critical care.

Caplan Model for Consultation

The Caplan model for consultation describes four types of consultations: (1) client centered, (2) consultee centered, (3) program centered: administrative, and (4) consultee centered: administrative[3] (Table 11–1). It is helpful to view the types of consultations as levels, with each subsequent level creating a greater distance between the patient and the CC-CNS. The goal of each consultation will determine which type is used. The CC-CNS is responsible for assessing the needs of the consultee to determine the type of consultation that is most appropriate. Knowledge of the organization and unit goals also influences the type of consultation selected. Anticipating future trends or organizational developments may guide the CC-CNS to educate and develop staff members instead of assuming direct patient care. Once a consultation level is determined the CC-CNS can implement the steps of the consultation process in a manner that best meets its goals.

Application in Critical Care. Caplan's model for consultation can be very effective for the nurse

TABLE 11-1 Caplan's Consultation Model

Type	Goal	Use
Client centered	Direct care by CC-CNS for specific problem	When consultee does not possess skills to provide care and problem is new, unique, or not seen frequently
Consultee centered	Direction and assistance to nurse caring for patient; indirect care provided by CC-CNS by assisting nurse with any phase of nursing process	When nurse needs direction for common clinical problems
Program centered: administrative	Provide clinical expertise for developing or supporting new or existing program	When clinical expertise is needed to guide unit or organization
Consultee-centered: administrative	Provide direction to consultee regarding process issues in relation to organization	When guidance is needed to work effectively within organization

Handwritten annotation next to "Consultee centered": "Include in LoS"

consultant in critical care. It can be used to structure and clarify consultations, or it can be used to organize all aspects of the CC-CNS practice. Clarifying the type and goals of a consultation can also help the CC-CNS determine which components of patient care are best assumed by the CC-CNS or the staff nurse.

The type of consultation in Caplan's model will vary depending on (1) the nurse caring for the patient, (2) the type of problem identified, (3) the unit or organizational goals, and (4) the expertise of the CC-CNS. *Client-centered,* or type 1, consultations are used if the nurse lacks the necessary skills to care for a specific patient problem such as managing a patient with an intraaortic balloon while awaiting transfer to a tertiary-care facility. In this consultation the CC-CNS may need to assume direct care for the patient. A *consultee-centered,* or type 2, consultation is selected when the problem is one that the nurse will see frequently. The goals of this consultation are met through CC-CNS demonstration of care or guidance while the nurse performs selected nursing interventions such as a complex dressing change. This type of consultation provides the expertise of the CC-CNS and prepares the nurse to face a similar problem in the future.

Frequent consultation for the same problem should direct the CC-CNS to move to the next level of consultation, *Program-centered consultation,* or

type 3. The CC-CNS has the ability to assess, develop, implement, and evaluate the efficacy of a project or program as it relates to patients. Examples of these are standardization of hemodynamic monitoring and preoperative teaching programs. This type of consultation requires the CC-CNS to work with other departments or committees or teach new information.

Caplan's last type of consultation, *consultee-centered: administrative,* or type 4, occurs when the CC-CNS is asked to provide guidance to individual nurses or groups as they work within an organization. The expertise of the CC-CNS in this type of consultation is not clinical content but expertise in the "process" of accomplishing a goal. As an example, a nurse manager may ask the CC-CNS to guide a unit-based continuous quality improvement program as they evaluate care. The goal of this type of consultation is not for the CC-CNS to chair the group or do the quality assurance, but rather to guide other nurses unfamiliar with group dynamics or the quality assurance and improvement process.

Caplan's model for consultation can be used to organize the multiple roles of the CC-CNS. This consultation framework clarifies the direct and indirect patient care roles of the CC-CNS and distinguishes advanced practice from that of the staff nurse. The model also demonstrates how formal and informal teaching occurs within the role of the

CC-CNS.[1] The CC-CNS provides education as an activity within the consultant role. This differs from the role of educator, whose major focus is to prepare nurses for practice in a variety of areas. Caplan's model also allows the CNS to categorize activities such as program and staff development within the administrative type of consultations. In summary, Caplan's model can guide CC-CNSs to structure their practice. It provides a framework for the multiple roles of the CC-CNS as a reflection of the unique contribution the CC-CNS makes as a consultant in critical care.

Content vs. Process Consultation

Another way to provide structure for consultation is to evaluate a consultation according to process or content criteria. A content consultation is one where the consultee recognizes unique knowledge possessed by the CC-CNS that will help solve a particular problem. The goal of a content consultation is to have the CC-CNS resolve the problem since the consultee lacks the necessary knowledge and skill. When providing a content consultation the CC-CNS has responsibility for resolving or referring the problem such as a skin ulcer, which may be addressed by a CC-CNS or referred to an enterostomal therapist.

A process consultation occurs when the consultee asks the CC-CNS assistance so that the individual can solve the problem. A subtle but important distinction exists between a process and a content consultation. The goal of a process consultation is to have the consultee manage the problem with guidance from the CC-CNS. The CC-CNS's expertise may guide the nurse in one or more areas of the nursing process but is not primarily responsible for the outcome of the problem. An example is when a nurse requests assistance to clarify outcomes for a complex critically ill patient.

Application in Critical Care. The CC-CNS is often faced with requests for assistance. Clarification of the problem and the kind of assistance needed is essential in using the process vs. content framework. Clarification of the problem will help the nurse determine if one has the necessary skills to provide care or if it is necessary for the CC-CNS to provide care. The CC-CNS may find that the nurse has adequate knowledge and skills to manage the care but may need assistance at some point in the nursing process. Clarifying whether the consultation is a content request or the nurse is requesting help to process knowledge in a difficult clinical problem will help the CC-CNS provide the appropriate level of support. A frustrated nurse may approach the CC-CNS and state, "I don't know what else to do with this patient; he keeps bucking the ventilator, and the physician won't answer my page" or "Can you look at this patient and tell me what you think?" Questions such as these should prompt the CC-CNS to clarify the situation by asking open-ended questions such as "What do you think the problem is?" or "What do you wish would happen?" This gives the nurse the opportunity to clarify the situation and identify if the request from the CC-CNS is to fill a knowledge need or help the nurse to process the assessment information. In this case the nurse knew what was required but sought validation of her assessment and backing in obtaining physician support.

As discussed in application of the Caplan model the CC-CNS may also be asked to provide direction to work groups. The content vs. process framework can also help the CC-CNS with this type of consultation. Asking whether the consultee expects the CC-CNS to produce a specific outcome for a project because of the CC-CNS's expertise (content consultation) or the consultee requests the CC-CNS to develop a group so they can deal with similar problems again (process consultation) is important. Clarifying expectations of the consultee will direct the CC-CNS's approach to the consultation.

Using the process vs. content model to clarify a consultation can help the CC-CNS clearly plan interactions with staff and meet the goals of the consultee. Since the CC-CNS is asked to engage in consultation for a variety of patient and system problems the content vs. process framework may be a useful tool to consider when a consultation is made.

Diffusion of Innovation Consultation

The diffusion of innovation model is useful to the CC-CNS when asked to provide consultation for change in the clinical area.[14,15] This model incorporates general principles of change theory but also details the role and contribution of the consultant. It is particularly useful since it can be applied to both internal or external consultation (Table 11–2).

The CC-CNS is often asked to provide consul-

TABLE 11–2 Stages for Adoption of Innovations and Consultant's Role

Stage	Consultant's Role
Initiation	
Agenda setting	Identification of need for innovation
Matching	Examination of alternatives
	Recommendation of appropriate innovation
	Planning of strategies for diffusion process
Decision to adopt implementation	
Redefining/restructuring	Identification of internal consultant
Clarifying	Collaboration for strategies and programs
Establishing routine	Evaluation of progress of diffusion
	Setting of support strategies
Exit	

From Barker ER: Use of diffusion of innovation model for agency consultation, *Clin Nurse Specialist* 4(1):164, © by Williams & Wilkins 1990.

tation for changes in practice or technology. The innovation model separates the consultation process into two phases: (1) the initiation phase and (2) the implementation phase.[14] During the initiation phase the CNS's clinical expertise allows for identification of the innovation, evaluation of alternatives, and recommendations of which innovation is most appropriate for a clinical area. Following selection of the specific innovation the CNS can plan strategies for the innovation to be introduced and diffused into practice. In phase 2, or the implementation phase, the CC-CNS decides how to introduce the innovation to the staff. The CC-CNS may select an outside consultant, such as an educator or a company representative, or may personally introduce the innovation. The CC-CNS needs to evaluate the progress of the diffusion and then develop support strategies to maintain the diffusion. Once the diffusion has occurred, the CC-CNS is no longer tied to the innovation and the consultation is complete.

Diffusion of any change requires evaluation of four elements: innovation, communication channels, time, and the social system.[15] The CC-CNS's position in the organization provides an understanding of these elements as they relate to the culture of the unit or organization. The CC-CNS's presence in the clinical area is critical for monitoring the innovation's progress and for providing support for staff until the innovation is diffused. The CC-CNS must make certain that processes are in place for maintenance of the innovation.

Although similar to the other models for change, the innovation model is unique in that it focuses on the role of the consultant in the change process. Since CC-CNSs are frequently consulted to evaluate and assist with change this model can guide the CC-CNS with this type of consultation.

Application in Critical Care. The CC-CNS may be asked to plan for a new documentation system. As a consultant the CC-CNS can clarify why the current system is ineffective and what alternatives may be helpful. Knowledge of the patient's needs, document requirements, and nurses' charting style could result in specific recommendations. The CC-CNS can then identify the steps needed for developing the system, obtaining approval, and producing the product. Once the system has been accepted the CC-CNS may work with the education department to do an in-service program for the staff and the quality assessment and improvement group to evaluate the system and plan for corrective action.

RELATED RESEARCH AND LITERATURE
Research on CNS Consultant Role

Studies evaluating the CC-CNS consultant role are limited. This may be related to the difficulty in differentiating the CC-CNS subrole of consultant from the other roles in the CNS practice. Related research about the CNS as consultant can be divided into (1) studies that evaluate the consulting role in CNS practice and (2) those that evaluate the outcomes on staff and patients when the CNS is present and practicing within all the subroles.

Studies that have evaluated the consultant role in the CNS practice show that the predominant consultation activities were those of informing, prescribing, questioning, and assessing.[16] Most consultations were aimed at clinical problems, and instructing the nurse on patient care was the activity most often performed during the consultation.[16] Other studies show that consultation consumes approximately 8% of the CNS's practice.[17] Examination of the activities within the practitioner role, however, reveals that many of the activities described as practitioner may also be interpreted as consultative activities. Since 47% of the activities were described within the role of practitioner it is clear that the role of consultant consumes a significant portion of the CNS practice. Further studies have demonstrated this high percentage of time allocated to clinical practice and consultation.[4] This study also shows that consultant activities increase with number of years of experience in the CNS role.

The second category of research studies has focused on the impact of the CNS's presence on staff and patients. Several studies have shown positive effects on staff nurses' clinical insights, intershift reporting, and documentation.[18-20] Again, the CNS consultant role was not evaluated separately. Recent studies have focused on the effect of CNS practice on patient outcomes. These studies show CNS effectiveness in the care of tuberculosis patients, myocardial infarction patients, oncology patients, and low–birth weight infants.[19,21-24] Subsequent evaluation of the specific activities of the CNS in care of high-risk infants shows assessments and interventions that demonstrate the advanced practice of the CNS.[9] Clearly the use of the CNS as a consultant for direct care activities for a specific group of patients is an important aspect of the CNS role.

Further evaluation of the CNS role needs to be done to describe the consultation activities of the CC-CNS in the critical care environment. Research also needs to focus on the outcomes related to CC-CNS consultation such as rate of wound healing, family support, shorter hospital stay, and decreased resource utilization. Outcomes related to patients, staff, and the organization need to be evaluated since the CC-CNS impacts these areas when functioning as consultant.

Consultation Process

The steps of the consultation process are very similar to the steps of the nursing process and have been described by several authors: (1) initial request and data collection, (2) problem identification, (3) clarification of consultee expectations, (4) type of consultation determined, (5) plan developed, (6) activities delegated or assumed, (7) documentation, (8) evaluation, and (9) clo-

sure.[3,12,25-27] Each step of the consultative process should be evaluated by the CNS so that successful consultation occurs.

Assessment

During the assessment phase of consultation the CNS must gather data from the consultee about needs and how the consultant is seen meeting those needs. While assessing the needs, it is important for the CNS to look for hidden agendas. The CNS may be asked to make recommendations for a common wound care problem, because disagreement or inconsistency exists among the staff. Discussing the problem and the current care plan and clarifying what the consultee expects of the CNS may help identify the hidden agenda of a consultation. When clear expectations are met the consultation will be seen as successful by both the consultee and CNS.

Evaluation

The CNS next needs to evaluate what type of consultation will best meet the needs of the consultee. Careful evaluation of the goals of the consultation can guide the CNS in determining the type of consultation that will be most successful. The goal and level of consultation will then direct the CNS's activities. Assessment of the problem or patient can now proceed. Assessment with or without the consultee will be determined by the goal of the consultee, the skill of the consultee, and the limits of time. The CNS may be asked to evaluate a patient whose clinical condition is deteriorating. If the consultee is a novice nurse who is not able to integrate complex assessment data quickly, the CNS may engage in type 1 activities such as performing hemodynamic calculations. If the nurse is experienced, a type 2 consultation may be more appropriate where the goal of consultation may be validation of assessment information and treatment options with the nurse.

Recommendations

The CC-CNS next makes recommendations for solving the problem. The CC-CNS can only make recommendations since the consultee has the authority to accept or reject the recommendations of the consultant.[3] The CC-CNS will need to review the recommendations with the consultee and determine if they are seen as useful. If the recommendations are accepted, the CC-CNS needs to clarify who will assume responsibility for implementing them. Some recommendations may best be implemented by the CC-CNS because of advanced practice skills, whereas others may be within the scope of practice of the nurse. For example, when the CC-CNS is consulted to work with an angry family, the CC-CNS and nurse may arrange a family meeting and based on the outcome design a plan to call the family daily with progress reports. Because of the CC-CNS's expertise and role, the CC-CNS may conduct the meeting and develop a plan while the staff nurse assumes responsibility for making daily calls.

Documentation

The CC-CNS should then document the consultation and how the intervention will be evaluated. The CC-CNS clarifies when the CC-CNS and nurse will return to evaluate the recommendations or if the nurse will evaluate their effectiveness and contact the CC-CNS if the problem is not resolved. The consultation process can be evaluated when the CNS closes or terminates the consultation. Closure is important so the consultee understands that the consulting relationship is finished. Closure gives both the consultee and consultant an opportunity to evaluate the impact of the CNS's recommendations and the consultation process. Asking the consultant how she or he felt about the consultation and how it could have been more effective will aid in closure and also reinforce the worth of the CNS as consultant.

PRACTICE IMPLICATIONS
Formal vs. Informal Consultation

The CC-CNS may be asked to provide consultation on a formal or an informal basis. Although both occur regularly in practice, it is helpful to examine the advantages and disadvantages of each. Formal consultation occurs when a consultee specifically requests the involvement of the CC-CNS. Formal consultations validate the CC-CNS's expertise, since the CC-CNS is viewed as someone who is able to solve a particular problem. Formal consultations frequently occur when the CNS has developed a specific area of expertise and has communicated this to others in the organization. Formal consultation examples may be seen when the CNS is asked to assist a family to cope, manage a complex wound, or coordinate a long-term weaning of a patient. The CC-CNS can increase the frequency with which formal consultations are made by defining an area of expertise and unique contribution to patient care. Asking consultees to identify similar cases and recommend referral to others fosters a referral pattern.

Formal consultations can be generated by nurses, physicians, administrators, or persons in other disciplines. Clinical specialists who are new in practice or to an organization may not receive formal consultations until their expertise has been defined and demonstrated. A CC-CNS may want to establish an automatic referral for formal consultations. Automatic referrals demonstrate to others the type of patient care problems that can most benefit from a CC-CNS consultation. They validate the consultant role and free the staff nurse from continual evaluation of the need for a CC-CNS consultation. Automatic referrals can be developed from unit or patient criteria, such as patients with intensive care unit (ICU) stays greater than 3 days, all patients requiring paralysis to maintain oxygenation, or the use of extracorporeal oxygenation. Any ICU patient meeting these criteria would automatically be evaluated by the CC-CNS.

Formal consultations require that the CC-CNS complete all the components of the consultation process. Tracking the frequency of formal consultations helps the CC-CNS determine if the value of the consultant role has been effectively communicated.

Informal consultations occur frequently, and the availability of an expert in the clinical area to readily respond to staff's needs is a valuable role of the CC-CNS. Informal consultations continue to require the CC-CNS to be responsible for all the steps of the consultation process. The focus of an informal consultation is narrow, and feedback to the consultee is immediate. The CC-CNS may be asked to troubleshoot equipment problems, demonstrate use of new technology (e.g., peripheral nerve stimulator), or evaluate a pediatric patient who will be managed at home with a ventilator. Informal consultations can be developed by establishing a routine time when the CC-CNS is present and available on the unit, by helping nurses with care, and by making patient rounds.

The informal consultation is an excellent opportunity for the CC-CNS to demonstrate expertise to staff members who are unfamiliar with the consultant role. Informal consultations are often requested by nurses, nursing managers, or other CNSs as they address problems in patient care. The CC-CNS is often asked "what do you think" type of questions by the staff. This informal type of consultation allows the staff to process or validate patient care issues. Although valuable to the staff, informal consultations are usually not documented in the patient's chart and may be difficult to track. It may be helpful to track informal consultations with a log or checklist recording unit and activity. The CC-CNS should look for patterns from informal consultations, since frequently occurring consultations of one type may identify a recurring patient or staff problem that the CC-CNS can address.

External Consultation

The CC-CNS may also act as a consultant outside the institution to organizations or people seeking expertise in a given area. Requests for external consultation are varied, such as consultation for establishing an open heart surgical program, implementing case management, or developing a transfer procedure for a community hospital. Business, industry, education, and other health care facilities may also use the CC-CNS as a temporary consultant. CC-CNSs may think their skills are limited to the critical care environment, but the changing face of health care will require the skills of the critical care nurse in a variety of settings. As an external consultant the CNS has the opportunity to accept or reject a request for consultation and to negotiate the terms of the agreement. CC-CNSs should reject the consultation if they feel they do not possess adequate skills or knowledge to meet the client's needs or if a conflict of interest exists with the CNS's current employer. The CC-CNS may act as an external consultant representing the institution or be employed independently. The organization experiences several advantages by supporting external consultation by the CC-CNS: (1) the organization is seen as a source of expertise and sharing in the community; (2) the organization retains expert CNSs as they develop new roles; and (3) a referral pattern develops for the organization's services as a result of CC-CNS consultations. One disadvantage to the organization is using the CC-CNS's time, which may result in decreased attention to the needs and goals of the organization.

When acting as an external consultant the CC-

CNS needs to clarify if she or he is acting as an agent of the organization or independently. Since an external consultation is temporary, the CC-CNS may find sporadic employment difficult both financially and professionally and may wish to perform external consultations as part of or in addition to a CC-CNS position. When acting as an external consultant several points in the employee-consultant relationship need to be clarified: (1) Will the CC-CNS be paid additional monies for services provided outside the organization? (2) Is external consultation covered under malpractice insurance provided by the organization? (3) Who will own the product (i.e. education program, innovation): the CC-CNS or the organization? (4) Will services be prepared or provided during the CC-CNS's paid work time? and (5) Will the materials (i.e., copying, secretarial, travel, telephone) be provided by the organization? The CC-CNS who wants to begin external consultation should clarify the expertise and skills and identify a target audience. A proposal outlining the services, benefits, and fees should be developed. A marketing plan will vary depending on the potential clients. Use of an introductory letter, fliers, proposals, advertisements, or networking may be effective with different audiences. Special attention to organizational assessment, communication, and cost considerations can provide both the CC-CNS and the organization with positive results when providing expertise outside the organization.

Developing a Contract and Fee for Consultation

Developing a contract for consultation services is a way to formalize agreed on expectations.[30,31] Contracts can be used for both internal and external consultation.[32] Using contracts for internal consultation can formalize goals and expectations of the consultee and the CC-CNS. The CC-CNS may find it helpful to establish a contract with nurse managers for projects that have been requested by others.[32] Contracts can define time lines, set evaluation dates, provide a written account of commitments, provide a tool for time management, and prevent misunderstandings.[28,29] The contract may be informal and merely include the terms of the agreement, or in the case of consultation for developing new products or materials the use of a lawyer may be essential. Essential components of a contract include (1) the service, (2) where it is provided, (3) the date or time line, (4) what the consultee and consultant will provide, (5) liability, (6) ability and consequences for each party terminating the consultation, (7) compensation, and (8) additional expenses such as travel.[30] Both parties should sign the agreement and keep a copy.

Developing a fee for consultative services is essential to success. As an internal consultant the fee is your negotiated salary plus benefits. The organization provides the resources to perform your services. As an external consultant several factors need to be calculated and evaluated to establish a fee that is reasonable for the CC-CNS and the client. Prices can be established as an hourly rate or determined per project. An hourly rate needs to include the anticipated hours required for preparation and the number of hours actually involved in performing the service. In addition to the hourly rate the CC-CNS must also include the cost of any materials such as slides or handouts involved in performing the consultation and average overhead costs. Overhead includes secretarial support, office space, legal and accounting fees, office supplies, insurance, licenses, taxes, travel, professional development, dues, subscriptions, telephone, mail, and marketing. When the CC-CNS is acting as an external consultant for an organization these overhead costs need to be established by the organization so the true cost of services is realized. When the CC-CNS is acting as an independent consultant these costs are an important part of determining a fee that will result in actual profit to the CNS. It may be helpful to price services based on a project price instead of costing out the hourly rate plus supplies and overhead and allow the client to select which method is best.[33] The following is an example of an hourly rate fee calculation for an electrocardiogram (EKG) education and competency program.

Preparation	16 hr
Teaching	8 hr
Total time × rate	24 hr × $26/hr (includes 14% benefits)
Teaching cost	$624.00
Overhead	$125.00
Handouts	$ 90.00 ($3.00 per person × 30 participants)
Total price	$849.00

It may be helpful to determine what other consultants with similar skills and services charge in the same geographic area. This will provide a reasonable charge that can be used to evaluate the economic feasibility of providing consultative services. It is also important to note that profits will be assessed for taxes at both the federal and state levels. Consulting a tax accountant will be essential when performing services that can result in taxable income.

Documentation and Record Keeping

Documenting the consultation is an essential part of the formal consultation process. Documentation provides evidence of the consultation and demonstrates the contribution of the clinical specialist. Documentation communicates to other care providers the specialist's assessment and recommendations and also who will provide the planned interventions and evaluation. Documenting in the patient's chart will demonstrate the unique contributions of the CC-CNS and validate the CC-CNS's role in patient care. Record keeping also demonstrates the activities that the CC-CNS provides for both direct and indirect patient care and can help the CC-CNS evaluate time use.

Documentation of patient care consultations should be charted in the patient's record. The new CNS needs to evaluate the organization's method for documenting consultations. Some organizations may not be familiar with the use of a nursing consultant. This may require careful negotiation and clarification before the CC-CNS begins to document. Discussions with nursing administrators, managers, medical records personnel, and physicians can clarify requirements necessary to meet documentation standards in an organization. These preliminary discussions can serve to prepare others for CC-CNS documentation and allow questions about the CNS role to be answered. Placing the nursing consultation in a place on the chart where other consultations are recorded validates the role of a nurse consultant.

When asked to consult on a patient care problem the CC-CNS needs to clearly document the assessment components that are completed independently or with the patient's nurse. The CNS should also detail the recommendations and document who will implement and evaluate them. The CC-CNS may want the nurse to complete a care plan for the patient. The CC-CNS may use this as an opportunity to work with the nurse to develop skills in preparing a care plan. If developing skills in care planning is not the nurse's goal the CNS may want to add to the care plan for problems assessed and make recommendations. Sometimes the CC-CNS may feel that the assessment or recommendations for care were not unique. However, the CC-CNS consultation may have been helpful to the nurse in evaluating or processing a patient problem. The CC-CNS may simply document that "the case and plan of care were reviewed with primary nurse." This provides evidence of CC-CNS participation and evaluation without redundancy.

Record keeping for the CC-CNS consultant is essential to assist in validating the CNS practice. Record-keeping tools can be developed in many ways to provide a concise record of the CC-CNS consultations.[34–37] It is generally helpful to keep a record of the (1) patient's or project's name, (2) referral source, (3) unit, (4) dates of visits, (5) time spent, and (6) type or level of consultation. The CC-CNS can use this information when completing quarterly reports as a reflection of her or his activities. Monitoring the referral source unit and level of consultation can help the CC-CNS cluster and evaluate patterns of consultation. Recording the type of consultation will allow the CC-CNS to use the same record-keeping tool for all aspects and activities of the role. Frequent consultations from a particular unit or about a recurring problem should direct the CNS to move involvement from a client-centered (direct care) to a consultee-centered (indirect care) to an administrative-centered consultation. Units with infrequent consultations may prompt evaluation by the CC-CNS. Strategies to increase consultations in these areas may include performing a needs assessment with the staff, evaluating the staff's perceptions of the role and effectiveness of the CC-CNS, increased presence on the unit, and mutual goal setting with the manager and staff.

CASE STUDY

When the CC-CNS came to the medical intensive care unit on daily rounds the charge nurse told her that the unit had not been busy except for the postoperative patient from late last night. The patient had "really been giving us a tough time and this is someone you should see." The CC-CNS entered the patient's room to find the patient intubated, four point restrained, and agitated. The nurse looked exasperated. The CC-CNS began the initial assessment of the consultation by asking the nurse what she thought was wrong and if there was anything the CC-CNS could do. The nurse described the patient as an 82-year-old woman who had an emergency operative bowel resection. The patient had been so agitated during the night that she was unable to maintain her oxygen saturation. Repeated doses of morphine did not help the patient's behavior so the patient was restrained. The nurse stated she felt frustrated because she wanted to avoid the use of paralyzing drugs but was concerned for the safety of the patient and the inability to adequately oxygenate the patient. This was the first time the nurse had cared for this patient, and she had a new admission coming from the emergency room. She hoped that the CC-CNS could help her "figure out what to do next." The CC-CNS asked questions about the patient's electrolytes, arterial blood gases, recent chest x-ray film, amount and frequency of suctioning, doses of morphine, and response to assess the patient for physiologic causes for the agitation. She then assessed the patient, who would not respond to commands but was continually attempting to get out of the restraints. The CC-CNS and staff nurse next reviewed the patient's chart, and they noted the patient had been admitted to the general care floor 5 days ago and had demonstrated increasing agitation, which had been attributed to abdominal pain. Before admission the patient had been a resident in a long-term care facility. Review of the transfer sheets showed that the patient had received haloperidol (Haldol), 2 mg twice daily, for several years. The patient had not received any medication since admission, because she was being given nothing by mouth.

The clinical specialist recommended several options for the patient's acute problem of agitation and oxygen desaturation. She also recommended that the nursing care facility be contacted to discuss the patient's behavior before admission. The nurse was willing to try the recommendations but needed the physician to prescribe the medications such as midazolam (Versed). The CC-CNS discussed whether the nurse or the CC-CNS would talk to the physician. The nurse felt comfortable discussing the recommendations with the physician if the CC-CNS could write clear indications for prescribing and the name of the medication. She wanted the CC-CNS to call the nursing home, since she was busy. The CC-CNS wrote a consultation note and left it on the front of the chart for rounds. Before leaving she asked the nurse if she wanted her to return to evaluate how the patient was doing. The nurse agreed that having the CC-CNS assist her in evaluating the patient in 2 hours would be helpful. The CNS returned to find the patient sleeping and well oxygenated on a midazolam drip. The nurse was grateful for the CC-CNS's assistance, and they agreed that the nurse could incorporate the other recommendations into the patient's care plan.

Commentary

This case study demonstrates how a CC-CNS can provide bedside consultation within a consultative framework. Routine daily rounds resulted in a patient consultation. The CC-CNS assessed the nurse's needs first and determined a type 2 consultation would meet the goal of the nurse and patient. Together the nurse and CC-CNS evaluated the current problem and potential precipitating factors. A series of recommendations were developed from the content expertise of the CC-CNS. The CNS also provided a process consultation by assisting the nurse in evaluating her own assessment information and developing a care plan. Because of time constraints the nurse and CC-CNS agreed who would complete each part of the plan and the evaluation. Documentation was completed to provide a record of the CC-CNS consultation and recorded for tracking of CNS consultations.

SUMMARY

This chapter discussed the unique role of the CC-CNS as a consultant. Consultation models were

presented as well as clinical examples of the CC-CNS as an internal and external consultant. Finally, a case study was presented with practical examples of documentation that can be utilized by CC-CNS consultants.

References

1. Chisholm M: Consultation, *Clin Nurse Specialist* 3(4):197, 1989.
2. Girourd S: The role of the clinical specialist as change agent: an experiment in preoperative teaching, *Int J Nurs Studies* 15:57-65, 1978.
3. Caplan G: *The theory and practice of mental health consultation,* New York, 1970, Basic Books.
4. Burge S et al: Quantifying clinical nurse specialist role development: quantifying actual practice over three years, *Clin Nurse Specialist* 3:33-36, 1989.
5. Fenton M: Identifying competencies of clinical nurse specialists, *J Nurs Admin* 15(12):31-37, 1985.
6. Hamric A: History and overview of the CNS role. In Hamric A, editor: *The clinical nurse specialist in theory and practice,* ed 2, Philadelphia, 1989, WB Saunders Co.
7. Hamric Λ: Role development and functions. In Hamric Λ, editor: *The clinical nurse specialist in theory and practice,* Orlando, 1983, Grune & Stratton.
8. Kohnke M: *Case for consultation in nursing: designs for professional practice,* New York, 1978, John Wiley & Sons.
9. Noll M: Internal consultation as a framework for clinical nurse specialist practice, *Clin Nurse Specialist* 1:46-50, 1987.
10. Sparacino P, Cooper M: The role components. In Sparacino P, editor: *The clinical nurse specialist: implementation and impact,* Norwalk, Conn, 1990, Appleton & Lange.
11. Cherniss C: The consultation readiness scale: an attempt to improve consultation practice, *Am J Comm Psycol* 6(1):15-21, 1978.
12. Barron AM: The CNS as consultant. In Hamric A, editor: *The clinical nurse specialist in theory and practice,* Orlando, 1983, Grune & Stratton.
13. Sneed NV: CNS power: its use and potential for misuse by nurse consultants, *Clin Nurse Specialist* 5:58-62, 1991.
14. Rodgers E: *Diffusion of innovation,* New York, 1983, The Free Press.
15. Barker E: Use of diffusion of innovation model for agency consultation, *Clin Nurse Specialist* 4:163-166, 1990.
16. Beyerman KL: Consultation roles of the clinical nurse specialist: a case study, *Clin Nurse Specialist* 2(2):91-95, 1988.
17. Boyd JN et al: The merit and significance of clinical nurse specialists, *J Nurs Admin* 21(9):35-45, 1991.
18. Ayers R: *The clinical nurse specialist: an experiment in role effectiveness and role development,* Duarate, Calif, 1971, City of Hope National Medical Center.
19. Georgopoulos BS, Jackson MM: Nursing Kardex behavior in an experimental study of patient units with and without a clinical specialist, *Nurs Res* 19:196-218, 1971.
20. Georgopoulos BS, Sana JM: Clinical nursing specialization

and intershift report behavior, *Am J Nurs* 15:538-545, 1971.

21. Brooten D et al: A randomized clinical trial of early hospital discharge and home followup of very low birthweight infants, *N Engl J Med* 315:934-939, 1986.
22. Little DE, Carnevali D: Nurse specialist effect on tuberculosis, *Nurs Res* 16:321-326, 1967.
23. McCorkle R: *The complications of early discharge from hospitals. Proceedings of the Fifth National Conference on Human Values and Concerns,* 1987, American Cancer Society.
24. Pozen MW et al: A nurse rehabilitator's impact on patients with myocardial infarction, *Med Care* 15(10):830-837, 1977.
25. Barron AM: The CNS as consultant. In Hamric A, editor: *The clinical nurse specialist in theory and practice,* ed 2, Philadelphia, 1989, WB Saunders Co.
26. Blake P: The clinical nurse specialist as consultant, *J Nurs Admin* 7:33-36, 1977.
27. Laureau SC: The nurse as clinical consultant, *Topics Clin Nurs* 2:79-84, 1985.
28. Beare P: The ABC's of external consultation, *Clin Nurse Specialist* 2(1):35-38, 1988.
29. Malone B: The CNS in a consultation department. In Hamric A, editor: *The clinical nurse specialist in theory and practice,* ed 2, Philadelphia, 1989, WB Saunders Co.
30. Johnson SH: *Developing consulting or private practice skills: health update, 1981,* ed 2, Lakewood, Col, Suzanne Hall Johnson Communications.
31. Manion J: *Change from within: nurse entrepreneurs as health care innovators,* Kansas City, Mo, 1990, American Nurses' Association.
32. Jones A: Gaining control of the CNS role through written contracts, *Clin Nurse Specialist* 5(2):102-104, 1991.
33. Flanagan L: *Earn what you're worth: a nurse's guide to better compensation,* Kansas City, Mo, 1989, American Nurses' Association.
34. Howell L: The pediatric surgical clinical nurse specialist in a university hospital setting. In Sparacino P et al, editors: *The clinical nurse specialist: implementation and impact,* Norwalk, Conn, 1990, Appleton & Lange.
35. Minarik P, Sparacino P: Clinical nurse specialist collaboration in a university medical center. In Sparacino P et al, editors: *The clinical nurse specialist: implementation and impact,* Norwalk, Conn, 1990, Appleton & Lange.
36. Robichaud AM, Hamric AB: Time documentation of clinical nurse specialist activities, *J Nurs Admin* 16(1):31-36, 1986.
37. Welch-McCaffrey D: The oncology clinical nurse specialist in a tertiary care referral center. In Sparacino P et al, editors: *The clinical nurse specialist: implementation and impact,* Norwalk, Conn, 1990, Appleton & Lange.

The Critical Care Clinical Nurse Specialist Role in Ethical Dilemmas

Deborah Caswell, RN, MN, CCRN
Anna Omery, RN, DNSc

Critical care units today are permeated with ethical issues from admittance (allocation of resources) to treatment (informed consent) to death (resuscitation, withdrawal of life support). Critical care health practitioners are now faced with the dilemma of rationing health care resources, as well as with issues of human dignity.

Bedside clinicians are confronted with these issues every day. Critical care clinical nurse specialists (CC-CNSs) are in a unique position to be especially beneficial in resolving these issues. In fact, by role definition the CC-CNS is mandated to identify and assist in the clarification and resolution of ethical problems in the intensive care unit (ICU). The American Association of Critical Care Nurses' (AACN's) *Competence Statements for Critical Care Clinical Nurse Specialists* state:

The CC-CNS demonstrates mastery of the advanced knowledge and skills required for critical care nursing. The CC-CNS is responsible and accountable for the development and application of standards, quality assurance mechanisms and research to enhance the quality of care to the critically ill patient and the patient's family. As an advanced practitioner, the CC-CNS is essential for the management of complex patient and system related problems.[1]

Critical care knowledge and skills for the advanced practitioner encompass much more than the ability to titrate medications or analyze laboratory data. The situation in critical care today is such that the CC-CNS must be able to identify and facilitate problem solving of a variety of ethical dilemmas, with patients and staff both benefiting. Often the staff nurse is too overwhelmed by maintaining physiologic functioning of the patient to have adequate time for resolving ethical disputes. The CC-CNS is essential in this regard to assist the staff, health care team members, and the patient in coming to a satisfactory solution for those involved.

THEORETIC PERSPECTIVES

Moral standards are the organizing principle of a professional community.   *Author Unknown*

Common sense, caring, and the desire to do the right thing are often not enough when critical care nurses are faced with ethical dilemmas in their practice. Ethical decision making requires an understanding of what constitutes an ethical dilemma as well as an understanding of ethical language, ethical theories, and the process of making an ethical decision. This knowledge provides the tools by which each nurse can address those ethical dilemmas most central to clinical practice.

Distinguishing Ethical from Nonethical Practice Issues

Many issues are of concern in critical care nursing practice. Determining whether they are clinical or ethical issues can actually be quite simple. Clinical issues are raised when the question to be addressed focuses on what or how, such as "What can we do here?" or "How do we do this procedure?" The nurse who begins to include "should" or "ought" in the question has moved from a clinical to a moral or an ethical focus. The questions "What should we do here?" or "Ought we do this procedure?" almost always involve ethical knowledge.

Defining the Ethical Domain

Ethics is the critical normative analysis of how to live with one another.[3] That is, ethics is concerned with determining and monitoring minimally acceptable standards of human behavior. Behavior that meets these standards is ethical; behavior that does not meet these standards is unethical.

Neither completely art, nor completely science, ethics is better described (as is nursing) as an art-science.[4,5] Ethics is like an art in that it involves an intuitive sense of connection with the real world as it is lived with all its uncertainties about what is right or wrong in any given situation. It is like a science in that it uses method to weigh, assess, analyze, and study relationships in that real or empirical world. The task of this art-science is to find the meaning in human behavior by discriminating the "ought" or "should." Bioethics becomes, then, that art-science that seeks to clarify and bring understanding to the moral issues related to human life.

Whereas ethics reflects the "ought" or "should," morality is thought to reflect the "is." Morality is the focus of descriptive ethics. Descriptive ethics is a type of ethics that describes what one does and the actual reasons given as to why one ought to do so in any specific ethical situation. Nurses, psychologists, and others who are involved in descriptive ethics describe the actual moral dilemmas and moral reasoning of nurses.

Moral reasoning is the mental process that intervenes between recognition and reaction to a moral dilemma. It is the decision-making process by which the nurse chooses among moral values to come to some decision as to the appropriate response to some moral dilemma.[3] It is the process by which a moral conclusion or judgment is reached. For example, when a nurse comes to a decision that to withdraw life support is the right choice for the patient because it is what the patient wishes, that is moral reasoning. Although the exact nature of moral reasoning remains uncertain and controversial,[6] two models of moral development (which document different stages in moral reasoning) have had a profound impact on descriptive ethics in nursing. These are Lawrence Kohlberg's and Carol Gilligan's models of moral development.

Although both models are founded in cognitive developmental theory, Lawrence Kohlberg's is the most popular.[7,8] It has six stages organized into three levels (Table 12–1). CC-CNSs who are interested in further discussion of this model are referred to Kohlberg's articles listed in the References. In testing Kohlberg's model, one recurring phenomenon was the apparent arrest of most females at stage 3. At stage 3, "right" is doing what is expected by people close to you or what people generally expect of people in your role. Kohlberg felt that this arrest was a reflection of the state of interaction of the female and her social world. As long as females feel they are adequately resolving their moral dilemmas at the lower stages, Kohlberg felt they would never proceed up the model to higher stages of moral reasoning.

Carol Gilligan interpreted female stage arrest differently.[9,10] She argues that instead of being deviant or arrested, feminine moral reasoning is simply but importantly different from masculine moral reasoning. Gilligan feels that females, in order to survive in a world where they lack power, have had to develop a sense of responsibility based on

TABLE 12–1 Kohlberg's Model of Moral Judgment

Level	Stage	Focus
I: Preconventional morality	1: Heteronomous morality 2: Instrumental morality	Self
II: Conventional morality	3: Mutual morality 4: Social systems morality	Society
III: Postconventional morality	5: Social contract morality 6: Universal ethical morality	Universal

TABLE 12–2 Gilligan's Model of Moral Judgment

Stage	Focus	Moral Imperative
Level I: orientation to individual survival	Self	Individual survival
Transition: from selfishness to responsibility		
Level II: goodness as self-sacrifice	Society	Consensual judgment
Transition: from goodness to truth		
Level III: morality of nonviolence	Universal	Care of self and others

the universal principle of caring. Table 12–2 gives Gilligan's model of moral judgment.

These two models of moral judgment provide a way of describing nursing's moral world, yet these models are not without limitations and controversy, such as an alleged gender bias and methodologic flaws.[11,12] Several current nursing studies have indicated that nursing's moral world cannot be understood as only a psychodymanic phenomenon and that nurses' moral judgments are an interaction of both moral knowledge and their assessment of factors in the practice environment.[13-15] The end result of the dialogues that surround the controversies in descriptive ethics will hopefully be a comprehensive normative ethic in which the nurse is able to leave the patient with the nurse's own moral integrity intact.

The final branch of ethics is normative ethics. Normative ethics asks questions directly related to the criteria and standards of right or wrong action, what things are good and evil, and moral conduct in general. Normative ethics uses ethical theories to determine what we ought to do.[2] Philosophers and ethicists apply ethical theory in doing normative ethical inquiry.

Ethical Theory

Two types of ethical theory have been most prominent in bioethical discussions: teleologic theory and deontologic theory. Increasingly, two other types of theory (care theory and virtue theory) are

being used to justify normative decisions in nursing ethics.

Teleologic Theory

All teleologic theory focuses on consequences. Nurses who use teleologic theories as their ethical justification support the belief that consequences alone determine the rightness of an act.[16] Teleologists regard the question "What is good?" as logically before the question "What should be done?" It should therefore be answered first. Right and duty are defined in terms of goods or that process that produces goods.[17] Axioms associated with this type of theory are "the greatest good for the greatest number" and "the ends justify the means."

Deontologic Theory

Deontologic theory maintains some acts are right and some are wrong independent of their consequences.[17] Deontologists maintain that the concepts of duty and obligation are independent of and have priority over any good that might result. That is, right actions are not determined exclusively by desired consequences. Ethical dilemmas arise when there are conflicting duties or obligations. Principles prescribe and justify the appropriate normative behavior in this conflict.[18]

Principles are universal directives that express a value judgment about what befits or does not befit the behavior of human beings. They are relevant generalizations about the normally valuable.[18-19] Certain principles (autonomy, beneficence, nonmaleficence, and justice) are more frequently used in the nursing literature to justify an ethical decision. They are not, however, the only principles available to the deontologist. Which principles will be appropriate to apply in a specific ethical dilemma will depend on the specific facts.

The principle of autonomy focuses on the right of persons to self-determination. Autonomy is a form of personal liberty of action where the individual determines his or her course of action in accordance with a plan by himself or herself. The autonomous person is one who not only deliberates about and chooses such plans, but also is capable of acting on the basis of such deliberation.[17,20] This principle is founded in and yet different from the principle of respect for persons in that it entails respect for self-determined choice of action.[21]

Beneficence and nonmaleficence are closely related principles. Beneficence is the duty to help others when we can do so with minimum risk to ourselves.[17] Nonmaleficence is the duty not to inflict harm on others.[22] It includes both actual harm and the risk of harm. Nonmaleficence is not violated when there is no intent to harm. For example, a critical care nurse may suction a patient, causing the patient discomfort and potentially even harm; but the intention was not to harm but to do good. As such, the principle was not violated.

Justice is the duty to act with impartiality and equality. Justice can be individual, distributive, and social.[23-25] Individual justice occurs when a person has been given what is due or owed and thus what he or she deserves and can legitimately claim. Distributive justice refers to the justified distribution of benefits and burdens in a society. Social justice proclaims the equal worth of all persons and backs that proclamation with various legal guarantees.

Other important principles that have been or could be implemented to justify a moral position are fidelity and veracity. Fidelity is the duty to be faithful to one's patients, with promise keeping as one aspect. It is the moral covenant between individuals in a relationship.[23,26] Veracity is the duty to tell the truth and not to lie or deceive others.[17]

The American Nurses' Association's (ANA's) Code of Ethics[27] is also founded in deontological theory. Each of the statements of the code can be thought of as a principle or professional rule that is meant to provide a minimally acceptable standard of behavior for the nurse.

Care Theory

Care theory is the newest of the normative theories. It originated in women's studies but has now moved past a gender focus. An ethic of care is a moral point of view that maintains that normative behavior can only be justified in the context of the human encounter or connection.[28] In this theory the fundamental obligation is maintenance of the human encounter (i.e., the relationship), and the affected response is basic.[29] The greatest and most universal obligation is to care for both self and others. Care is the obligation rooted in receptivity, relatedness, and responsiveness. Ethical inquiry in an ethic of care emphasizes the concrete situations, networks of relationships, interpersonal communications, caring, and responsibility. Normative behavior is the result of dialogue and negotiation of engaged participants who operate from the center of a web of relationships in order to maintain that network of interconnected relationships.[18]

Virtue Theory

Virtue theory is probably the oldest of the ethical frameworks and in some ways the most problematic. Virtues are habits, dispositions, traits, or character that a person may possess or desire to possess. Moral virtues are acquired habits or dispositions to do what is morally right or praiseworthy.[17] One becomes virtuous as a result of integrating acceptable virtues into one's self. The sources of these virtues are professional or community ideals. The premise is that if a person is virtuous (i.e., they integrate acceptable virtues), their acts will be morally acceptable.

In any specific ethical dilemma the application of one theory over the other can result in a different ethical choice. There are no algorithms in ethical knowledge. No one type of ethical theory is necessarily more effective or more efficient than another. Which theory will be acceptable in any given dilemma depends on the individuals involved in the situation and their relationships. The best theory will be the one that leaves all of the participants with the least moral distress at the conclusion of the situation.

RELATED RESEARCH AND LITERATURE
Ethical Decision Making in Critical Care

One of the most common discussions in the nursing ethics literature seems to be descriptions of ethical decision-making models. Models have both been borrowed from other disciplines and developed by nurses. What all of these decision-making models have in common, however, is that they are problem-solving models. Where ethical decision-making models differ from other models is that at some time in the decision-making process, the participants are required to examine the moral values that are integral to the process.[3] What any nurse needs to keep in mind is that these models are guidelines. A model that is ineffective in guiding ethical practice should be abandoned.

The ethical nursing process (Table 12–3) is one such decision-making model. It was developed to be integrated into the decision-making process that is common to most nurses. The intent is to dem-

TABLE 12–3 The Ethical Nursing Process

ASSESSMENT
I. Clinical parameters
   A. Identify all significant nursing and medical factors and facts in the case. What is the clinical status of the patient involved? What are the likely outcomes?
   B. What are the human factors in the case, such as patient's age, attitudes, occupation, family situation, behavioral history, and value orientation.
II. Participants
   A. Who are the participants in the dilemma? Who beside the patient is involved? What other health care providers are involved in the case?
   B. What are the judgments, extent of care, treatment or counsel, and formal or informal reports known to be held by the participants? Which of these constituents are currently unknown but desired to be known?
   C. Who owns the problem and the solution?
III. Ethical issues
   A. What are the sources of conflicts, if any, in this case? Articulate clearly the issues on both side of the conflict, such as quality of life vs. longevity, therapeutic or experimental, patient's interest and well-being and allocations of limited resources, learning research value of case, and primary concern for the patient.
IV. Ethical norms and values of participants
   A. Cost/benefit (consequences/outcomes)
   B. Principles
   C. Caring

NURSING DIAGNOSIS
Specific ethical response

NURSING GOAL
To maintain ethical integrity

INTERVENTIONS: (consider)
I. Personal-focused interventions
   A. Consultation
      1. Peer
      2. Professional
         a. CNS/ethics
         b. Medical ethicist
   B. Review of previous ethical analysis
II. Unit-focused interventions
   A. Unit forums
   B. Unit rounds
   C. Interdisciplinary or family conferences
   D. Standards of care
III. Institutional-focused interventions
   A. Ethics committee
      1. Institutional
      2. Nursing
      3. Medical
   B. Policies and procedures
      1. Institutional, e.g.
         a. DNR policies
         b. Durable power of attorney for health care
         c. Withdrawal or withholding of life-sustaining treatment
      2. Nursing policies, e.g., nurses' role in institutional policies

Table continued on following page

TABLE 12–3 The Ethical Nursing Process *Continued*

INTERVENTIONS: (consider) *Continued*

IV. Professional-focused interventions
   A. *ANA Code of Ethics*
   B. Position statements
      1. American Association of Critical Care Nurses
      2. American Nurses' Association
   C. Laws
      1. Federal laws, such as Patient Self-Determination
      2. State laws, such as California Natural Death Act

EVALUATION

 I. Is your moral agency or integrity intact?
 II. Would you make the same decision again? Why or why not?

onstrate that no special process is necessary to make "good" ethical decisions. Rather, ethical decisions can be the result of integrating additional considerations into the decision-making process that is already fundamental to established critical care nursing practice.

The nurse implements the ethical nursing practice as she or he begins to recognize that the clinical situation has the components of an ethical dilemma. Ethical dilemmas are those interpersonal situations in which an individual must chose between two mutually incompatible choices related to right or wrong. These choices may be equally "hard" choices characterized by equally disadvantaged or undesirable options. At this point the nurse begins the assessment phase.

Role of CC-CNS in Resolving Ethical Dilemmas

Making treatment decisions that are in the patient's best interest has been named the most important ethical issue that confronts critical care nurses.[30-32] This dilemma is testimony to the conflicting role of nurse as patient advocate. It has been said that nurses, by virtue of their place in the health care hierarchy, are not able to be autonomous moral agents.[33] It has also been said that nurses, as bedside clinicians, are in the best position to assist the patient in making treatment decisions because of their contact with the patient and family.[34] By the very nature of their work, nurses tend to know a lot about what being sick really means to the patient.[35] The CC-CNS as advanced practitioner is integral in assisting the bedside clinician in achieving some moral autonomy by role

modeling, consulting, and facilitating problem solving.

Nurse and CNS as Patient Advocates

"The nurse's primary commitment is to the client's care and safety. As an advocate for the client, the nurse must be alert to and take appropriate action regarding any instances of incompetent, unethical, or illegal practices."[27] Advocacy is defined as active support of an important cause.[21] The role of the advocate in the health care setting is to look out for the patient's best interest, to maintain autonomy, and to preserve human dignity. In nursing school, nurses are taught that their primary commitment is to the patient. In patient advocacy, one becomes a partisan in conflicts and assumes responsibility for presenting the rights and interests of the patient.[36,37]

The role of advocate is not new to nursing. Florence Nightingale, in her book *Notes on Nursing, What It Is and What It Is Not*, stated that nurses had the responsibility to "put the patient at the best possible state for nature to act upon him."[38] This is indeed that most basic form of advocacy, acting to ensure that the patient benefit from the care and the environment or, at least, that the patient not be harmed from these. Today, in the critical care environment, the line between benefit and harm is nebulous. The bedside nurse frequently must balance treatments with care. Nursing beliefs of the past, rooted in unquestioning obedience to the physician, have given way to an ethic of advocacy for the patient.[35]

If one subscribes to the covenantal relationship

of nursing, the balancing of a higly technical environment with the patient at its center becomes even more significant. Covenantal relationships are those in which a covenant or promise is understood at the beginning of that relationship by one or both parties involved. The covenantal relationship in nursing makes the promise that the nurse will act to maintain the nurse-patient relationship. A covenantal relationship, with fidelity at its core, becomes the driving force for advocacy as a role of the nurse. By entering into the covenantal relationship, the caregiver has made a commitment or promise to protect human dignity.[39] This goal becomes difficult to achieve and maintain in the technologic climate of modern ICUs. The ability of the bedside nurse to continuously act in the patient's best interest and thus to keep the covenant becomes compromised as the acuity and therefore the machinery surrounding the patient skyrocket. The priority for the nurse necessarily becomes maintenance of physiologic functioning. Decisions regarding treatment may be made without the informed consent of the patient or family. The technologic imperative manifests itself then around the patient and the nurse. As a result the line between benefit and harm becomes fuzzy or nonexistent.

PRACTICE IMPLICATIONS

The CC-CNS is mandated as an "expert practitioner" to come to the aid of not only the patient but also the bedside nurse. The motivation for assisting the patient should be evident. The need for supporting the nurse may not be so apparent to those unfamiliar with the critical care setting. If the nurse is genuinely seeking to serve as patient advocate, the inability to foster and maintain patient autonomy and to abide by the professional nurse-patient bond can become the basis for burnout. It is at this point that the benefit of the consultation and educator role of the CC-CNS becomes more evident. Relying on her or his expertise, the CC-CNS should be able to decipher the issues, clarify the values, initiate consultation, and facilitate collaborative decision making. By doing so, the CC-CNS is acting as not only a patient advocate but also a staff nurse advocate.

Acquiring Knowledge and Skill Development

The ability to filter through the plethora of issues that encompass an ethical dilemma in critical care is a skill that comes with experience and education.

The first step in achieving proficiency at deciphering and resolving ethical disharmony is for the CC-CNS to clarify her or his value system. For example, does the CC-CNS believe in the sanctity of life or in the right to die? This may be a difficult process but one that is essential if one hopes to assist in clarification of ethical issues at the bedside.

The next step for the CC-CNS is to become knowledgeable in bioethics content. Numerous references in the form of textbooks, articles, and journals are available to the interested student of nursing ethics. Many critical care journals feature ethics articles on a regular basis written by experts in biomedical or nursing ethics. Nursing research in the area of ethical dilemmas and management is present in almost any nursing research journal. The body of knowledge in the area of biomedical ethics is growing daily, and much of this knowledge is coming from nurse experts who are conducting research into ethical conflict or decision making.

Most advanced-degree curriculums also include ethics content as an integral part of the clinical concepts and theories presented. Some universities employ nurse ethicists as well. These experts are an excellent source of information for the neophyte CC-CNS.

Conferences on ethical issues in critical care are no longer scarce. In fact, many critical care seminars feature ethics content. The AACN presents ethics content in their National Teaching Institute held each year. In addition, a yearly conference on the ethical issues in critical care is held by the AACN in conjunction with the Society of Critical Care Medicine. These conferences are an excellent means to enhance one's knowledge regarding this subject. The ability to network with other critical care practitioners with similar interests or dilemmas is an added bonus. Many times unique approaches can be discussed that have been tried with success at other institutions.

Professional organizations such as the AACN or the ANA have prepared position statements on a variety of ethical issues. For example, the AACN's task force on ethics in critical care formulated a position statement on ethics in critical care research.[40] The California Nurses' Association has a prepared statement on withdrawal of life-sustaining treatment.[41] A Society of Critical Care

Medicine task force has written several position papers on ethics-related topics including foregoing life-sustaining treatment.[42]

Managing Ethical Conflicts

Several strategies can be used with a clinical ethical dilemma. It is important to remember that there is not a right answer for these struggles, but there will be a best answer for each patient and situation. The role of the CC-CNS is not only to facilitate arriving at that best answer, but also to assist the health care team to accept the decisions made.

One useful strategy for the CC-CNS is daily bedside collaborative rounds that incorporate patient condition, treatment plan, and long-term goals. Conversations with the staff nurse caring for the patient and with the primary physician can alert the CC-CNS to ethical difficulties that may ensue. Knowledge of the patient and the patient's condition and situation as well as familiarity with the family can greatly aid the CC-CNS. Having someone such as the CC-CNS who the patient and family trust and see as an expert can be a great comfort in making life and death decisions. These rounds also help to establish the CC-CNS as the expert practitioner in more than just clinical applications. Role modeling by the CC-CNS in dealing with these conflicts is an excellent means to assist staff members in acquiring the confidence to deal with these issues.

An offshoot of bedside rounds is bedside ethics rounds. These can be facilitated by an ethics consultant. Rounds of this type can be solely nursing staff members or interdisciplinary. This type of rounds serves two purposes: prevention and education.[43] This type of rounds may also evolve into a unit-based ethics committee enabling staff members to deal more effectively with ethical issues and thereby alleviating the need for outside consultation such as ethicists or institutional ethics committees. Issues such as resuscitation decisions, withdrawal of life-sustaining treatment, or conservator appointment may be foreseen in either type of rounds and thus a crisis prevented. "In clinical practice, the best ethics is sound preventative ethics."[43]

A fundamental component of the CC-CNS role is staff education. Knowledge of ethical principles

and problem solving not only will help prevent burnout but also will help the staff to feel empowered in clinical situations. Frequently the bedside clinician feels caught in the middle. Ordinarily nurses are not self-employed and are obliged to abide by institutional policies. Also, they are expected for the most part to follow the medical treatment plan. At the same time nurses feel that their primary commitment is to the patient. Nurses, by virtue of their advocacy mandate, are expected to act in the best interest of the patient, operating from a patient-oriented rather than a medically oriented perspective. Conflicts of this nature are an increasing source of moral anguish for nurses.[35] Nurses who are educated in ethical principles and processes are more likely to initiate and participate in ethical discussions regarding patient care. All health professionals must learn methods of reasoning through ethical dilemmas so as to approach these situations rationally:

While righteous indignation has its place, nurses need to move away from such reactions, for at least two reasons. First, they need to think about ethical issues rather than react emotionally so that they can understand their own ethical positions. Second, they need to reason through these often profound and emotion-laden dilemmas so as to be able to explain their thinking to others.[44]

Classes on ethical principles and conflicts are one way to assist staff members in gaining knowledge in this area. However, classes of this nature, unless mandatory, may not be well attended by critical care nurses who are typically interested in the physiologic processes. Ethical topics can be incorporated into longer classes or seminars on physiologic topics such as transplantation or new technology. Short in-service programs can be effective at reaching more staff members and are appropriate choices for this forum. Again, bedside rounds with discussion of ethical topics are invaluable in transferring knowledge to the staff nurse and to the physician team.

The CC-CNS role in research and research utilization can be an effective mechanism to identify sources of ethical conflict as well as solutions. Much exists in nursing research journals in the area of ethical issues that can be applied or replicated at the bedside by the CNS.

CC-CNS's Role in Identifying, Developing, and Utilizing Resources

The CC-CNS must have knowledge of the workings of ethics in a hospital or medical center. These can take many forms, including institutional ethics committees, institutional review boards, ethics grand rounds, bedside ethics rounds, and nursing ethics committees.[43] The CC-CNS can play a key role in the function or initiation of such groups. Being at the hub of the critical care unit where many ethical problems are encountered, the CC-CNS can be invaluable to the committee as well as to the patients and staff.

Estimates indicate that 60% of hospitals nationwide have ethics committees.[45] Ethics committees are cited frequently in court decisions and federal guidelines.[46] Many health care institutions have nursing ethics committees as well. Although these committees' functions may overlap, they are distinct.

The institutional ethics committee is the most common method of institutional review. These committees should be multidisciplinary. Historically these committees have been made up of physicians, with other departments, such as nursing, periodically invited as nonparticipatory guests. However, the 1992 Joint Commission on Accreditation of Health Organizations's hospitals manual[47] states: "When the hospital has an ethics committee or other defined structures for addressing ethical issues in patient care, nursing staff members participate." Institutional ethics committees (IECs) tend to be medical staff committees or hospital administration committees that convey some degree of influence.

Nursing ethics committees (NECs), although as common as institutional ethics committees are growing rapidly in number at health care institutions. These committees are not duplicates of IECs but are formed to investigate issues unique to nursing. Issues typically addressed in NECs and not in IECs are such things as staffing patterns, allocation of an individual nurse's time among the patients assigned, a nurse's refusal of an assignment, continued admissions where beds or nurses are lacking, and creation of medical subspecialty units where attention has not been given to nursing staffing needs.[43] Even though these issues can be appropriately brought to the IEC, many nurses find

it less intimidating to present the case to the NEC, a council of their peers. If necessary, the case can then be brought to the attention of the IEC by members of the NEC.

Bylaws of both types of committees usually direct the function of the committee to three major areas: education, policy development, and case review or consultation. Education is the least threatening function for a neophyte committee as well as the most obvious. Self-education is the primary goal for the first years of a committee's existence. The members of such a committee must feel competent and comfortable with their knowledge of ethical principles and conflict resolution. Despite the pressures that any such committee might feel to deal with specific issues, prematurely doing so can have devastating consequences. It is estimated to take approximately 2 to 3 years of persistent study for an ethics committee to be able to take on the issues of the institution.[43]

After the education of the committee is well underway, the education of the institutional staff should begin. This can be accomplished in a variety of ways, including seminars, rounds, newsletters, and consultations. Some committees also take on community education as the next step in the process.

Development and utilization of policies and procedures addressing ethical issues are seen by some as the primary functions of the ethics committees. These committees assist health care professionals in establishing and maintaining patient-centered standards of care. Effective policies will support patient autonomy and competent decision making at all levels of the organization in which patient care issues are addressed.[46] These policies can be viewed as preventive ethics. The development of the policies by an interdisciplinary committee can initiate a collaborative effort at the bedside as well. Policies such as withdrawing and withholding life-sustaining treatment or not resuscitating, for example, are multidimensional in the practice implications they hold for health care professionals. The individual perspectives of each profession should be assimilated into the policies.

Many resources are available for the development of these policies. Professional organizations frequently have developed statements on life-sustaining treatment or on issues of resuscitation, among others. The President's Commission for the Study of Ethical Problems in Medicine and Biomedical Behavioral Research has published several documents on ethical issues.[48] Many health care institutions have developed policies and are willing to share these with other IECs or NECs that are beginning their policy development phase.

The case review or consultant aspect of the IEC or NEC is the most controversial of the functions. Concerns are mainly twofold: that the members of the IEC or NEC lack the clinical expertise to understand the intricacy of a particular case and that the decision-making authority will be usurped from the clinician by the committee.[46] However, the literature does not support these fears. Ethics committees serve in an advisory capacity, review for due process, or suggest options.[46] The clinician is then left with the ultimate decision-making power in the case. Committees with consultation services do have an impact on physicians. Ethics rounds, consultations, and conferences have been shown to help health professionals make decisions, understand personal values, identify ethical issues, improve patient care, and plan patient management.[49–54]

The consultation assistance provided by the IEC or NEC can take the form of either a group review or a review by a designated participant who is well versed in ethical principles. The presence of an institutionally based clinical ethicist is becoming more common. These specialists can be philosophers, lawyers, advanced-degree nurses, clergy members, or interested practitioners who have studied the field of bioethics as part of their educational preparation. These specialists may consult as a representative of the committee, or they may serve in an advisory capacity only. Either way, these specialists are a valuable resource to the bedside practitioner. Although overlapping in their concerns, nursing and medicine differ in their goals, values, and procedures.[44] Establishment of active and interactive IECs and NECs can only help to resolve the differences and assist in eliminating many of the conflicting perceptions that are common at the bedside in critical care.

The CC-CNS is integral in initiating, organizing, and participating in ethical forums. Ethics rounds, either unit-based or grand rounds, are effective tools for the practitioner. Grand rounds usually are an educational tool. These are typically done in the case review format, with the case being presented by either the nursing staff members responsible for the patient or by an interdisciplinary team. The physiologic and pathophysiologic data and the psychosocial information are briefly reviewed. The case is then discussed with an analysis of the ethical dilemmas that are present. Possible resolutions or options are deliberated by the audience. This format is a common one used by NECs for staff education. In those institutions that do not have a functioning NEC, this type of rounds may be a part of the clinical grand rounds.

Conflicts that arise between the health care team members are best dealt with directly. It is important to remember the value system that each member is bringing to the situation. Team members may view the goal of treatment differently from each other and from the patient. Establishing collaborative goals, with patient and family participation, can alleviate many conflicting feelings. Assisting all members of the health care team (including nurses) to realize that nurses are in a unique position to contribute pertinent information about burdens and benefits of treatment plans on a particular patient is pivotal in staff satisfaction and quality care.

Ethical Issues Common to Critical Care

The successful development of a critical care nursing ethic depends on an accurate appraisal of the issues that are common to nursing practice. Table 12–4 lists the ethical issues in nursing practice that were identified as the result of an ongoing survey in the southern California area since 1986. From 1986 to 1991, few changes occurred in the top 10 issues or practice situations listed. Indeed the only statistical difference demonstrated was greater numbers of subjects identifying organ transplant issues and quality of life decisions with each passing year.[32] Then in 1992 the top five issues shifted dramatically. The most frequently encountered ethical dilemmas identified by critical care nurses dealt with treatment decisions, cost to the patient, cost containment, allocation of resources, and pain management. Although this shift can probably be explained in terms of changing societal and economic trends, it points out dramatically that any critical care ethic must be dynamically ongoing, incorporating descriptive ethics into any con-

TABLE 12–4 Ethical Issues in Critical Care Nursing Practice

From 1986 to 1991[29] the top 10 issues or practice situations identified as sources of ethical dilemmas for critical care nurses were as follows:
1. Do not resuscitate decisions
2. Quality of life decisions
3. Organ transplantation
4. Dealing with difficult patients
5. Issues of beneficence
6. Conflict of interest
7. Cost of care to patient
8. Pain relief or management
9. Patient-physician-nurse relationship
10. Dying with dignity

In 1991[30] the top 5 issues or practice situations identified as sources of ethical dilemmas for critical care nurses were as follows:
1. Making treatment decisions in the patient's best interest
2. Pain management
3. Cost containment
4. Allocation of resources, such as beds and technology
5. Cost of care to patient

---

sideration of normative ethics if it is to be relevent to critical care nursing practice.

It is beyond the scope of this chapter to discuss all of the ethical issues found in the critical care area. Many excellent texts and journal articles examine these issues in depth. The neophyte clinical specialist would benefit from reviewing information on these issues. Some degree of familiarity with the commonly encountered issues will enable the CC-CNS to recognize and be better prepared to confront ethical conflicts as they arise.

Most CC-CNSs will be called on to deal with these issues in one way or another. Frequently the solution will not easy, or there may not be a satisfactory solution.

These problems are of obvious concern to more than critical care nurses, as evidenced by the steps the U.S. government has taken to assist in preventing or resolving these disputes. The federally mandated Patient Self-Determination Act requiring hospitals to provide patients with information regarding life support decisions may help alleviate some of the controversy at the bedside. However, most of the potentially burdensome treatments will still not be addressed by this mandate and will continue to present problems for critical care health care providers.

Treatment Decisions

The number one issue, making treatment decisions that are in the patient's best interest, encompasses concerns with resuscitation, invasive or painful treatments for severely ill patients, withdrawing or withholding life support, and informed consent. These problems confront the critical care nurse almost every day of practice.

Treatments such as dialysis, nephrotoxic medications, or line insertions are done habitually without informed consent in many or most institutions. The distress associated with these matters, as well as those mentioned previously, could generally be reduced if informed consent were obtained. However, this is frequently difficult in critical care for a number of reasons. The patients are typically very sick and therefore unable to provide any degree of informed consent for treatments. The nature of critical care is such that many decisions are made in emergency circumstances. Thus, frequently insufficient time exists to obtain consent from the patient or family. The degree of sophistication and technologic advancement of treatment options almost precludes attainment of informed consent from the majority of intensive care patients. In reality, informed consent may be a misnomer for what the patient or family is asked to provide. Sprung and Winick stated: "Physicians have described informed consent as a myth, a fiction, and an unattainable goal that has been transformed into a legal requirement."[55] This is because informed consent requires not only that the patient be competent to make a decision, but also that he or she be able to understand the treatment procedure and sequelae in order to make that decision.[56] It is difficult if not impossible to understand the technical and physiologic implications of most of the therapies provided in critical care. Such treatments as intubation and mechanical ventilation cannot be truly comprehended until experienced.[55] And as critical care practitioners know, anxiety and other emotional states associated with critical illness serve to decrease that ability of the decision maker to hear and understand the information being provided.

CASE STUDY

Lindsay was a 21-year-old woman who developed hepatic failure after taking a large amount of acetaminophen to relieve the discomfort of flulike symptoms during her finals. Lindsay underwent an emergency liver transplantation and did well postoperatively. Approximately 1 year after her transplant, Lindsay was readmitted with recurrent hepatitis, pain, and sarcoma. She was diagnosed as terminal with only a few days to live. She was awake, alert, and receiving large doses of morphine for pain control. She developed severe respiratory failure and was maintained on a ventilator. About 3 days into her critical illness, Lindsay requested that she be extubated to allow her to speak with her family. The nurse and the physician explained to Lindsay that this would mean certain death within minutes of extubation. Lindsay was cognizant of this and requested that no heroic measures be performed when she died. Lindsay had a very large and close family. A conference was held with the family to discuss Lindsay's request. Some of the siblings were reluctant when the end result of this withdrawal of support was presented. The sister to whom she was closest stated that Lindsay had mentioned similar wishes to her regarding life support measures a few months ago and that "she seemed to know that she was going to die soon." After the conference the family gathered in the hallway, Lindsay was extubated, and her family was called in. The family gathered around her bed, and Lindsay had her final conversations with her family in privacy. She died very peacefully a short time later holding the hands of her mother and father. All of the 15 siblings were around her bed at the time of death.

Role of CC-CNS The nurse caring for Lindsay called the CC-CNS when Lindsay communicated her request. The CC-CNS spoke with Lindsay. Lindsay was taking large doses of morphine for pain control, but this had not affected her ability to communicate her wishes by writing nor her ability to make rational decisions. The CC-CNS spoke with the attending physician regarding Lindsay's request. The physician

and the nurses, include the CC-CNS, were reluctant to go forward with this request. The CC-CNS, the physician, and the nurse caring for Lindsay had an informal conference to sort out the values influencing their feelings. Lindsay understood the consequences of her decision and was willing to accept these, thereby giving informed consent. All team members felt uncomfortable with this request but acknowledged that there was no other beneficial course of action and that to not follow Lindsay's wishes would have been to violate the principle of autonomy.

After the death the CC-CNS arranged a meeting for the staff, both physicians and nurses, with a facilitator to assist in clarifying the feelings and issues that seemed so overwhelming. All agreed that this death was as it should be. However, the actual withdrawal of life support such as the ventilator is such an obvious act that many of the health care team felt that this was actual participation in Lindsay's death and, in giving her large doses of morphine before the extubation, staff members may have even been responsible for the death. Resolution of these issues was achieved with the realization that there was no cure for Lindsay no matter what was done and that responsibility should naturally shift from a curative focus to comfort and allowing for a "healthy" death.[57]

After the death the CC-CNS arranged follow-up consultation with the family and the social worker to assist in dealing with any feelings of resentment and in assessing the need for grief counseling. Follow-up telephone calls were made to the family with information regarding the well-being of the family passed on to the staff.

Ethical Issue

Relief of suffering is a fundamental moral value for critical care nurses. Pain management and control are primary nursing goals. When clinical conditions are such that the nurse cannot meet these goals, the nurse feels morally compromised.

At least two kinds of pain management situations may result in the nurse feeling morally compromised. In the first situation the nurse may assess that the patient is in pain. This assessment will lead to a request of the physician to either begin or increase pain medications. When the physician refuses to do either, the nurse will experience moral distress. The principles of beneficence and nonmaleficence direct the nurse to do good and no harm, yet the political dynamic has placed the nurse in a situation where those principles cannot be acted on. The nurse cannot write the pain order. The nurse who continues to request the pain medication may jeopardize the relationship with the physician. If the nurse, operating from an ethics of care perspective, is committed to maintaining the relationship with the physician, an ethical dilemma results. The nurse can maintain the "good" relationship with the physician, leaving the patient in pain, or the nurse can challenge the physician, possibly sabotaging the relationship, yet achieving pain control for the patient.

The second situation results when the nurse and the patient define pain differently. In this situation the CC-CNS may first recognize that an ethical problem exists. The pain experience is a qualitative subjective phenomenon in a world of hard technical data. Many, if not most, of the assessments that the critical care nurse makes involve interpretations removed from the patient. Hemodynamic status, respiratory parameters, and even renal function assessments are based in objective, numeric readings from pieces of technology juxtaposed between the patient and the nurse. There is, however, no invasive line that will give a pain score. The nurse depends on the patient's interpretation of pain. The nurse who does not share the pain interpretation (i.e., the nurse does not believe that the behaviors exhibited by the patient mean or should be interpreted as pain) may deny the patient is in pain. In this case the CC-CNS must choose between an ethic of care (i.e., maintaining a relationship with the staff nurse) and the principles of beneficence and nonmaleficence.

CASE STUDY

Mr. Lark, a 56-year-old man, had been diagnosed with acute myelocytic leukemia some months earlier. He had originally been denied treatment for a facial melanoma because of the extent of the surgery required. Also, his oncologist believed that the leuke-

mia would be terminal before the melanoma caused significant health problems. Nevertheless, he and his family had traveled from Hawaii to seek treatment at a well-known teaching facility. A surgeon was found who would proceed with the treatment. The surgery entailed removal of almost the entire right side of his face and placement of a large graft taken from his left buttock. Approximately 12 hours postoperatively he developed hypotension and fever. He was mechanically ventilated but was experiencing severe respiratory failure. The plastic surgeon managing the patient in the ICU discontinued all pain and sedation medications. The patient was started on a paralytic agent to assist in ventilator management. No sedation was ordered. The physician, when questioned about the lack of pain medication and sedation, especially in association with the paralytic agent, stated that the hypotension precluded these even though the patient was paralyzed. The CC-CNS spoke with the physician regarding the concerns she and the staff were experiencing about the lack of pain and sedation. She suggested that the plastic surgeon consult the pulmonary team or some team accustomed to managing critically ill patients or at least assisting in pain management. The physician stated that he did not feel pain relief was important for this patient at this time. All suggestions were met with resentment and refusal. It soon became obvious that this patient was not going to survive and that the plastic surgeon was intent on managing him until the patients's death.

The CC-CNS confronted the physician with the feelings of horror that she and staff members were experiencing in regard to the total management of this patient. She explained that she had no recourse but to call the medical director of the unit. The medical director spoke with the attending physician, and it was agreed to administer 1 mg of morphine every 3 hours. This was not viewed as an adequate solution by the CC-CNS and the nursing staff. The nursing director was consulted and held a meeting with the medical director, the CC-CNS, and the nurse manager. The medical director did not feel comfortable assuming care for the patient but did feel that more action should be taken. The case was brought to the attention of the medical ethics consultant. The consultant wrote a note in the chart with strong recommendations that sedation be administered in conjunction with pain medication; otherwise, the principles of beneficence and nonmaleficence were being violated. This note did not achieve any change in treatment. The patient died that night.

Role of CC-CNS The CC-CNS was consulted early in this case for two reasons: first, because the attending physician was unaccustomed to caring for critically ill patients; and second, because the staff believed that this operation was inappropriate given this patient's medical history and therefore this death was not necessary. The CC-CNS, acting as patient advocate, used every possible resource to achieve what she believed to be basic care for the patient. The outcome of pain management was not attained even though all avenues were explored. The immediate need, to act in the best interest of the patient, was followed by the need to assist the nursing staff in dealing with this issue. The powerlessness felt by staff after a distressing case such as this one can damage morale of the unit. Staff members need to see that there are mechanisms in place to ensure that this type of incident will not recur.

The CC-CNS and the medical ethicist presented this case before the IEC at the next session. The IEC agreed that this was indeed a case of medical mismanagement and that the exclusion of pain and sedation medications was unethical. A letter containing a summary of the discussion and recommendations from the IEC was sent to the physician.

A quality assurance monitor was developed and implemented to assess the knowledge of the nursing staff regarding pain and sedation medication and to assess the patient's perception of pain relief during ICU stay. Unit-based standards for pain management and for management of a pharmacologically paralyzed patient were developed, using the results of the monitors. The unit director supported the standards as well.

In addition, the CC-CNS and the nurse manager wrote a letter to the chief of surgery detailing the incident. This began documentation of serious incidents that could have been prevented had there been an intensive care physician in the unit to oversee the care of these critically ill patients. The following year, a surgical intensive care physician was hired.

These scenarios demonstrate the difficulties facing CC-CNSs in dealing with ethical dilemmas. If feelings and issues are not resolved at the bedside with the health care team, resentment, powerlessness, and anger can develop with resultant burnout. One important point to remember is that not always is there immediate gratification from one's efforts. Through careful planning and knowledge of the workings of the institution one can eventually achieve the changes mandated by the moral values that are foundations of ethical nursing practice.

SUMMARY

The rapidly changing health care environment has brought with the changes new ethical dilemmas in health care. Allocation of scarce resources and issues of human dignity are daily events in the critical care setting. The CC-CNS must now possess knowledge of principles of ethical problem solving and be prepared to serve as a resource and support person to staff, patient, and family. This chapter has presented models of modern ethical thought that can provide a foundation for CC-CNS practice. Acting within these models, the CC-CNS is prepared to assist staff members in sorting through ethical issues and coming to terms with ethical interventions that meet the needs of all parties involved.

References

1. American Association of Critical Care Nurses: *Competence statements for critical care clinical nurse specialists,* Laguna Niguel, Calif, 1989, The Association.
2. Ladd D: The task of ethics. In Reich WT, editor: *Encyclopedia of bioethics,* New York, 1978, The Free Press.
3. Omery A: Values, moral reasoning, and ethics, *Nurs Clin North Am* 24:499-508, 1989.
4. Maguire D: *The moral choice,* Minneapolis, 1978, Winston Press.
5. Fargnoli A, Maguire D: *On moral grounds,* New York, 1992, Crossroads Press.
6. Foot P: Moral reasoning. In Reich WT, editor: *Encyclopedia of bioethics,* New York, 1978, The Free Press.

7. Kohlberg L: A reply to Owen Flanagan and some comments on the Puka-Goodpaster exchange, *Ethics* 92:513-528, 1982.
8. Kohlberg L, Levine C, Hewer A: *Moral stages: a current reformulation and response to critics,* Basel, 1983, S Karger.
9. Gilligan C: *In a different voice,* Cambridge, Mass, 1982, Harvard University Press.
10. Gilligan C, Ward J, Taylor J: *Mapping the moral domain: a contribution of women's thinking to psychological theory and education,* Cambridge, Mass, 1988, Harvard University Press.
11. Huggins E, Scalzi C: Limitations and alternative: ethical practice theory in nursing, *Adv Nurs Pract* 10:43-47, 1988.
12. Omery A: Moral development: a differential evaluation of the dominant models of moral development, *Adv Nurs Sci* 6(1):1-17, 1983.
13. Omery A: *Moral reasoning of nurses who work in the adult intensive care setting,* dissertation, Boston, 1985, School of Nursing, Boston University.
14. Cooper M: *Moral reasoning of nurses in critical care,* dissertation, 1987, School of Nursing, University of Virginia, Richmond.
15. Viens D: *Moral reasoning of nurse practitioners,* dissertation, San Diego, 1991, School of Nursing, University of San Diego.
16. Baier K: Teleological theories. In Reich WT, editor: *Encyclopedia of bioethics,* New York, 1978, The Free Press.
17. Beauchamp T, Childress J: *Principles of bioethics,* ed 2, New York, 1983, Oxford University Press.
18. Omery A: Culpability and pain management/control in peripheral vascular disease: using the ethics of principles and care, *Crit Care Nurs Clinics* 3(3):551-558, 1991.
19. Maguire D: *Death by choice,* New York, 1984, Doubleday.
20. Greenawalt K: Privacy. In Reich WT, editor: *Encyclopedia of bioethics,* New York, 1978, The Free Press.
21. Fry S: Autonomy, advocacy, and accountability. In Fowler M, Levine J, editors: *Ethics at the bedside,* Philadelphia, 1987, JB Lippincott Co.
22. Davis A: The boundaries of intervention: issues in the non-infliction of harm, In Fowler M, Levine J, editors: *Ethics at the bedside,* Philadelphia, 1987, JB Lippincott Co.
23. Bandman B: The human rights of patients, nurses, and other health professionals. In Bandman B, Bandman E, editors: *Bioethics and human rights,* Boston, 1978, Little, Brown & Co.
24. Feinberg J: Justice. In Reich WT, editor: *Encyclopedia of bioethics,* New York, 1978, The Free Press.
25. Veatch R: *A theory of medical ethics,* New York, 1981, Basic Books.
26. Ramsey R: *The patient as a person,* New Haven, Conn, 1970, Yale University Press.
27. American Nurses' Association: *ANA code of ethics with interpretive statements,* Kansas City, MO, 1985, ANA Publications.
28. Fry S: The role of caring in a theory of nursing ethics, *Hypatia* 4:85-89, 1989.
29. Nodding N: *Caring: a feminine approach to ethics and moral education,* Berkeley, Calif, 1984, University of California Press.
30. Omery A, Henneman E: Ethical issues in critical care nursing practice, *Heart Lung* 20(4):25A, 1991.
31. Omery A, UCLA Nursing Ethics Committee. *Ethical issues in critical care nursing practice,* unpublished paper, 1992.
32. Omery A, Henneman E, Billet B: A survey of the ethical issues faced by nurses in practice and the resources desired by nurses to address them, manuscript under review.
33. Yarling R, McElmurry B: Autonomy in nursing, *Adv Nurs Sci* 8(2):63-73, 1986.
34. Murphy C: The changing role of nurses in making ethical decisions, *Law Med Health Care,* pp 173-175, 184, Sept. 1984.
35. Theis E: Ethical issues: a nursing perspective, *Engl J Med* 315(19):1222-1224, 1986.
36. Jameton A: *Nursing practice, the ethical issues,* Englewood Cliffs, NJ, 1984, Prentice-Hall.
37. Benes R, Bronst K: Defining quality in ethics consultation: first steps, *Quality Review Board* 18(1):33-39, 1992.
38. Nightingale F: *Notes on nursing, what it is and what it is not,* New York, 1969, Dover Publications.
39. Gadow S: Nurse and patient: the caring relationship. In Bishop AH, Scudder J, editors: *Caring, curing, coping: nurse, physician, patient relationships,* University, Ala, 1985, University Press.
40. American Association of Critical Care Nurses: *Statement on ethics in critical care research,* Newport Beach, Calif, American Association of Critical Care Nurses, 1985.
41. California Nurses' Association Ethics Committee: *Statement on the nurse's role in withholding and withdrawing life sustaining treatment,* Sacramento, Calif, 1987, California Nurses' Association.
42. Task Force on Ethics of the Society of Critical Care Medicine: Consensus report on the ethics of foregoing life-sustaining treatments in the critically ill, *Crit Care Med* 19(12):1435-1439, 1990.
43. Fowler M: Nursing ethics committees, *Heart Lung* 17(6):718-719, 1988.
44. Davis A: Helping your staff address ethical dilemmas, *J Nurs Admin,* pp 9-13, Feb 1982.
45. McIver G, Kimbrough K: Ethics committees: how they are doing, *Hastings Center Rep* 16(3), 1986.
46. Bartels D: Ethics committees and critical care: allies or adversaries? *Perspect Crit Care* 1(2):83-90, 1988.
47. Joint Commission on Accreditation of Health Organizations: *Accreditation manual for hospitals,* vol 1. *Standards,* Chicago, 1991, The Commission.
48. President's Commission for the Study of Ethical Problems in Medicine and Behavioral Research: Washington, DC, 1983, U.S. Government Printing Office.
49. Carson R, Curry R: Ethics teaching on rounds, *J Fam Prac* 11:59-63, 1983.
50. Self D, Lyon-Loftus G: A model for teaching ethics in a family practice residency, *J Fam Prac* 16:355-359, 1983.
51. Lo B, Schroeder S: Frequency of ethical dilemmas in medical inpatient service, *Arch Intern Med* 41:1062-1064, 1981.
52. Levine M, Scott L, Curran W: Ethics rounds in a children's medical center: evaluation of a hospital-based program for continuing education in medical ethics, *Pediatrics* 60:99-102, 1977.

53. Sun T, Self D: Medical ethics programs in family practice residencies, *Fam Med* 17:99-102, 1985.
54. Perkins H, Saathoff B: Impact of medical ethics consultations on physicians: an exploratory study, *Am J Med*, pp 761-765, Dec 1988.
55. Sprung C, Winnick B: Informed consent in theory and practice: legal and medical perspectives on the informed consent doctrine and a proposed reconceptualization, *Crit Care Med* 17(12):1346-1353, 1989.
56. American Hospital Association: *The patient's choice of treatment options: policy and statement,* 1985, The Association.
57. Omery A: A healthy death, *Heart Lung* 20(3):310-311, 1991.

The Critical Care Clinical Nurse Specialist as Researcher

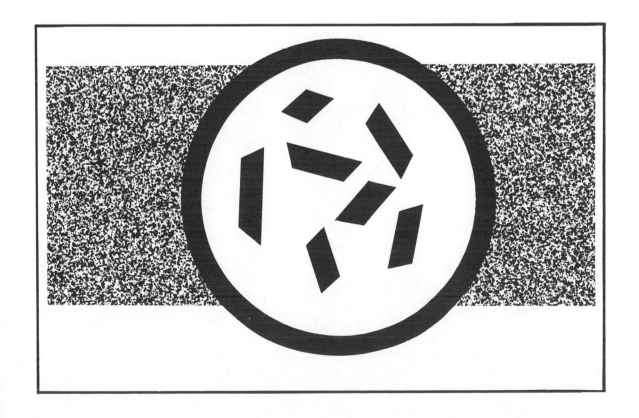

The Role of the Critical Care Clinical Nurse Specialist in Critical Care Research

Patricia A. O'Malley, RN, MS, CCRN

Clinical research in nursing has been historically linked with the clinical nurse specialist (CNS) role.[1] Ideally, research roles of the critical care CNS (CC-CNS) complement the roles of expert practitioner, educator, consultant, and leader. Pragmatically, research efforts are often last on a long list of projects and responsibilities. This chapter provides practical information for the CC-CNS on ways to fulfill research responsibilities inherent in the role of the CNS. It also reviews the benefits of research for practice, education, and leadership.

The CC-CNS is in a unique position to promote research in the clinical setting. Daily contact with clinical problems, quality assessment and improvement activities, and program and policy development all create an excellent impetus for research activities. Lack of time and administrative support, emphasis on the roles of educator and practitioner, and differing levels of research knowledge included in graduate programs are all forces inhibiting research by the CC-CNS.[2,3]

THEORETIC PERSPECTIVES

According to Fawcett,[4] research consists of three different activities: generation, dissemination, and utilization. Conducting research as a primary or coinvestigator is an example of generation. Presenting research through publications or at conferences, seminars, and staff meetings is an example of dissemination activities. Incorporation of research findings in policies, procedures, or stan-

dards of care is an example of utilization of research. The choice of activities by the CC-CNS depends on the role responsibilities defined by the organization, the CC-CNS, and the educational preparation and experience of the CC-CNS.

Whereas organizational expectations of CC-CNS research responsibilities affect choices of research activities, educational preparation and experience profoundly affect the process of those activities. As research in nursing has changed, demonstrated by increasingly sophisticated designs, methods, and analyses, so have the expectations of research activities related to educational preparation. In 1989 the American Nurses' Association Cabinet of Nurse Researchers prepared a landmark report describing the relationship of educational preparation and corresponding activities in nursing research. The report provides practical recommendations to decide what research activities are appropriate based on educational preparation. This report is helpful not only for the CC-CNS in deciding appropriate research activities but also for assisting others in selecting levels of participation in the research process. Table 13-1 describes research activities related to degree preparation.[5] Each level of educational preparation offers a unique preparation for the research process. Choosing research activities congruent with educational preparation and experience may result in fewer problems reported in critical care nursing literature such as inadequate linking of theory and method, biased and small samples, inappropriate use of sta-

TABLE 13–1 Relationship of Educational Preparation and Research Activities in Nursing

Educational Preparation	Research Activities
Associate degree (AD)	Identifies clinical problems in practice
	Assists in data collection protocols
Bachelor's degree (BSN)	Reads research critically
	Uses existing standards to determine readiness of research utilization in practice
	Identifies clinical problems in research
	Assists investigators to gain access to research sites
	Participates in data collection and implementation of findings
Master's degree (MS, MN)	Active member of research team
	Clinical expert, collaborating with investigator in proposal development, data collection, analysis, and interpretation of results
	Appraises clinical relevance of research findings in relation to quality assurance and nursing care
	Creates climate in practice setting that supports inquiry and scientific investigation of clinical nursing problems
	Integrates research findings into practice
Doctoral degree (PhD, DNS)	Conducts research and theory generation and theory testing
	Independently designs studies as well as assists other researchers

Reprinted with permission from *Education for Participation in Nursing Research,* © 1989, American Nurses' Association, Washington, DC.

tistics in analyses, and premature generalizations to practice.[6]

RELATED LITERATURE AND RESEARCH
Recommended Research Activities of CC-CNS

The American Association of Critical Care Nurses (AACN) published a position statement defining the roles of the CC-CNS.[7] Research roles are clearly defined and include the following. First, the CC-CNS expands the scientific base of critical care nursing by using, facilitating, and conducting research. Second, the CC-CNS disseminates research findings relevant to critical care practice, which includes presenting and publishing research. Finally, the CC-CNS assures legal and ethical practices in the conducting of research. The CC-CNS is the clinical expert for all phases of the research process in that the CC-CNS provides leadership in research utilization, evaluation of clinical relevance of research, and creating an environment conducive to research.[8-10]

Status of Critical Care Nursing Research

Before presenting methods CC-CNSs can use to generate research, it is necessary to examine the status of critical care nursing research. Critical care

research has been influenced by increasingly sophisticated technology, an increased ability to sustain life, and development of the intensive care unit (ICU) environment.[11] From 1975 to 1985, research topics focused on the structure of critical care units, the process of nursing, and predictions of patient outcomes. A particular focus concerned patient stress and the impact of critical illness on families and nursing staff. The majority of the research was atheoretic and descriptive in nature. Research concerning the relationship of patient outcomes to nursing care was done most often by disciplines other than nursing. Unfortunately, these studies lacked a nursing orientation and as a result findings concerning patient outcomes had a medical model perspective and interpretation.[11,12] Despite nearly 20 years of research in critical care, very little is known about nursing's contribution to patient outcomes in critical illness.

In another analysis of critical care practice research from 1979 to 1988,[6] 129 studies were examined, and the identified gaps in critical care research were similar. Individual topics were the most prevalent focus of concern (41.5%) followed by studies concerning stress or anxiety (11%) and effects of positioning on hemodynamics (11%).

Other content areas included family members' needs (8.5%), cardiac output measurements (8%), effects of suctioning (7%), coagulation studies (5%), teaching (3%), chest tube care (2%), and sleep deprivation (2%). Few studies examined ethical dilemmas inherent in critical care nursing or research on the psychologic effects of the intensive care environment.[6]

Despite the gaps in existing research, there has been progress, generated with a movement from just describing critical care nursing phenomena to explanation and prediction. Because critical care nursing is illness oriented and so highly integrated with technology, there is a constant danger in adopting a medical model perspective in selection of research questions.[12] Therefore selection of topics for research by the CC-CNS should reflect critical care nursing's concern. Research should expand the scientific base for the practice of critical care nursing to improve practice and patient outcomes.[6,13]

Recommendations for Research in Critical Care

The complexity of critical care nursing phenomena makes it difficult for the CC-CNS to prioritize areas of concern for research. This problem was addressed in 1991, when the AACN sponsored the Research Priorities Consensus Conference. Fifty critical care nurse experts from across the United States met and developed an agenda for future critical care research based on areas of concern defined from nationwide survey data. Research topics were identified and prioritized into two categories: clinical practice and the context within which critical care nursing takes place. Table 13-2 describes the priorities established for future nursing research in critical care.[14] These priorities for research can assist the CC-CNS in the selection of research activities. The priorities provide direction for all critical care nurse researchers that may result in building nursing knowledge for critical care. This will certainly help develop nursing knowledge more quickly, which will benefit critical care nurses and patients.

CNS as Researcher

The CNS roles in critical care research have not been well defined in the literature. This is related to a lack of consensus concerning the research activities of the CC-CNS. As a result the research

TABLE 13-2 AACN Research Priorities for 1991

PRIORITIES FOR CLINICAL PRACTICE RESEARCH

Techniques to optimize pulmonary functioning and prevention of pulmonary complications

Weaning of mechanically ventilated patients

Effect of nursing activities and interventions on hemodynamic parameters

Techniques for real-time monitoring of tissue perfusion and oxygenation

Nutritional support modalities and patient outcomes

Interventions to prevent infection

Pain assessment and pain management techniques

Accuracy and precision of invasive and noninvasive monitoring devices

Effects of nursing activities, environmental stimuli, and human interactions on intracranial and cerebral perfusion pressure

PRIORITIES FOR RESEARCH ON CONTEXT WITHIN WHICH CRITICAL CARE NURSING TAKES PLACE

Incorporating research findings into practice

Levels of nursing competence (e.g., certification) and effects on patient outcomes

Occupational hazards (e.g., human immune virus [HIV], noise, substance abuse, premature delivery)

Ethical issues related to initiation, maintenance, and withdrawal of life support technology (e.g., living wills)

Patient care delivery models for critical care

Collaboration and communication among health care professionals

Role of critical care nurses in decisions regarding resuscitation status of critically ill patients

Used with permission from the American Association of Critical Care Nurses: *AACN announces research priorities. Press release,* Aliso Viejo, Calif, Nov 21, 1991.

roles of the CC-CNS have been described differently.[15]

Activities of the CC-CNS researcher include promoting collaborative research, preparing protocols, gathering preliminary data, and implementing research projects.[16] Factors identified that facilitate research by the CC-CNS include a centralized nursing research committee as well as a unit-based committee, access to literature and statistical services, and ability to obtain expert assistance from doctorally prepared nurses with experience in conducting research. Lack of time to do research is a commonly identified problem, and strategies such as creating research interest groups and building collaborative relationships to enable research have been presented as possible solutions.[17]

Research roles of the CC-CNS are also influenced by personal and organizational factors. What are the responsibilities related to research activities identified in the CC-CNS job descriptions? How are research activities perceived in the organization; are they considered an integral part of the CC-CNS role or an additional activity after the roles of teacher and practitioner? Further research is needed to describe CC-CNS research activities and how the roles of researcher are best integrated with roles of practitioner, educator, and consultant.

PRACTICE IMPLICATIONS

Assessment of Research Environment

Assessment of the research environment should not be a one-time activity for the CC-CNS. Organizations are fluid and change over time. At best, assessment should be done before any research activity is attempted. Research takes place in context; therefore the research process is influenced by the research environment, which consists of the organizational environment, human resources, and available support.

Organizational Assessment

Assessing the organizational environment is the most complex part of the process. First, is the planned research focus consistent with the mission and values of the organization?[18] For example, if the mission of the organization is to provide only basic care for admitted trauma and provide for subsequent transfer to a level I trauma center, a study focusing on the long-term outcomes of trauma care by the CC-CNS would probably be inappropriate. The CC-CNS must also consider what activities of the organization potentially promote or limit nursing research. If the organization is undergoing structural or financial reorganization, implementing a research project may be difficult. There are strategies that the CC-CNS can use to initiate research in this type of situation, such as designing a study to address issues related to reorganization.

For example, a division of nursing decides to redesign the care delivery model by changing the skill mix of caregivers in the critical care units to reduce salary expenditures. The CC-CNS could design a variety of studies to examine issues such as nurse-patient satisfaction, nurse retention and recruitment, patient outcomes, and financial outcomes. The research would benefit the organization because needed information would be obtained, and the information would benefit others considering skill mix redesign if the information was published. Knowledge of organizational goals and activities can only help the CC-CNS make the best decision regarding the focus of planned research and enable the CC-CNS to develop a more accurate assessment of the feasibility of the research project.[18,19]

The history of research in the organization and in the critical care unit is also an important factor the CC-CNS must consider. If clinical research has been accomplished only within the departments of medicine or pharmacy in the critical care area, the CC-CNS can be a pioneer in establishing nursing research activities. The CC-CNS in this circumstance will likely have to establish a foundation to legitimize research by developing multidisciplinary collaborative relationships and nursing-based protocols for inclusion in approved proposals. For example, a CC-CNS discovers a research proposal is being prepared by a multidisciplinary group examining the efficacy of a pharmacologic agent in individuals experiencing shock. The CC-CNS's research interest is patient respiratory outcomes in shock. The CC-CNS could develop a protocol that *complements* the intended project and provides data that could benefit all the researchers involved. Subsequently, research by nurses in the organization is legitimized.

This process can also be done with approved nursing studies. For example, a CC-CNS is interested in pain management in individuals with chest trauma. The CC-CNS finds out a protocol is being prepared to examine pain management in thoracic surgery patients by the nurse researcher. The CC-CNS could meet with the nurse researcher and explore implementing the protocol examining pain in the chest trauma population as well. This process can be a good way for a new CC-CNS to begin conducting research. It eliminates the need for preparing multiple proposals for approval that examine similar phenomena or populations and fosters development of collaborative relationships.

Part of organizational assessment should include evaluation of committees charged with the approval and monitoring of research proposals. Federal guidelines for protection of human subjects require that research with human subjects be reviewed by a committee of peers. In most organizations this committee is known as an institutional review board (IRB). Some organizations designate this group a department review committee (DRC).[20,21] Many organizations also have a nursing research committee that complements the IRB committee.

The IRB or DRC and the nursing research committee should have written documents describing the purposes and functions of the committee, responsibilities of members, member selection criteria, and reporting procedures. The CC-CNS should review these documents and make contacts with members from both committees. Also important is to review guidelines for proposal submission. Nearly all review committees have written procedures for proposal submission, and these will help the CC-CNS in planning a research project. Finally, the CC-CNS must assess the relationship of the review committees with quality assessment and improvement groups and education. There should be some interface among these three committees, since data collection can be a shared process and findings can be a basis for future research.[18,22-24]

When evaluating the nursing research committee, check whether the committee is centralized or decentralized. Centralized committees usually have one committee in which all research interests are addressed. Decentralized committees have subgroups, usually by practice specialty, that communicate with a central committee. Whether committees are centralized or decentralized, their authority and credibility depend on group efforts and not the qualities of the individual members.

Purposes of the nursing research committee include development of a research mission or agenda, reviewing requests to conduct research, establishing policies and procedures for research in the clinical setting, providing educational programs concerning research, and maintaining records of research projects completed and in progress.[18] Guidelines should exist on how proposals should be submitted to the committee, how the committee interfaces with the IRB, and responsibilities of members.[18,22,23]

The strength of the committee is built on the committee's knowledge and interest in research,

effective written and verbal communication skills, and commitment to use research in practice.[23] The CC-CNS planning to conduct research should seek early membership in formal research committees by contacting members and the chair of the committee. Membership not only provides an avenue for networking and learning, but also increases the credibility of the CC-CNS as researcher. The nursing research committee can also benefit by the membership of the CC-CNS.

Finally, assess whether market factors exist that support the development of a systematic program of research.[19] For example, the CC-CNS in cardiovascular nursing discovers that the organization has decided to develop a program to provide implantation of automatic implantable cardioverter defibrillators (AICDs). Certainly this offers unique opportunities for the CC-CNS for a variety of research activities. Possible research activities could include standards development based on existing research (utilization), education of staff (dissemination), and development of evaluation of care protocols on patient outcomes (generation).

Human Resources Assessment

Assessment of human factors is necessary in any evaluation of the research environment. First, the CC-CNS must consider the case mix in the critical care unit. Case mix characteristics can be determined by examining unit and division quality assessment and improvement records. What are the common admission diagnoses and average length of stay? Acuity information can also be helpful in determining patient population characteristics and the intensity of nursing care required. This information will be necessary to assess whether adequate sample size can be obtained if the intended research examines a specified population.[13]

The CC-CNS must also consider the care delivery model used in the critical care unit. Is the care model primary (in which the only caregiver is a nurse) or segmented (in which a mix of caregivers provides services)? Consider also if staffing in the unit is adequate. If the unit has persistent short staffing or the majority of staff members are novice nurses, involving staff in the research process will be difficult but possible. Whereas patient characteristics of diagnosis, acuity, and length of stay will impact the choice of research activities by the CC-CNS, care models, staffing factors, and available patient populations will affect the feasibility of the research project.

Staff knowledge of and experience with the research process are important factors as well. These factors are difficult but not impossible to assess. Depending on the number of staff members, data can be obtained through informal discussion, open meetings, or questionnaires to all or a sample of individuals.[19]

A survey of staff should be designed to provide the CC-CNS data on perceived support of research in the clinical area, research needs and interests, educational preparation, past research activities, and expectations of clinical research. Surveying management as well as all levels of the clinical ladder is necessary to obtain an accurate assessment. Particularly important is to determine the extent to which nursing administration supports staff participation in clinical research and if staff members desire participation in the research process.[19,25]

Of all the methods, questionnaires yield the most substantive information. A helpful text that describes questionnaire development options, scaling, and formatting is Mueller's *Measuring Social Attitudes*.[26]

Access to university faculty or a doctorally prepared nurse with experience in conducting research is certainly a favorable factor.[18,27] Assess whether the organization has a formal or an informal relationship with a university. If a formal relationship does not exist, the CC-CNS can develop relationships with faculty through planned meetings, development of research groups with faculty interested in clinical research, or membership in organizations such as Sigma Theta Tau. University faculty members are generally eager to establish collaborative research relationships with a CC-CNS. This professional relationship is a powerful one in generating relevant research, since each person brings unique resources to the relationship.[27]

Another resource is the *Sigma Theta Tau Directory of Nurse Researchers*. This directory contains names, addresses, and research interests of hundreds of nurse researchers and can be obtained through the national office. The address is Sigma Theta Tau, 1100 Waterway Blvd., Indianapolis, IN 46202.

Finally, the CC-CNS must assess the availability of support services. The importance of having accessible word processing, copying, and data management services cannot be underestimated. Although seemingly insignificant compared to organizational and human factors, they are necessary, and in some organizations, the CC-CNS will have to negotiate with nursing administration to obtain the necessary services.[18,19,28]

Technical Support Assessment

Evaluation of available technical supports is the least difficult part of assessing the research environment. First, determine if space is available for meetings and storage of information and data.[18] Having a designated area within the unit or organization available for researchers to meet and store data, references, or equipment helps in legitimizing nursing research in the organization or in the critical care unit.

Identifying available statistical services is essential before any research project is planned.[28,29] Statistical consultations should be obtained before data collection, at the midpoint of data collection, at the end of data collection, and during analysis of data. Statistical services are most likely available through any university. Faculty can also assist in choosing appropriate statistical packages. The key in choosing the best statistical program is well-defined variables for study. Also, assess what statistical programs are available within the organization. Programs such as D-base and Lotus are often available in health care organizations and are very useful for data management. It is wise for the CC-CNS intending to conduct research to develop a relationship with the statistical services provider early to facilitate the process of future consultations.

Library resources are particularly important. Find out what periodicals are available and whether computerized data base services are accessible. Obtain from the librarian what services are available for researchers and costs. Some libraries will obtain articles for a fee.

The CC-CNS should be aware of what equipment is used in the critical care unit to obtain biophysical measures. Assess the feasibility of available equipment's use in research. It is appropriate for the CC-CNS to meet with biomedical services personnel and vendors to discuss future research possibilities. They can provide valuable information for research planning.

Nearly all organizations have designated persons or departments to manage extramural funding. Find out who in the organization manages external funding and the extent of assistance available such as locating funding and grant application assistance. Finally, do not forget to look outside the formal organization for supports. Sigma Theta Tau, AACN, the American Nurses' Foundation, and hospital consortium groups can all help the CC-CNS in research activities. These groups offer financial support, feedback, and networking opportunities.[27] They also offer an excellent medium to share research ideas and findings.

Table 13–3 summarizes factors the CC-CNS should consider when assessing the research environment. The questions provided are not exhaustive but do provide a framework to assess both the positive and negative aspects of the research environment.

Creating a Climate for Research

The CC-CNS's attitude toward research is a powerful influence and affects perceptions of administration and staff. Enthusiasm for nursing and nursing research is a powerful influence in promoting participation in the process. If staff members sense that the CC-CNS dislikes research or perceives little benefit from research, they will be less likely to support research in the critical care area.[30,31]

The CC-CNS must dispel any ivory tower perceptions of researchers by participating in every aspect of the research process and involving staff in all areas as well.[30] Consider the following example.

A CC-CNS decides to measure predischarge anxiety of patients moving from ICU to a stepdown unit. The CC-CNS receives approval for the proposal and subsequently meets with nursing staff. The CC-CNS informs the staff of the study and requests staff to provide tools before discharge to subjects who have consented to participate. Staff members are instructed to return the tool to a designated box on the unit. They are not asked to give feedback concerning the proposal, nor are they asked to present perceived problems of administering the tool in the ICU. Subsequently, the CC-CNS is not seen for 3 weeks after the designated start date for the study. The CC-CNS returns to obtain completed tools and wonders why only two surveys have been completed.

Designing a project without considering the demands of the protocol on the clinical site and without opportunities for participants' feedback will negatively impact the research process, since research activities will be perceived as another layer of work added to clinical responsibilities.[32] If the CC-CNS is not visible and accessible for staff during the research process, there will be greater numbers of errors and considerable animosity toward the CC-CNS and the research project. Attention by the CC-CNS to all phases of the research process will create a perception that the research is important and worthwhile.[31]

Finally, the CC-CNS must be politically astute to work effectively within the power structures of the organization.[30] To facilitate nursing research in the critical care area, it is necessary to have favorable and supportive relationships with nursing, medicine, and allied health services. Research is too complex to be done alone.[33]

Legitimizing Research in Critical Care

Legitimizing research in critical care depends on early articulation of what research can and cannot do. Research goals are not necessarily concomitant with clinical goals, which are usually more immediate in nature.[30] Research takes time, which is problematic, since legitimization depends on producing results; and even producing research results may not legitimize research efforts since the data may not be desired data or it may not be clearly interpretable.[30]

Once assessment of the research environment is completed, the CC-CNS should set clear goals concerning research activities. Flexible, realistic goals based on practical timetables will foster legitimization in the critical care area. Goals should be based on staff and administrative feedback and evaluation once completed. A very helpful method is to post for staff the projected research goals for the year and request feedback. Another technique is the Delphi technique in which group consensus is achieved through successive rounds of questionnaires. The first round focuses on obtaining topics for research, and subsequent rounds focus on rating the importance of the proposed topics. This technique is attractive in that staff identities are protected.[34] In this way, all participants in the critical

TABLE 13-3 Assessment of Organizational, Human, and Support Factors Affecting Clinical Nursing Research

Factor	Questions
Organizational	Does the organizational mission support research activity?
	What organizational activities potentially promote or limit clinical research?
	Does the philosophy of the division of nursing support research in nursing?
	What is the organization's history of research?
	Is there an organizational body to approve and monitor research projects (e.g., IRB, nursing research committee)?
	Is the nursing research committee centralized or decentralized?
	What is the relationship between nursing quality assurance and nursing research?
	Do market factors exist that support a systematic program of research?
Human	What is the case mix in the critical care units?
	What is the care delivery model in the critical care units?
	What are the nursing staff members' experiences in clinical research?
	Do investigators have adequate educational background, experience, and interest in clinical nursing research?
	Does nursing administration support nursing staff participation in clinical research?
	Is there support from medicine and allied health disciplines for nursing or multidisciplinary research?
	Is there access to university faculty for consultation and collaborative research?
	Is secretarial support available?
Technical	Is space available for meetings and storage of data records?
	What resources are available for statistical analysis?
	What equipment is available in the clinical areas for research requiring biologic measures?
	What library resources are available (e.g., periodicals, computer data bases)?
	What department in the organization manages extramural funding?
	Who are the local professional nursing organizations (e.g., AACN, Sigma Theta Tau)?

care unit clearly know what will be done in the following year. Staff can also be asked to sign up for projects of interest.

A unit-based research interest group is a powerful medium to develop goals and integrate research activities into the critical care area.[2] The chair of such a committee may be a CC-CNS or staff nurse mentored by the CNS. The committee can be structured depending on the needs of the unit, research experience of members, and goals of planned research activities. The best time to develop a research interest group is after evaluation of the research environment, since the results can be used to set goals and plan activities.

Membership should be open to all interested nurses in critical care including staff nurses, educators, managers, and faculty. In some groups other disciplines such as medicine and allied health may also be members.[32] A good method to begin is to schedule open meetings close to the critical

care area at times that all staff members can attend. Invite all persons to attend who are interested in research in critical care. This forum provides a means to find nurses who have similar research values and interests and permits the critical care area to develop a research consciousness.[32] Initial meetings should focus on members' interests and expectations and then sharing of the results of the CC-CNS's assessment of the research climate. After several meetings, goals for the group, responsibilities of members, and meeting times can be planned for the coming year. The group should meet at least monthly. The group's activities should be evaluated yearly.

The purposes of research interest groups vary depending on membership and experience of the group. A group may decide to focus on utilization activities (see Chapter 14). Purposes of this group may then include literature reviews related to nursing interventions, continuous quality improvement issues, or standards of practice.[2,23] Another focus a group may choose is staff education regarding research topics in critical care nursing or dissemination activities. The group may plan a research day or a poster presentation concerning research methods or a specific area of research such as family needs or suctioning.[35] The possibilities are unlimited.

Groups with members who have adequate education and experience in research may decide to focus on conducting research or generation activities. The research interest group provides an excellent medium to foster collaborative research that will be explored later in this chapter. Whatever activities are chosen by the group, they should be congruent with members' knowledge, experience, and goals.

Meetings should be held at a designated time, preferably in the same location. The agenda should be mailed to all members 1 week before the meeting, and minutes summarizing the meeting should be reviewed at each subsequent meeting. It is also helpful to post meeting minutes for nonparticipating staff so that they are aware of research activities taking place in the area. This is a way to recruit future members.[13] An excellent text that presents additional strategies to develop practice setting research groups is Stetler's *Nursing Research in a Service Setting*.[36]

Creating a climate that is conducive to research depends on an accurate assessment of the research environment, involving staff and management in goal setting and research activities, and knowledge that research activities take time. The remainder of this chapter explores methods the CC-CNS can use to identify clinical topics for research activities, locate related literature, and prepare proposals and other related research activities.

CONDUCT OF RESEARCH IN CRITICAL CARE
Clinical Problem Identification

Identification of clinical problems for research activities is not easy. The complexity of critical care practice makes it difficult to decide which problem area to research first.[37] The best advice is to limit the focus of concern as much as possible. Too often areas are chosen for research that are too large and too complex, which results in frustration and failure to complete the research activity. For example, a research committee and CC-CNS de-

cide to explore possible outcomes of a family support group led by an ICU nurse that is held weekly for family members of critically ill patients. After several meetings, committee members decide many possible variables could be assessed such as anxiety, stress, and concerns with nursing care. Members find multiple tools that potentially measure the variables of interest, and the committee finds that so many variables and tools are identified that potential subjects would be saturated if all variables of interest were measured. The committee wisely decides to focus on one variable: concerns with nursing care. Narrowing the focus of study also will facilitate data management and analysis and will permit an in-depth examination of the variable of interest.

Patient care problems identified by staff should be the starting point. Identification of problems for research can be accomplished through various processes. Brainstorming with peers or in a research interest group meeting is a good place to start. What do staff members perceive are the problems in practice? Problems could be identified related to patient care, procedures, or families.[38,39] Whatever topic is chosen, it must be perceived as significant and worthwhile to maintain interest over the life of the project.[13]

The literature is another excellent source. A review of the literature can help the CC-CNS define a problem area and place the problem in perspective. No research activity should be attempted unless a literature review is completed in the problem area. The CC-CNS should pay particular attention to studies previously done. The CC-CNS may wish to replicate a study that can result in less time spent for proposal preparation and perhaps promote greater generalization of findings in the problem area.[12,33,40-42] A good review of the literature not only will assist the CC-CNS in defining the problem area but also will help the CC-CNS make decisions concerning the purpose of the research activity, defining the variables of concern and design, sampling, and instrumentation issues.[42]

Another helpful source to identify possible research problems is awareness of research priorities designated by the AACN.[14] Attending national, regional, or local professional meetings where research is presented is also an excellent way to increase awareness of what has been done and what is being done in the problem area. Even if the CC-

CNS cannot attend, the CC-CNS can request from AACN or another sponsoring organization copies of abstracts and written copies of proceedings.

Personally contacting a researcher in the problem area can help as well. Nearly all published research or proceedings from meetings have addresses listed where researchers can be contacted. Before contacting the researcher, have specific questions ready and be familiar with what has been published. Generally, researchers are eager for contact with clinicians interested in the same problem area and can give valuable advice on how to approach a problem.

Reviewing the Literature

The most common question associated with a review of the literature is, "Where do I start?" First, assess library resources. This includes available periodicals, journals, and computerized data bases. Computerized data bases have many advantages over printed indices. They are timesaving and current, and they give more options for searching the literature in that one can search by subject, journal name, publication year, or specific concepts.[43] Table 13–4 lists printed indices and Table 13–5

lists computerized data bases the CC-CNS can use.[42-44] Costs vary for computerized data base searches, and the librarian can suggest ways to reduce costs such as limiting the search to a particular period or a specific number of journals. Check with the librarian about what data bases are accessible and if they can be accessed through CD-ROM. A short class is generally required to learn how to search a particular data base through CD-ROM, and once this class is completed, the CC-CNS can search the literature with minimal expense.[44] Finally, consider the costs and benefits of purchasing access to a computerized data base for the nursing department.

Several excellent resources are available that give practical information on locating data in both printed indices and computerized data bases and how to manage information found:

1. *A Basic Guide to On-Line Information Systems for Health Care Professionals* by RG Albright[45]
2. *Information Sources for Nursing: A Guide* by J Shockley[46]
3. *Library Research Guide to Nursing* by K Strauch, R Linton, and C Cohen[44]

TABLE 13–4 Printed Indices for Review of Literature

Title (City, Organization)	Focus
Social Sciences Citation Index (SSCI), 1961-present (Philadelphia, Institute for Scientific Information)	Indexes 2500 social science journals
Psychological Abstracts, 1927-present (Washington, D.C., American Psychological Association)	Indexes 1400 periodicals on psychology and psychologic topics in nursing and medicine
Social Sciences Index (SSI), 1974-present (New York, Wilson)	Indexes 260 journals in all social sciences including sociology, law, social service, and public policy
Cumulative Index to Nursing and Allied Health Literature (CINAHL), 1961-present (Glendale, Adventist Medical Center Publication Services)	Indexes 300 nursing, allied health, biomedical, social, business, education, and popular literature; also indexes American Nurses' Association (ANA) and National League for Nursing (NLN) publications
International Nursing Index, 1966-present (New York, *American Journal of Nursing*)	Indexes 200 nursing journals and related articles in *Index Medicus*
Index Medicus, 1960-present (Bethesda, Md., National Library of Medicine)	Indexes 2600 journals in all languages
Abridged Index Medicus, 1970-present (Bethesda, Md., National Library of Medicine)	Indexes 100 journals; use for information not found in nursing literature
Hospital Literature Index, 1955-present (Chicago, American Hospital Association)	Indexes English language journals only

Data from Strauch K, Linton R, Cohen C: *Library research guide to nursing,* Ann Arbor, Mich, 1989, Pierian Press.

TABLE 13–5 Computerized Data Bases for Review of Literature

Data Base	Literature Accessed
Medline	Medical literature, *International Nursing Index,* and *Index Medicus*
Nursing and Allied Health	*Cumulative Index to Nursing and Allied Health Literature* (CINAHL)
Psychinfo	*Psychological Abstracts*
Social Scisearch	*Social Sciences Citation Index*
ERIC	Current index to journals in education and resources in education
Cambridge Compact	CO-ROM program with medical and nursing literature

Data from Hutchinson,[42] Sinclair,[43] and Strauch et al.[44]

Another resource is a telephone service available to AACN members for a nominal fee. The service, called "STAT Reference Service," is operated by the Glendale Adventist Medical Center Library. AACN members receives a printout of up to 35 citations on a requested topic and information on how to request copies of articles. Questions concerning the service can be directed to 1-800-359-STAT, 9 to 5 PM (Pacific time) Monday through Thursday and Friday 9 to 3 PM (Pacific time).

Everyone organizes information differently. A practical way to organize related literature is to create a summary on 5 × 7 inch or larger index cards. The card should contain the title of the article, author, data, and journal name. Include a brief summary of the purpose, variables of study, design, sample, instruments, results, and an overall evaluation of the paper. When needed, the cards can be accessed quickly for information. This will save money in copying multiple articles, and cards are more manageable than large numbers of copied articles.

Developing Research Questions

A problem well stated is a problem half solved.
Charles F. Kettering

A good review of the literature should yield a new perspective of the problem selected for research. What is known and what is not known about the problem are the key questions to ask *before* designing any research question.

Research design emerges from the research question; therefore the question is the foundation of the research proposal. Questions that begin with "what" generally result in exploratory or descriptive research designs, whereas "when" results in associational or correlational designs. Interventional or experimental designs are related to "what would happen if" type of questions. Finally, if one asks, "How can I make a particular event happen?" prescription testing designs usually result.[41,42,47] Therefore the CC-CNS should word research questions carefully. Particularly important will be specifically defining the variables for study and how they will be measured. Unless this is done, subsequent research activities will be difficult.

Preparing the Research Proposal

A research proposal is a written summary of what the researcher plans to do and why. The proposal is a tool that helps the CC-CNS to plan, implement, and report the intended research.[41] Although proposal formats vary among organizations, the critical elements for evaluation are the same. The research should have scientifically sound design, which includes valid and reliable instruments to measure the variables of interest. There also must be evidence of protection of human subjects.[20] The proposed research must not be incongruent with established policies and procedures of the organization.[13] Before beginning to write the research proposal, obtain guidelines from the organizational IRB. Particularly helpful is to also contact a member of the organizational IRB for assistance and advice during proposal preparation.[20,48]

The primary purpose of IRB review of any research proposal is to ensure protection of human subjects, the basis of which is informed consent.[3] Informed consent is based on the rights of human subjects: the right not to be harmed, the right of self-determination, the right to privacy, and the right to obtain services.[41] Ten required elements for informed consent must be addressed in any proposal (Table 13–6).[3,20,23,41,49]

Achieving informed consent in vulnerable populations such as the critically ill may be a challenge for the CC-CNS. Implicit in informed consent is the autonomy of the subject, but factors associated

TABLE 13–6 Required Elements for Informed Consent

1. Statement of purpose, procedure, and duration of the study
2. Description of emotional and physical risks and discomfort
3. Description of benefits for subject and researcher
4. Description of alternatives that might benefit the subject
5. Protection of privacy: how confidentiality will be assured
6. Statement of compensation for participation or if injury occurs
7. Who can be contacted for questions and who will monitor the safety of subjects
8. Assurance that participation is voluntary and no penalty exists for refusal to participate and that withdrawal can occur anytime after consent is given
9. How informed consent will be documented and how records will be maintained
10. Participation in the protocol does not interfere with treatment

Data from Parker et al.,[3] Tething,[20] Lieske,[23] Seaman,[41] and Lawson.[49]

with critical illness can limit autonomy. The subject's physical, social, and psychologic status can dependence on the researcher for information to make a decision on participation limit autonomy. The illness may interfere with the subject's abilities to evaluate the risks and benefits of participation in research. Subjects may give consent just to please caregivers and to decrease a sense of vulnerability.[3,50] Therefore the CC-CNS researcher must make sure the 10 elements of informed consent are met for each subject. Statements of informed consent must be clear, simple, easy to understand, and at an appropriate reading level. If the CC-CNS believes that the subject is not giving informed consent for any reason or if the subject experiences negative consequences, the CC-CNS must remove the subject from the study immediately.[22]

Assessment and recruitment of subjects for research are affected not only by informed consent issues but also by the nature of the problem being studied. The more common the problem and the less stringent the criteria for subject selection, the greater the number of subjects that will be available. The more unique the problem or if there are multiple numbers of measures, the fewer the number of subjects that will be available. When possible, consent should be requested in advance. For example, if a study is designed to compare noninvasive and invasive methods of assessing cardiac output in cardiovascular surgery patients, informed consent could be requested in advance during preoperative teaching rather than seeking consent from subjects or families after surgery. Researchers generally underestimate the time needed to recruit subjects because of failure to address the impact of consent and design issues.[48] As a result, researchers obtain an insufficient number of subjects, which negatively impacts the results of the study.[51]

Finally, the CC-CNS should consider the element of competing research projects in the critical care area.[48] Multiple simultaneous studies of one patient population are never appropriate. It is stressful for patients and for staff, and it is nearly impossible to monitor the impact of the individual research projects. This element should be addressed in the proposal in that the CC-CNS should specify the time period subjects will be approached for consent and over what time period the proposal will be implemented.

Design and Methods Considerations

The research design presented in the proposal must be congruent with the research question, and the methods of data collection must be clinically realistic.[3,13] Even if the proposed methods are feasible, implementation and control of the research protocol may be compounded by the generally short length of stay in critical care units, consent issues previously presented, and lack of control over variables in the clinical setting.[6,9,52] Both the nature of the question and review of the literature will influence the type of design chosen.

The research design is defined as the plan, structure, and strategy of the investigation.[53] Choices concerning the sample, instruments, procedures, and data analysis are influenced by the choice of design for the study.

Depending on the nature of the question, the CC-CNS should consider using a *retrospective* design. This design is good for descriptive studies, particularly ones that address outcomes of nursing interventions. Multiple data sources can be used, including the clinical record, staff, and patients. Generally, accessing data is not time bound, but remember that variables not present or assessed in the clinical record may have actually impacted outcomes, which is a threat to validity in this design. *Concurrent designs* are helpful to describe an ongoing situation and may yield more accurate information than retrospective designs, but concurrent designs are time bound and affected by multiple variables in the clinical setting such as caregivers, familiarity with the research protocol, scheduled and unscheduled procedures or tests, subject characteristics, and availability of the researcher. *Prospective designs* are longitudinal in nature and good for correlational research studies examining patient outcomes. In a prospective design, one can generally use a broader range of questions, but data collection must be timed to accurately reflect changes. This design is the most difficult to implement in the critical care setting related to length of stay and variable acuity issues.[3,6]

Descriptive studies are exploratory in nature and are useful when little is known about a particular phenomenon. Correlational studies are useful to evaluate possible relationships among variables. True experimental designs require manipulation of an independent variable, random assignment to an experimental or control group, and use of a control group for comparison. When it is not possible to meet the three requirements of true experimental design, the study is considered quasiexperimental.[53]

Qualitative designs are useful when research questions focus on the meaning or subjective experience of an event.[54] Some qualitative approaches include phenomenologic grounded theory and ethnography. These approaches can also provide a basis for future quantitative research by identifying important aspects of a particular phenomenon or experience.

Whatever design is chosen, a research protocol must be developed for the design and methods section of a clinical research proposal. The protocol should list sequentially what exactly happens and in what order before and after consent is obtained. The protocol should describe who will be approached for consent, who will obtain informed consent, who will collect data, the sequence of data collection, and what will happen to data after collection. The protocol must also describe any potential events that may affect data collection and exactly how each event will be addressed. For example, you are studying perceptions of stress in stable myocardial infarction subjects in the coronary care unit. You decide only to approach subjects who have been pain free for 48 hours, are not receiving narcotics, and have no evidence of complications such as heart failure. Based on the population characteristics of the myocardial infarction patient, you must address in the proposal what you would do in the event that the subject begins having chest pain or an arrhythmia. An appropriate response would be that data collection would be stopped and the primary nurse would be notified immediately. In summary, the population of study characteristics must be carefully considered and any potentially intervening variables must be addressed in the protocol. A good rule to follow is to expect all possible responses or events and account for them in the research protocol.[55]

Instrumentation Issues

Selection of instruments is a critical aspect when preparing the research proposal. Depending on the variables of interest, measures may be psychosocial or biophysical. Whatever instrument is selected, the CC-CNS should evaluate it carefully. Criteria to evaluate psychosocial instruments will be presented first followed by considerations in selection of biophysical measures.

Psychosocial Instruments

Psychosocial instruments measure complex phenomena of psychologic characteristics or social behaviors. Methods to measure psychologic phenomena include observation, interviews, and questionnaires.

Selection of a psychosocial measure is a difficult process when the population of interest is critically ill persons. Clear definition of the variable to be measured is essential. Written questionnaires offer ease in coding and management of data but may be difficult for the critically ill subject to complete. The subject's illness, treatment, visual problems, anxiety, or shortened attention span will all affect the reliability of the instrument. Selection of a structured or semistructured interview is attractive in that it is possible to obtain richer data and it affords the subject an opportunity to describe the illness experience, but this method is time consuming and data obtained are difficult to analyze and interpret. Observation techniques may be chosen to describe a particular phenomenon. The problem with observation techniques involves the bias of a single observer and the reliability issues concerning use of multiple observers.[3]

Whatever choice the CC-CNS makes, it is better to use multiple measures of the variable of interest rather than a single measure to decrease bias and to obtain a more accurate representation of the phenomenon of interest. For example, a CC-CNS decides to measure perceptions of pain in postoperative open heart surgery patients before and after a biofeedback protocol. Rather than using only one measure of pain (e.g., a 10-item questionnaire), the CC-CNS decides to also use a visual analog scale. Use of both measures will enable the CC-CNS to obtain a multidimensional perspective of the phenomena of interest.

Existing measures for the variable of interest can be found in several areas. A primary source is the literature in the area of interest. Although instruments are rarely presented in totality in a research report, the CC-CNS can contact the researcher and request a copy of the instrument for evaluation. Another source is published texts of psychosocial instruments. Table 13–7 describes resources the CC-CNS can use to locate psychosocial instruments.[56] The Frank-Stromborg text[57] is particularly helpful in that the described instruments measure phenomena specific to nursing such as functional state, self-care, pain, dyspnea, skin integrity, and mental status. This text provides a summary of each instrument that includes reliability and validity characteristics and how the tool has been used in research. Other sources to locate instruments include textbooks, peers, and research conferences.[58]

When evaluating psychosocial instruments for use in research, the CC-CNS has many factors to evaluate. First, how are the variables measured defined by the author, or does the tool measure the variables you intend to study? Second, consider the nature of the measure or the type of data obtained by the tool. Third, consider first the instrument's appropriateness for use in the critically ill population. Very few instruments measure psychosocial phenomena in the critically ill population, since the majority of available instruments have been de-

TABLE 13–7 Resources for Psychosocial Instruments

1. *Annual Review of Nursing Research,* New York, 1983-1988, Springer Publishing Co.
2. Reeder LG, Ramacher LG, Gorelink S: *Handbook of scales and indices of health behavior,* Pacific Palisades, Calif, 1976, Good Year Publishing Co.
3. Ward MJ, Linderman CA: *Instruments for measuring nursing practice & health care variables,* vols 1 and 2, DHEW (HRA-78-53 & 54), Washington, DC, 1978, US Government Printing Office.
4. Mitchell MJ, editor: *The 9th mental measurement yearbook,* Lincoln, 1985, University of Nebraska Press.
5. Mitchell MJ, editor: *Tests in print 3,* Lincoln, 1983, University of Nebraska Press.
6. Frank-Stromberg M, editor: *Instruments for clinical nursing research,* Norwalk, Conn, 1988, Appleton & Lange.

Data from McLaughlin FE, Marascuilio LA: *Advanced nursing and health care research quantification approaches,* Philadelphia, 1990, WB Saunders Co.

veloped in populations other than the critically ill. However, this does not mean the tools cannot be used in critical care research. It is necessary to assess the instrument's psychometric properties of reliability and validity in the critically ill population.

Table 13–8 describes elements the CC-CNS should consider before selecting a tool.[58-61] Using the checklist can help the CC-CNS make a better decision concerning instrument selection. Once the CC-CNS decides to use a particular instrument, permission must be obtained. Generally, authors of instruments are delighted to give permission. The CC-CNS should write a short letter to the author requesting permission to use the tool. In the letter, briefly describe the purpose of the study. It is appropriate to ask the author for recent information concerning the tool. Be aware that the author may place conditions on the use of the tool, and if this occurs, the CC-CNS is obligated to fulfill those conditions in the project. A condition the author may request could be limits on copying of the tool, requiring purchase of tools from a publisher, or requiring copies of data obtained for future psychometric evaluation.[59]

TABLE 13–8 Evaluation Checklist for Psychosocial Instruments

1. What variable does the instrument purport to measure?
2. What is the level of measurement (nominal, ordinal, interval, or rational data)?
3. What is the purpose of the tool (description, screening, diagnosis, or prediction)?
4. Who is the intended population for use?
5. What type of response is sought from the subject (judgment, knowledge, affect, feeling, or preference)?
6. How does the tool reflect the variable of interest?
7. Do the items of the tool reflect the variable of interest?
8. What is the reported reliability of the instrument (stability, equivalence, or internal consistency)?
9. What are the reported validity measures (face, content, criterion, construct)?
10. What are the associated costs in using the instrument?
11. Can permission be secured to use the tool?
12. What are the author's qualifications related to the development of the tool?

Data from Jacobson,[59] Larochelle,[60] Rempusheski,[61] and Waltz, Strickland, and Lenz.[58]

The difficulty encountered in locating appropriate, reliable, and valid instruments may result in the temptation to develop one's own instrument. This choice is strongly discouraged for several reasons. Instrument development is a research activity in and of itself and not a part of a research project. Instrument development takes much time related to theory and item development, scaling and scoring issues, and establishing psychometric properties of reliability and validity. Very few CC-CNS positions allocate the time necessary to complete such a project. The better choice is to choose existing measures and assist doctorally prepared researchers in the development of future measures.

Biophysical Measures

Biophysical instruments measure information that cannot be ascertained by the five senses.[62,63] They are attractive measures in that they are vigilant and objective and do not become distracted or bored.[64] Variables that can be detected with biomedical instruments include electrical potentials, pressure, mechanical waves, temperature, and gases.[63]

Biophysical instruments measure a physiologic event by changing or conditioning signals so that they can be seen as output. The output may be in the form of scatter plots, graphs, waveforms, numbers, or sounds. Data may be stored as photographs, as written notations, or on a computer disk.[63,64] Data may be obtained invasively or noninvasively.

Selection of biophysical instruments should be done in collaboration with a biomedical engineer. Only then can instruments be chosen that are appropriate to measure the variable of interest. Additional sources of information concerning biophysical measures can be found in instrumentation texts, review articles, published research, equipment catalogs, and exhibits at professional meetings.[62]

The CC-CNS should evaluate a biophysical instrument in relation to how well the measure reflects the variable of interest. Factors to consider are the accuracy, precision, and amount of error in the measure. Consider also the availability of the equipment, the level of data obtained, and the cost associated with use.[62]

Whatever instrument is chosen, it must measure what it is designed to measure. In the research proposal the sensitivity or the ability to detect change must be reported as well as the range of measures that can be ascertained.[65] The CC-CNS must also describe the procedures that will be used and report the available safety information.

Improper use, failure to calibrate, failure to follow established procedures, and clerical error in reporting results are the most common reasons for unreliable or invalid biophysical measures.[59,64,65] Other factors include noise, signal drift, and failure to let the equipment warm up. Development of a protocol that describes calibration procedures and exactly how biophysical data will be collected will improve the accuracy of the measurement.

Remember that most biophysical instruments used in the clinical setting usually do not provide real-time data. Data such as heart rates, blood pressures, or pulmonary artery pressures are reported as average values computed over a fixed time, such as 6 seconds. This characteristic will affect data analysis and interpretation of results, particularly in intervention studies.

Finally, increasing numbers of personal computer–based (PC) packages can be used to record and store real-time biophysical measures. The biomedical engineer can help the CC-CNS locate equipment that can interface with preexisting biophysical instruments. As more PC packages become available, it will be easier to measure and interpret biophysical data in the future.

Analysis of Results

Every research proposal must describe how the results will be analyzed. Before presenting statistical packages available to aid in the analysis of data, some theoretic considerations must be addressed.

The CC-CNS must make sure any findings are interpreted in terms of clinical significance as well as statistical significance. Statistically significant results are not necessarily clinically relevant. The CC-CNS should identify any rival or alternative explanations for results that may not be apparent to explain findings.[9]

The CC-CNS must also consider in the interpretation of findings interactions of all possible intervening variables. This is particularly important in patient outcome research. Research concerning patient outcomes in critical illness is an attractive subject for CC-CNS researchers, but it is deceptive in its apparent simplicity.[66] Patient outcomes can be operationalized in measures of morbidity, mortality, physical, or psychologic indices, but the criteria for each of these outcomes must be exact. The CC-CNS must remember that patient outcomes are influenced by treatment, iatrogenic complications, environmental conditions, subject characteristics, care providers, and the interaction of all these variables.[66,67]

Interpretation of findings will be based in part on the quality of the data. If the data collected are incomplete, missing, or coded incorrectly, the results will be suspect. Therefore the integrity of the research protocol must be maintained throughout the study. The CC-CNS can build into the research protocol methods to monitor the quality of the data. For example, data collection forms could be checked for completeness daily or weekly. Never wait till the conclusion of the protocol to find out that data are missing. Coding of data from data collection forms requires an exact protocol as well. The coding protocol should be developed before data collection and tested for accuracy.[68]

The CC-CNS should consult with the statistician during the research protocol preparation. The value of preplanning the analysis cannot be overstated. The best time for the consultation is after the variables for study have been defined and potential instruments have been chosen. This will enable the statistician to help you decide which instruments to use and suggest methods to establish reliability of the tool's use in the critically ill population. Statisticians can be accessed through university faculty, university research centers, or private consulting firms found in the telephone directory.[69]

A statistician can help the CC-CNS determine the number of subjects needed and provide guidance for the coding of acquired data. During the consultation, statistical tests for analyses should be chosen and an estimate of costs should be provided. Costs should reflect charges for program entry, cleaning data, running sequential analysis, printouts, storage of data, and consultation fees.[70]

Mainframe statistical packages most commonly used for analysis include (1) Statistical Analysis System (SAS), (2) Statistical Package for Social Sciences (SPSS), and (3) Biomedical Data Programs (BMDP). PC statistical analysis packages, such as CRUNCH, MINITAB, or SYSTAT, are available.[68] For further information regarding statistical packages and software options, consult the chapter titled "Computers and Data Processing in Nursing Research" in Wilson's *Research in Nursing*.[71]

Pilot Studies

A pilot study is a trial run of a research protocol. It can test the feasibility of the proposed methods and instruments in the critical care setting and can help the CC-CNS revise the research protocol accordingly. A pilot study can also identify hidden costs and unforeseen problems in implementing the protocol, coding, and analysis procedures.[72]

During pilot studies, it is helpful to also interview the participants in the research process. Subjects and staff members can report valuable subjective information useful in revising the research protocol, particularly in reference to the recruitment of subjects, instruments, and data collection forms. The pilot study is also valuable in assisting the CC-CNS to determine a time line for the study.

Funding Research

Part of planning any research activity is consideration of associated costs. The success of any project depends on accounting for expenses, particularly the hidden costs. Only when costs have been specified for the project can the CC-CNS begin to seek funding.

Table 13–9 describes costs the CC-CNS should account for, and Table 13–10 gives a sample budget. Total costs will depend on the number of subjects required and the projected time line for the study. Never overestimate associated costs. Funding agencies can detect inflated estimates when monies are requested. When estimating costs, also write a list of what the organization contributes to the research process such as a library, office space, secretarial support, or clinical access.[73]

Sources for funding research include private foundations, corporations, nursing specialty organizations, or the federal government. AACN has a brochure, "Grants in Support of Research," that describes funding opportunities for the novice or expert researcher and can be obtained from the Department of Research at the national office in Aliso Viejo, California. Grant applications can also be obtained from AACN. Also consider seeking

funding from the American Heart Association, the American Lung Association, or the American Cancer Society. Whatever source is used, you must follow the funding agency's request guidelines exactly. Be open-minded about offers of support other than monies. Often agencies can offer equipment or other resources (e.g., preparation of presentation media) free for use in research.

The crucial element in requesting support is convincing the funding agency that you can do the research. This can be accomplished by presenting your curriculum vitae and a history of previous work done in the problem area. The most powerful evidence for the agency is results of a pilot study in the problem area.[73]

When presenting your case for funding, describe exactly the purpose of the research, the problem the research will address, and the long-term usefulness of the research.[73] Presenting gaps in previous literature and how your research will address those gaps is helpful as well.

Grant applications fail for a number of reasons (Table 13–11).[73,74] One must also consider that as research becomes more prevalent in nursing, the competition for funds will only increase. The CC-CNS should not become discouraged if the grant application fails. Instead, contact the funding agency and find out what would have made the grant application stronger. Remember that the basis of a sound grant application is a well-written research proposal. Excellent sources for preparing proposals and funding applications are Ogden's *Research Proposals: A Guide to Success*[74] and the AACN's *Writing that Winning Research Proposal*,[75] which can be obtained from the national office.

Collaborative Research

Collaborative research is one of the most desirable strategies for accomplishing the goals of research. Usually more work can be accomplished and a larger program of research can be attempted. Combining different talents and experiences facilitates mentorship of both experienced and novice investigators.[13,24,76,77]

Collaborative relationships often solve problems related to limited resources, particularly time, money, and access to subjects. Collaborative research is more likely to be funded than single investigator studies. In short, a collaborative research

TABLE 13–9 Costs in Funding Research

Personnel Participation	Wages, Benefits, and Insurance
Consultant services	Statistician fees
	Biomedical engineers
	Statistical analysis of data
Nonpersonnel costs	Space
	Rental, lease, or purchase of equipment
	Consumable supplies
	Travel
	Telephones
	Postage
	Mailing and addressing
	Copying and paper supplies
Personnel costs	Salaries

TABLE 13–10 Sample 12-Month Budget (Direct Costs Only)

Personnel	Position Title	Time	Salary ($)	Amount Requested ($)
Statistician	Consultant	6 meetings	50.00/hr	300
Graduate student assistant		10%	12.50/hr	6200
			TOTAL	6500

EQUIPMENT	
Rental SVo₂ monitor and cables	1000

SUPPLIES ($)

Paper = 500.00
Cart = 125.00
Office supplies = 350.00   975

OTHER ($)

Laboratory expenses = 10,000.00
Photocopying = 200.00
Travel = 300.00   15000
                                    TOTAL DIRECT COSTS $23,475.00

effort is a powerful way to overcome the obstacles inherent in clinical research.[33,78]

There are four different types of collaborative relationships: (1) nursing service and nursing education, (2) within and between organizations, (3) researcher and clinician, and (4) multidisciplinary. The combination of academic researcher and practitioner is probably the most powerful in that research is more likely to be funded and the resulting research is more likely to have strong design features and clinical relevance.[9,13,33]

Collaborative research is not without problems. Elements that can undermine the benefits of collaborative research include power, trust, and status issues.[78] Individual visibility is sacrificed in a collaborative relationship in the interest of group goals. Individual competition for rewards and recognition within the group at the expense of group goals may destroy any positive benefit of the collaborative arrangement. Therefore agreement on the purpose, expected benefits, and rules should be established before any research activity is attempted.[76,78]

Before planning the research project, the group should meet and discuss the positive and negative aspects of the collaborative agreement. In the beginning the group should specify responsibilities of members and the conditions for publication and authorship. A person should take responsibility for the role of primary investigator.

Authorship rules vary from group to group. Generally, the order of authorship is related to who takes major responsibility for proposal preparation and writing of the research report. Subsequent authors are listed in the order of their contribution to the paper or project. Some groups decide on listing authors alphabetically following the primary investigator's name. The method chosen by the group must be decided before the research is started. The

TABLE 13–11 Why Grant and Funding Applications Fail

1. The problem is not important.
2. The research will not produce new or useful information.
3. The problem is too complex or too many elements are being investigated at one time.
4. A pilot study has not been done.
5. The design or method is not congruent with the problem.
6. The proposed time schedule for the project is inappropriate.
7. The investigator is poorly trained or inexperienced.
8. The proposal submission guidelines were not followed.
9. The budget for the project is poorly prepared.
10. The literature review was insufficient.

Data from Tornquist and Funk[73] and Odgen.[74]

group must also decide early what will be done if members fail to complete their responsibilities associated with the project. Generally it is acceptable to recognize members in a footnote if they were involved in the planning of the research but did not follow through in the project.[77] A good resource to determine authorship rules is the American Psychological Association's (APA's) *Publication Manual*.[79] This text provides multiple suggestions for determining authorship.

In the event that the collaborative research relationship is multidisciplinary, there are additional considerations. The group should agree early to multiple publications with different primary authors representing each discipline *but* to specify in each paper that the research was part of a larger collaborative project. For example, a CC-CNS is involved in a collaborative project examining weaning from mechanical ventilation in open heart surgery patients. Nursing, medicine, and university faculty members of the research group could all potentially publish papers in their area concerning different aspects of the project. As long as the larger study is recognized in the published works and all the members of the group are recognized in authorship credits, it is appropriate.

Regular meetings of the group and records of the meeting (minutes) are necessary to maintain collaborative relationships. Meeting minutes are a good way to record each member's contribution. In the event that a member has not fulfilled responsibilities, written evidence is available that is more powerful than memory. Since research takes time, records are necessary, because members may forget what they agreed to do in the research project. Minutes also provide members a way to gauge progress as the research progresses.

Dissemination of Results

Communication of research results is certainly one of the benefits of doing research. Sharing results is not only advantageous for the researcher but for the profession as well. Sharing research expands knowledge concerning nursing phenomena, encourages interaction between investigators and colleagues, and provides an opportunity for feedback and constructive criticism.[30,80]

Results can be shared in many formats. Publication of research benefits the writer, the profession, and the patient. Even if the results are not significant or if the CC-CNS discovers that another method would have worked better, the research should be published. Researchers learn from the efforts of other researchers, and the growth of the profession depends on communication of ideas and projects. The research proposal is the foundation of the published article. Although writing research for publication takes time, the foundation for the effort is present that will help the CC-CNS get started. Excellent sources for the CC-CNS publishing research are the AACN's *Writing for Professional Nursing Journals* and *Writing Research Abstracts Successfully,* which can be purchased from the AACN national office.[81,82] These guides offer practical information on how to organize the manuscript and select journals, and they have extensive bibliographies of resources.

Results of research can also be shared in poster or paper presentations at professional meetings. Paper presentation is a more formal method of presenting research and provides opportunities to share results with a greater number of persons at one time than poster presentations, but the informal feedback and discussion associated with poster presentations are valuable. Whatever method is chosen to present results, follow the sponsoring organization's criteria for presentation exactly.

Whether publishing for the first or the tenth time, expect revisions or even rejection. Generally, journal reviewers will provide feedback that can be used to rewrite the paper. Then the paper must be resubmitted multiple times if necessary. Persistence is the key to publishing nursing research.

CASE STUDY

Lori was a newly hired CC-CNS for a surgical ICU in a community hospital. Responsibilities included education of staff, developing and maintaining a quality assessment and improvement program, and developing nursing procedures. The job description also required research activities in the clinical setting.

Lori spent the first 3 months completing an organizational assessment and establishing goals for the year. Based on data collected from the staff surveys, Lori decided that conducting clinical research was not possible in the first year. The staff members were unfamiliar with the research process and what research could do. Also, quality assessment and improvement data related to patient outcomes were lacking. Therefore Lori decided to focus on the following objectives:

1. Develop, implement, and evaluate a quality improvement program that would develop a data base concerning the patient population in the ICU. Based on outcomes, problems for clinical research could be identified.
2. Provide staff education in research in nursing. This process would be accomplished by development of a research interest group at the unit level. Goals for the group would depend on group consensus. The group would be a starting point for staff education, problem identification, and conducting research in the future.

The CC-CNS also decided to chair the research interest group for the first year.

The following year was successful. The research interest group met monthly, and membership was growing. The group sponsored two mini seminars on nursing research to increase staff knowledge and appreciation of research. The 2-hour seminars focused on the research process and how research could benefit nursing practice. Unit quality assessment and improvement outcomes were reported monthly to the committee for feedback. Negative outcomes were evaluated via literature reviews of existing research in the problem area, and procedures or policies were revised based on those literature reviews and committee recommendations. At the end of the year the CC-CNS obtained membership in the division of nursing research committee, thereby linking the two groups.

The second year found the committee more knowledgeable of research in nursing. The committee became more diverse in that educators and managers joined the unit committee. The CC-CNS made contact with a local university, and faculty members interested in critical care research joined the committee as well. The members became knowledgeable of the research process and as a result decided to conduct a project addressing a clinical problem identified by nursing staff committee members through analysis of quality assessment and improvement data.

A problem identified was an increasing frequency of reintubation within 4 hours of extubation in the open heart population. The CC-CNS and committee reviewed the data and decided that the existing protocol for weaning and extubation were insufficient and possibly contributing to the problem. The committee decided revision of weaning protocols and evaluation was necessary.

First, the research group explored the literature and surveyed staff for feedback concerning weaning procedures. Information was collected concerning intermittent mechanical ventilation (IMV) vs. continuous mechanical ventilation (CMV) weaning. Some committee members surveyed other hospitals to find out about their weaning procedures. Physicians were invited to meetings to share their knowledge. The committee and physicians decided to develop new weaning protocols and measure outcomes as a result of the intervention, since information obtained from the literature, staff, and surveys did not provide enough information to decide which protocol resulted in more favorable patient outcomes. The CC-CNS worked with the staff and surgeons, and based on acquired information, two protocols were developed. Two surgeons decided that they would use protocol A (IMV wean) for their patient population, and one surgeon decided to use protocol B (CMV wean).

Before the protocols were implemented, staff were given an in-service program by the committee. The problem was defined, the protocols were reviewed extensively, and information that must be documented in the clinical record was reviewed. Staff provided valuable feedback on data collection form construction. The committee decided that the majority of data (arterial blood gas results, weaning time, age, time on bypass, respiratory vital signs) would be from the clinical record; therefore accurate documentation was a must.

The CC-CNS and nursing staff prepared the IRB proposal and invited the participating surgeons to be coinvestigators as well as participating committee members. The university faculty members assisted the CC-CNS in proposal preparation, particularly with the data analysis section. Faculty members had access to statistical support that reduced related expenses of the project. The CC-CNS also met with nurse administrators and presented the project goals of reducing emergent reintubation. As a result, financial support was received for the project and provided salaries to members after completion of their shift. Secretarial support for the project was also provided. The protocols were tested on five patients. Staff and committee members critiqued the pilot process and outcomes, and the protocols and data collection forms were revised accordingly. The project was implemented with a goal of obtaining 50 patients during the first phase of the project. Subject consent was obtained by the CC-CNS during preoperative teaching.

The CC-CNS monitored the implementation of the protocol and outcomes daily. Data collection forms were returned to designated committee members who coded the data according to coding protocol developed with the statistician. All coded data were checked for accuracy by the CC-CNS and another committee member. Following data analysis, results were reviewed by the CC-CNS, university faculty, and the committee. It was determined that both protocols were equally effective and that reintubation rates decreased significantly with both protocols. Outcomes of both protocols were found not statistically or clinically different.

The committee decided to publish the results. The group prepared a draft of the paper according to specifications of the journals chosen for publication. The first draft was edited by the CNS and staff colleagues, and feedback was incorporated accordingly. The committee also decided to design a poster, and three conferences were chosen to present the study. Three committee members were elected to present at each conference. The final result was adoption of the weaning protocols for all surgical patients in the unit when results were presented in grand rounds.

When the research committee met to plan goals for the third year, members evaluated their research activities of the second year. Members expressed what they found favorable about conducting research in the clinical setting. Positive aspects included collaboration, networking, problem solving, publishing, and presenting findings to peers. They also agreed the research process positively impacted clinical practice and patient outcomes. Staff members were more aware of weaning processes and outcomes, and patient outcomes had improved. The committee also found that staff members were approaching members with other clinical problems that could be researched.

SUMMARY

This chapter presented the unique role of the CC-CNS in promoting research in the clinical setting. Both theoretic perspectives and practical information for ways to fulfill research responsibilities were presented. Finally a case study was discussed that exemplifies activities of the CC-CNS who works with staff in the conduct of critical care research.

References

1. Wabschall J: The CNS as researcher. In Menard SW, editor: *The clinical nurse specialist: perspectives on practice*, New York, 1987, John Wiley & Sons.
2. Gaits V et al: Unit based research forums: a model for the clinical nurse specialist to promote clinical research, *Clin Nurse Specialist* 3(2):60-65, 1989.
3. Parker BJ, Gift AG, Creasia JL: Clinical nursing research with patients in crisis: pitfalls and solutions, *Clin Nurse Specialist* 3(4):178-181, 1989.
4. Fawcett J: A topology of nursing research activities according to educational prep, *J Prof Nurs* 1(2):75-78, 1985.
5. American Nurses' Association: *Education for participation in nursing research*, Kansas City, Mo, 1989, The Association.
6. VanCott ML et al: Analysis of a decade of critical care nursing practice research: 1979-1988, *Heart Lung* 20(4):394-397, 1991.
7. American Association of Critical Care Nurses: *The critical care clinical nurse specialist: role definition. AACN position statement*, Aliso Viejo, Calif, 1987, The Association.
8. Ryan-Merritt M, Mitchell C, Pagel I: Clinical nurse specialist: role definition and operationalism, *Clin Nurse Specialist* 2(3):132-137, 1988.
9. Nail LM: Involving clinicians in nursing research, *Oncol Nurs Forum* 17(4):621-623, 1990.
10. Houston S, Luquire R: Measuring success: CNS performance appraisal, *Clin Nurse Specialist* 5(4):204-209, 1991.
11. Dracup K: Critical care nursing. In Fitzpatrick JJ, Taunton RL, editors: *Annual review of nursing research*, vol 5, New York, 1987, Springer.
12. Fonteyn M: The need for nurse involvement in critical care research, *Crit Care Nurs Q* 12(4):1-4, 1990.

13. Tyler DO et al: Strategies for conducting clinical nursing research in critical care, *Crit Care Nurs Q* 12(4):30-38, 1990.

14. American Association of Critical Care Nurses: *AACN announces research priorities: press release,* Aliso Viejo, Calif, 1991, The Association.

15. VanBree Sneed N: Collaboration as a means to achieving the clinical nurse specialist research role expectations, *Clin Nurs Specialist* 1(2):70-74, 1987.

16. Medoff-Cooper B, Lamb AH: The clinical specialist-staff nurse research team: a model for clinical research, *Clin Nurse Specialist* 3(1):16-19, 1989.

17. Beavers F, Gruber M, Johnson B: A model for group research by master's degree RNs in advanced roles, *Clin Nurse Specialist* 4(3):130-135, 1990.

18. Bolton LB: Resources for research. In Mateo MA, Kirchoff KT, editors: *Conducting and using nursing research in clinical setting,* Baltimore, 1991, Williams & Wilkins Co.

19. Egan EC, McElmurry BJ, Jameson HM: Practice base research: assessing your department's readiness, *J Nurs Admin* 11(10):26-36, 1981.

20. Tetting D: Preparing for the human subject review, *Crit Care Nurs Q* 12(4):10-16, 1990.

21. *Protection of human subjects (45 CFR 46).* Code of Federal Regulations. Pub. 0-406-756, U.S. Department of Health and Human Services.

22. Howser D: Research committee membership: roles and responsibilities. In Lieske AM, editor: *Clinical nursing research,* Rockville, Md, 1986, Aspen Publishers.

23. Lieske AM: Basis of a research program: the committee structure. In Lieske AM, editor: *Clinical nursing research,* Rockville, Md, 1986, Aspen Publishers.

24. Grant M, Fleming I, Calvanico A: Research and quality assurance. In Mateo MA, Kirchoff KT, editors: *Conducting and using nursing research in clinical setting,* Baltimore, 1991, Williams & Wilkins Co.

25. Meade C: Conducting research in the acute care setting. In Lieske AM, editor: *Clinical nursing research,* Rockville, Md, 1986, Aspen Publishers.

26. Mueller D: *Measuring social attitudes,* New York, 1986, Teachers College Press.

27. Glass E: Importance of research to practice. In Mateo MA, Kirchoff KT, editors: *Conducting and using research in clinical setting,* Baltimore, 1991, Williams & Wilkins Co.

28. Nelson A: Application of micro computers in nursing research, *West J Nurs Res* 8(1):117-120, 1986.

29. Scheetz S, Wilson HS: Computers and data processing in nursing research. In Wilson HS, editor: *Research in nursing,* ed 2, Redwood City, Calif, 1989, Addison-Wesley Publishing Co.

30. Chance HC, Hinshaw AS: Strategies for initiating a research program, *J Nurs Admin* 10(3):32-39, 1980.

31. Foreman MD, Smeltzer C: Gaining support for the study. In Mateo MA, Kirchoff KT, editors: *Conducting and using nursing research in clinical setting,* Baltimore, 1991, Williams & Wilkins Co.

32. Davis MZ: Promoting nursing research in the clinical setting, *J Nurs Admin* 11(3):22-27, 1981.

33. Blichfeldt M, Deane D, Lancaster J: Facilitating research in critical care, *Dimen Crit Care Nurs* 6(5):284-292, 1987.

34. Fitzpatrick E et al: Clinical nurse research priorities: a delphi study, *Clin Nurse Specialist* 5(2):94-99, 1991.

35. Smith J, Diekmann J: Strategies for teaching nursing research fair—a strategy for rekindling research interest in nursing staff, *West J Nurs Res* 9(4):631-633, 1987.

36. Stetler CB: Nursing research in a service setting, Reston, Va, 1984, Reston.

37. Johnson BK: How to ask research questions in clinical practice, *Am J Nurs* 91(3):64-65, 1991.

38. Munro BH, Visintainer MA, Page EB: *Statistical methods for health care research,* Philadelphia, 1986, JB Lippincott Co.

39. Wilson HS: Writing a research proposal. In Wilson HS, editor: *Research in nursing,* ed 2, Redwood City, Calif, 1989, Addison-Wesley Publishing Co.

40. Reynolds M, Haller K: A case for replication in nursing. I, *West J Nurs Res* 8(1):113-116, 1986.

41. Seaman C: *Research methods: principles, practice and theory for nursing,* ed 3, Norwalk, Conn, 1987, Appleton & Lange.

42. Hutchinson SA: Getting started on a study. In Wilson HS, editor: *Research in nursing,* Redwood City, Calif, Addison-Wesley Publishing Co.

43. Sinclair V: Literature searches by computer, *Image* 19(1):35-37, 1987.

44. Strauch K, Linton R, Cohen C: *Library research guide to nursing,* Ann Arbor, Mich, 1989, Pierian Press.

45. Albright RG: *A basic guide to on-line information systems for health care professionals,* Arlington, Va, 1988, Information Resource Press.

46. Shockley J: *Information sources for nursing: a guide,* New York, 1988, National League for Nursing.

47. Diers D: *Research in nursing practice,* Philadelphia, 1979, JB Lippincott Co.

48. Diekmann JM, Smith JM: Strategies for assessment and recruitment of subjects for nursing research, *West J Nurs Res* 11(4):418-430, 1989.

49. Lawson S: Funding for research. In Lieske AM, editor: *Clinical nursing research,* Rockville, Md, 1986, Aspen Publishers.

50. Davis A: Informed consent process in research protocols: dilemmas for clinical nurses, *West J Nurs Res* 11(4):448-457, 1989.

51. Leidy N, Weissfield L: Sample sizes and power computation for clinical intervention trials, *West J Nurs Res* 13(1):138-144, 1991.

52. Topf M: Increasing the validity of research results with a blend of laboratory and clinical strategies, *Image* 22(2):121-123, 1990.

53. Beck S: Designing a study. In Mateo M et al, editors: *Conducting and using research in the clinical setting,* Baltimore, 1991, Williams & Wilkins Co.

54. Munhall P, Oiler C: *Nursing research: a qualitative perspective,* Norwalk, Conn, 1986, Appleton-Century-Crofts.

55. Woods NF: Testing theoretically based nursing care: necessary modification of the clinical trial, *West J Nurs Res* 12(6):777-781, 1990.

56. McLaughlin FE, Marascuilo LA: Advanced nursing and health care research quantification approaches, Philadelphia, 1990, WB Saunders Co.

57. Frank-Stromborg M, editor: *Instruments for clinical nursing research,* Norwalk, Conn, 1988, Appleton & Lange.
58. Waltz CW, Strickland O, Lenz E: *Measurement in nursing research,* ed 2, Philadelphia, 1991, FA Davis Co.
59. Jacobson S: Evaluating instruments for use in clinical nursing research. In Frank-Stromborg M, editor: *Instruments for clinical nursing research,* Norwalk, Conn, 1988, Appleton & Lange.
60. Larochelle D: The selection and development of psychosocial instruments. In Wilson HS, editor: *Research in nursing,* ed 2, Redwood City, Calif, 1989, Addison-Wesley Publishing Co.
61. Rempusheski V: The proliferation of unreliable and invalid questionnaires, *Appl Nurs Res* 3(4):174-176, 1990.
62. Lindsey A, Stotts N: Collecting data on biophysical variables. In Wilson HS, editor: *Research in nursing,* ed 2, Redwood City, Calif, 1989, Addison-Wesley Publishing Co.
63. Stone K: Biomedical instrumentation. In Mateo M, Kirchhoff K, editors: *Conducting and using nursing research in the clinical setting,* Baltimore, 1991, Williams & Wilkins Co.
64. Abbey J: Development of instruments to measure physiological variables in clinical studies, *Crit Care Nurs Q* 12(4):21-29, 1990.
65. Gassert CA: Reliability and validity of physiologic measurement, *Crit Care Nurs Q* 12(4):17-20, 1990.
66. Jennings BM: Patient outcomes research: seizing the opportunity, *Adv Nurs Sci* 14(2):59-72, 1991.
67. Ferraris V, Propp M: Outcome in critical care patients: a multivariate study, *Crit Care Med* 20(7):967-976, 1992.
68. Gillis C, Kulkin I: Monitoring nursing interventions and data collection in a randomized clinical trial, *West J Nurs Res* 13(3):416-422, 1991.
69. McElroy M, Gonyon D: Analyzing the data. In Mateo MA, Kirchhoff KT, editors: *Conducting and using nursing research in clinical setting,* Baltimore, 1991, Williams & Wilkins Co.
70. Slichter M, Hanson C, Gortner S: Researchmanship: computer costs for research grant planning, *West J Nurs Res* 6(1):133-135, 1984.
71. Wilson HS: Discovering research problems in clinical practice. In Wilson HS, editor: *Research in nursing,* ed 2, Redwood City, Calif, 1989, Addison-Wesley Publishing Co.
72. Lindquist R: Don't forget the pilot work! *Heart Lung* 20(1):91-92, 1991.
73. Tornquist E, Funk S: How to write a research grant proposal, *Image* 22(1):44-51, 1990.
74. Ogden T: *Research proposals: a guide to success,* New York, 1991, Raven Press.
75. American Association of Critical Care Nurses: *Writing that winning research proposal #3031,* Aliso Viejo, Calif, 1988, The Association.
76. Jackson NE, Driever M: Anticipating and evaluating the collaborative research process, *West J Nurs Res* 8(1):110-112, 1986.
77. Hanson S: Collaborative research and authorship credit: beginning guidelines, *J Nurs Res* 37(1):49-52, 1988.
78. Buckwalter K: Collaboration with medical structure. In Lieske AM, editor: *Clinical nursing research,* Rockville, Md, 1986, Aspen Publishers.
79. American Psychological Association: *Publication manual,* ed 3, Washington, DC, 1983, The Association.
80. Kirkpatrick H, Martin M: Communicating nursing research through poster presentations, *West J Nurs Res* 13(1):145-148, 1991.
81. American Association of Critical Care Nurses: *Writing for professional nursing journals: a guide,* Aliso Viejo, Calif, 1990, The Association.
82. American Association of Critical Care Nurses: *Writing research abstracts successfully #3032,* Aliso Viejo, Calif, 1989, The Association.

Chapter 14

Research Utilization in the Critical Care Setting

Anna Gawlinski, RN, DNSc, CS, CCRN
Elizabeth A. Henneman, RN, MS, CCRN

Developing a scientific basis for nursing practice is essential for quality patient care and advancement of the nursing profession.[1] Until recently, most nursing research was done by nurses in academia rather than in the practice setting. Today more research is being generated by nurses in both clinical and academic settings.

Although research productivity has increased in the last decade, a large gap still exists between the discovery of research-based clinical knowledge and its utilization in practice. One promising development in nursing with the potential to counter this gap is the emerging field of clinical specialization.[2] With advanced preparation at the master's level, nurses learned the foundations of the research process and are viewed as critical thinkers who can analyze the applicability of research findings in practice.

The literature supports the notion that the clinical nurse specialist (CNS) is in a unique position to bridge the gap between research and practice.[3] However, the reality is that numerous barriers exist to using research as the basis of practice. Lack of skill in research analysis[4-8] and poor communication between researchers and clinicians are just a few.[9-11] Additionally, in critical care the lack of replicated research studies is also a barrier to applying research to practice. If the critical care CNS (CC-CNS) is to be the driving force for research utilization, the CC-CNS must develop strategies to overcome these barriers.

This chapter presents an introduction to research utilization (RU) in nursing and discusses the CC-CNS's role in both the process of RU and techniques for establishing an RU program. Theoretic perspectives of RU and practice implications in critical care are presented. Critical care case studies are used to guide the CC-CNS in the process of using research findings to improve practice.

THEORETIC PERSPECTIVES

Research consists of three interrelated activities: knowledge generation, dissemination, and utilization.[12] Knowledge generation is the process of conducting nursing research as a principal investigator or coinvestigator. Knowledge dissemination is the process of sharing research findings via activities such as citing relevant research during patient conferences, at staff meetings, or while making clinical rounds. Knowledge utilization is the process of incorporating research findings to verify current practice or to change practice.

RU is the process through which research findings are critiqued, implemented, evaluated, and disseminated.[13] Horsley[14] described RU as the act of using methods and products of research to expand knowledge and verify or change nursing practice.[13,14] It has also been defined as the process through which scientific substantiation of nursing activities take place.[13,15] Consequently the utilization of nursing research refers in general to the findings of research.[16] RU includes the process of critically reviewing scientific statements or descriptions (explanation or causation of nursing phenomena that are substantiated by a set of data) to judge whether a change in practice is warranted. RU differs from research dissemination in that RU requires planned change. The systematic use of planned change begins with the identification of a clinical problem and ends with maintenance of the research-based practice.

In the nursing literature, application and utilization are two words often used synonymously, although some authors make distinctions between them. For example, according to Krueger,[16] application of research implies a temporary change in knowledge, attitude, or behavior; like a bandage application, the change may be easily removed and discarded.[17] On the other hand, Stetler and Marram[18] use application to denote a permanent change that occurs on one of two levels, the second of which is synonymous with utilization as defined by Krueger.[16,17]

According to Stetler and Marram, the first level of application is cognitive, the process of filing a piece of information for later use in practice. The second level of their two-level conceptualization of research application is direct application—actual use of the filed information at the appropriate time and after careful evaluation. Thus direct application or utilization implies evaluation of the existing research, implementation, clinical use, and modification of clinical practice based on research findings.[17]

Nurses as Users of Research

Theoretically the CC-CNS is the consumer in the utilization of research. The nursing research consumer, according to Phillips,[19] "is a role that is enacted by any nurse-clinician who desires to use nursing research and nursing theory as the basis for the nursing care delivered."[17] Rempusheski[17] states "The necessary requirements for the nursing research consumer role are knowledge and skill in both clinical practice and the research process." Clearly, the CC-CNS has the potential to play an important role as a consumer of nursing research. The CC-CNS's consumer role can take many forms, including that of facilitator (assisting with removal of barriers for the conduct of research and use of research results in practice), advocate (supporting the efforts or activities), activist (speaking out for the cause), risk taker (attempting to do something rather than nothing), learner or educator (learning or teaching the skills), innovator (introducing new ways of thinking and doing), coordinator of planned change, negotiator (mediating between the believers and the nonbelievers), collab-

orator (establishing a stronger front with partners), and evaluator of clinical costs and benefits of innovations.[17]

Phillips[19] identified five role activities of the nursing research consumer: (1) evaluation, which begins with evaluating one's own practice and moves on to evaluating practice within the setting; (2) translation from scientific research terminology to clinically used terms; (3) interpretation of the language and results incorporated into practice; (4) dissemination, which entails spreading the word (through publication conferences, discussions, informal meetings, or committees) and citing existing literature; and (5) application or utilization by writing critical care standards of practice based on what is gathered from the research literature specific to a critical care procedure, population, or issue.[17] The CC-CNS plays an integral role in each of these activities.

Theories of Knowledge Utilization

"Most people believe that a good idea will 'sell itself'—the word will spread rapidly, and the idea will quickly be used."[20] However, this is seldom true. Many ideas that are regarded as exceptional are not always immediately accepted. For example, the pacemaker was first conceived in 1928 but was not in practice until 1960. Table 14-1 presents examples of ideas and the span of time between the idea's first conception and initial utilization.[21] This table indicates that the average length of time between discovery and utilization is 19 years.[20]

It is not clearly understood why some findings require more time than others to implement. The time required for implementation is influenced by historical events, attitudes toward the researcher and research in general, and the necessity with some innovation to change attitudes and values before the findings can be accepted and utilized.[20]

In the early 1970s a group of experts in the area of RU was convened by the government to examine issues related to the lack of utilization and to propose strategies to improve this situation. From the work done by this group, a field of study evolved that examines the process of utilization. Researchers and theorists from various disciplines began addressing the problem. What has since emerged are three theories about utilization, diffusion, and adoption of innovations: Rogers' theory of diffusion of innovation, Havelock's theory of linker sys-

TABLE 14-1 Time Between Idea and Utilization

Innovation	Year Conceived	Year of Realization	Duration (yr)
Pacemaker	1928	1960	32
Input-output economic analysis	1936	1964	28
Hybrid corn	1908	1933	25
Electrophotography	1937	1959	22
Magnetic ferries	1933	1955	22
Hybrid small grains	1937	1956	19
Green revolution: wheat	1950	1966	16
Organophosphorous insecticides	1934	1947	13
Oral contraceptive	1951	1960	9
Videotape recorder	1950	1956	6
			AVERAGE DURATION 19.2

From Glaser EM, Abelson HH, Garrison KN: *Putting knowledge to use,* San Francisco, 1983, Jossey-Bass.

tems, and Lewin's force field theory, which describes the process of change.[20] CC-CNS knowledge of these theories is important, since they provide the framework for most of the research in the area of knowledge utilization. In addition, these theories provide the CC-CNS with a means of planning strategies to increase utilization of research in critical care nursing.

Theories of Utilization, Diffusion, and Innovation

Rogers[22] developed a theory of the process of adoption of innovation. His theory provides a framework with which the CC-CNS can understand the dynamics of knowledge utilization within critical care nursing. According to Rogers, diffusion is the process by which an innovation is communicated through certain channels. Communication occurs over time and among the members of society.[22] Rogers considers dissemination synonymous with diffusion. The main elements of diffusion are (1) the innovation, (2) communication channels, (3) time, and (4) the social system. Rogers describes an innovation as an idea, practice, or object perceived as new by an individual or group. Characteristics of an innovation that determine the probability and speed of its adoption include relative advantage, compatibility, complexity, and "trialability." Relative advantage is the extent to which the innovation is perceived to be

better than current practice. Compatability is the extent to which the innovation is perceived to be consistent with current norms, past experience, and priority of needs. Complexity is the degree to which the innovation is perceived to be difficult to understand or use. Trialability is the extent to which an individual or agency can implement on a limited basis with the option of returning to previous practices.[20,22] The CC-CNS involved in RU needs innovations that have great relative advantage, are compatible, have flexible trialability, and are not complex. These will be adopted more quickly than innovations that do not meet these criteria.[20,22]

Communication channels are also factors that affect the diffusion of an innovation. Communication may include one-to-one communication, one individual communicating to several others, or large-scale communication such as that accepted by the mass media. Interestingly, face-to-face communication is the most powerful determinant of individual innovation use. The communication is also more effective when the two interacting individuals are similar in such characteristics as beliefs, values, education, social status, and profession. Rogers refers to these individuals as near peers.[20,22] This has important implications for the CC-CNS. A doctorally prepared nurse scientist may not be the most effective person to discuss adopting an innovation with a staff nurse. Rather, the CC-CNS, because of close contact with the staff, clinically would be the best link between research and its utilization in practice.

Innovativeness

Innovativeness is the degree to which an individual or group adopts new ideas earlier than other members of the system.[22] Rogers uses five categories to describe adopters based on their degree of innovativeness: (1) innovators, (2) early adopters, (3) early majority, (4) late majority, and (5) laggards (Fig. 14–1).[23] Innovators actively seek information about new ideas. Innovators cope with higher levels of uncertainty related to an innovation than other adopters do and are usually the first to adopt a new idea. Early adopters tend to be leaders in organizations. They tend to learn of new ideas quickly, utilize them, and then serve as role models in their use.[20] By the nature of critical care nursing, innovators and early adopters are attracted to the clinical setting. Members of the early majority rarely are leaders but are active followers. They will follow willingly in the use of a new idea. Members of the late majority are skeptical about new ideas and will adopt them only if group pressure is great. Laggards tend to isolate themselves without a strong support system. They are security oriented and cling to the status quo. By the time a laggard adopts a new idea it is considered by most to be an old idea.[20,22]

The rate of adoption is an important concept for the CC-CNS. First, it helps to explain why changing nursing practice based on research is not an easy process. It requires patience and persistence.

In addition, it stresses the importance of knowing which groups to target when introducing an innovation. For example, the CC-CNS should not spend a lot of time on laggards, since change will be resisted by this group. However, the CC-CNS can target the late majority, who are willing to change if group pressure is great. Understanding that the essence of the diffusion process is imitation by potential adopters of their near peers can help the CC-CNS in the process of RU.

Havelock's Theory

Havelock[24-26] added another dimension to the current knowledge of utilization theory by proposing the development of the linker system. This linker system transfers new knowledge, skills, or products (innovations) from the resource system (researchers and their publications) to the user system (the practitioners) for dissemination. The linker is an individual who serves as a connection between the user system (practitioner) and the resource system (the researcher).[20]

Havelock suggests the linker takes the new idea and develops practical ways to use it. The linker has a broader range of knowledge of research findings and strategies for implementing them and could serve as an advisor to the user system in implementing new ideas.[20,27]

The CC-CNS is clearly the linker in RU. The CC-CNS translates the research innovation for use in practice. The CC-CNS prepares the nursing research findings for utilization. In addition, the CC-CNS also communicates the practitioners' needs to the researcher. Thus the CC-CNS functions as a linker in the RU process.

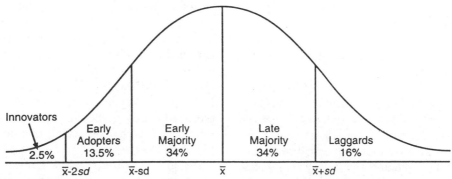

Figure 14–1 Adopter categorization on basis of innovativeness. (Reprinted with the permission of The Free Press, a Division of Macmillan, Inc. from *Diffusion of innovations*, Third Edition by Everett M. Rogers. Copyright © 1962, 1971, 1983 by The Free Press.)

Change Theory

RU ultimately requires a change for all persons involved, and resistance to change is a normal human response. Lewin's force field theory[28,29] describes the strategies necessary to successfully achieve change. According to Lewin, behavior in any institutional setting is not a static pattern. Rather, it is a dynamic balance of forces that tend to increase the possibility for change or movement (driving forces) and forces that tend to depress change or movement (resisting forces).

Change theory also incorporates the concept of the change agent, that is, an individual or group who imitates and facilitates the change process (see Chapter 16). The CC-CNS is the change agent in the process of RU. In attempting to change a situation and move behavior to a new level the CC-CNS needs to (1) increase the driving forces by adding new ones or strengthening existing ones, (2) reduce or remove the restraining forces, or (3) translate one or more restraining forces into driving forces. Careful plans are made by the CC-CNS as change agent to facilitate, strengthen, and promote those factors facilitating change. The CC-CNS as change agent seeks to diffuse the innovations through the system and, working through leaders, modifies attitudes toward the change and implements the findings into the routine practices of the system.[20]

RELATED RESEARCH AND LITERATURE

To date, there is a lack of research on the process of knowledge utilization specifically related to critical care. However, several projects and models have been developed to attempt to increase utilization of nursing research findings. Table 14–2 lists various projects and models that CC-CNSs can use with staff in clinical practice.

Projects

WICHEN Project

In 1975 the first large-scale project for nursing RU was sponsored by the Western Interstate Commission for Higher Education (WICHEN) Regional Program for Nursing Research Development. WICHEN, composed of deans and directors of nursing graduate programs in 13 Western states, with its network of 163 educational programs in nursing and 69 agency representatives, seized the opportunity to link nursing research and clinical practice.[16,36]

The aim of the project was to improve patient care by increasing utilization of nursing research through a series of workshops for educators and clinicians. WICHEN described five components necessary to a model for the utilization of research, components that nurses would need before they could effect change: (1) access to innovative research findings, (2) ability to evaluate critical research findings before implementing change, (3) preparation in change theory and the management of change, (4) strategies for coping with problems of risk taking, and (5) planning for introducing change and criteria for evaluating its effect on the health care system.[16,19]

The outcome of this project was the development and implementation of information systems such as the Delphi survey to determine research priorities in nursing. A list was also compiled of nurse researchers by interest and expertise.[13]

CURN Project

The Michigan State project for the utilization of nursing research resulted in the Conduct and Utilization of Research in Nursing (CURN) Project. This project developed and tested a model to facilitate the use of scientific nursing knowledge in clinical practice settings.[30]

Guidelines delineating the parameters of safe nursing RU did not exist; therefore the CURN Project established three parameters for the development and testing of nursing RU. First, nursing RU should be based on a series of replicated studies (minimum of three studies), because frequently the findings of a single research study may be insufficient or inconsistent. Indirect replication of a group of studies to extend and validate a defined area of nursing research where the relationships among variables are similar was the second parameter for the project. Results from indirect replication must correlate, extend, or define one another. Last, the nursing innovation should result in the predicted outcome of the research base. The measure of evaluation included a minimum of one dependent variable used by the original investigators.[19,37] The CURN Project identified six phases of the research utilization process (Table 14–3).[30]

TABLE 14–2 RU Strategies in Nursing: Projects and Models

Author or Project	Type	Description
Havelock[24] (1974)	Theory	Person who identified clinical practice issues linked with nurse scientist
WICHEN[16] (1978)	Project	Initiated collaborative effort among nursing service and education settings to design research studies and utilization plans on mutually identified problems
CURN[30] (1983)	Project	Designed to enhance use of research in clinical practice; 10 areas identified that had sufficient quality research to warrant implementation in practice
NCAST[31] (1981)	Project	Provided educational program directed at individual practicing nurse via satellite communication system; communication was directly from researcher to practitioner
OCRUN[32] (1989)	Project	Provided RU networking and education program to nursing organizations; targeted nursing staff, designated organizational links and nursing executives
Stelter and Marram[18] (1976)	Model	Evaluates research findings for applicability in practice; tool included for evaluation of applicability of research in practice; research critiqued, findings evaluated for clinical feasibility, and decisions on utilization are made
Dracup and Breu[33] (1977)	Model	Describes a framework used to meet a problem in clinical practice through utilization of current research findings
Krueger[34] (1979)	Model	Systematic evaluation of quality and relevance of research; provides for generalizations for use in practice, dissemination, planned use of research, need for replication and new research
Goode[35] (1979)	Model	Represent concepts for conduct and utilization of clinical nursing research; uses input, throughput, output, and feedback

As a result of the CURN Project 10 clinical areas were identified that had sufficient quality research to warrant implementation in practice (Table 14–4).[30] CC-CNSs should be aware of these protocols from the CURN Project, since they provide the basis for research-based practice. For example, the CURN protocol that deals with deliberative nursing interventions for pain can be useful during CC-CNS rounds or in a clinical conference for patients in pain. This intervention states that

the use of deliberative nursing—an approach of skilled communication that allows the nurse to effectively ascertain the patient's real need—results in speedier and more complete relief of patient's complaints of pain and the use of fewer pain medications[38]

Directions for research-based practice that can be applied to critical care are provided for patients with tube feedings, decubitus ulcers, and closed urinary drainage systems. These are an excellent

TABLE 14–3 CURN Project Steps in Using
Nursing Research

Since the CURN Project was based on the diffusion
of innovations and planned change theory model,
they list these steps in using nursing research:

* Systematically determining patient care problems
* Finding and assessing research-based knowledge
  to solve those problems
* Adopting and designing nursing practice innovations that come from the research-based knowledge
* Conducting a clinical trial and evaluating the innovation
* Deciding whether to adopt, alter, or reject the innovation
* Developing the means to extend the new practice
  beyond the trial unit
* Developing mechanisms to maintain the innovation over time

From Horsley JA et al: *Using research to improve practice: a
guide,* New York, 1983, Grune & Stratton.

source of research-based innovations that CC-
CNSs can use as they begin their RU process.

NCAST Project

In a series of research use projects, King et al.[31]
developed a model for the diffusion and utilization
of a research-based nursing innovation. The Nursing Child Assessment Satellite Training (NCAST)
projects emphasized translation of research findings for practicing nurses. Each project built on
findings from previous projects and integrated components of Rogers' diffusion framework. The
model consisted of four interacting components:
(1) recruitment, (2) translation, (3) dissemination,
and (4) evaluation.

Practicing nurses were taught assessment procedures that identified and evaluated the animate
and inanimate environment of the infant. A satellite
communication system was used to send the information to various sites across the United States.
The teaching was provided through on-site satellite
communication systems. The communication was
directly from the researcher to the practitioner.[20]
Barnard[39] reported that 85% of nurses exposed to
the protocols adopted the assessment procedure.
Four years after the program was initiated, the high
adoption rate has continued.[20]

OCRUN Project

The Orange County Research Utilization in
Nursing (OCRUN) Project created a regional network of 20 participating nursing organizations and
six schools of nursing with the goal of providing
research use networking and continuing education
to nursing service organization. The OCRUN Project uses a regional network and exposes assigned
nursing staff, the organization's designated "link-
ers," and nurse executives to a three-tiered continuing education curriculum that increases use of research by the organization and individuals.[32]

Models for Research Utilization

A model for RU is a systematic plan and an
organized strategy for facilitating the use of clinical

TABLE 14–4 Outcomes of Clinical Research

Scientific basis now exists to warrant application of
the following principles in clinical nursing practice:

* Structured preoperative teaching by nurses reduces postoperative complications.
* A lactose-free diet reduces the incidence of diar-
  rhea from tube feeding.
* Sensory information given to patients before a
  stressful, complex, or high-technology procedure
  reduces stress during the procedure.
* Sensory information given by nurses to patients
  undergoing a stressful procedure enhances the recovery rate.
* Periodic nonsterile urinary catheterization reduces
  costs of frequent sterile catheterization and does
  not increase the number of infections.
* Nursing interventions can prevent catheter-associ-
  ated urinary tract infections.
* Changing intravenous cannulas (tubes) can reduce
  the incidence of infections acquired in the hospital.
* Nursing care measures such as small shifts in
  body weight can prevent decubitus ulcers (bed-
  sores).
* The patient is much more likely to reach specific
  health-related goals when nurses and patients
  work together to attain them.
* Nursing actions can produce effective pain management.

Reprinted with permission from *Research in nursing,* © 1987,
American Nurses' Association, Washington, D.C.

research as the basis for individual and institutional nursing practice.[17] Table 14–2 lists several models that the CC-CNS can use as a framework for the RU process. As CC-CNSs we have found the Stetler-Marram model particularly useful, since it provides both a model and tool for the actual evaluation of the applicability of research for practice.

Stetler-Marram Model

The Stetler-Marram model guides the nurse in deciding whether and how to use nursing research findings in practice. This model suggests before the current practice is modified, three phases of critical thinking must be considered: validation, comparative evaluation, and decision making (Fig. 14–2).[18]

Validation is the identification of the study's strengths and weaknesses to determine if the weaknesses invalidate the findings. Each step of the research study should be closely scrutinized, especially if the study is an unpublished document. If the results are invalid, no further consideration should be given to the study.[19]

The second phase, comparative evaluation, focuses on four critical issues: substantiating evidence, fit of setting, basis for practice, and feasibility. Can the results be substantiated in other empiric studies in similar settings? Similarity of the characteristics of the sample needs to be examined to determine if the characteristics will prevent achievement of the same results as those of the study. Environment should also be examined in

relation to setting, organization, staffing patterns, technology, and time for implementation.[19]

In the comparative evaluation phase the third issue of concern is the examination of the theoretic base for practices in the setting. For example, the current nursing practice may be based on sound theoretic knowledge. Therefore it is important to evaluate the new research findings in relationship to the theoretic soundness of current practice. It is essential to be able to place the findings of the study in the context of the practice setting. In addition, analysis of the nurse's current mode of behavior is necessary to the project's potential success. The final issue of the second phase is determining the feasibility of the utilization of the nursing research findings in the practice setting in relation to legal and ethical risks, constraints, rewards, time, effort, and costs.[19]

The final phase of the Stetler-Marram model is decision making. Based on the review of activities in phase 2, the nurse has three choices: termination, cognitive application, or direct application. Cognitive application is the use of research findings as additional information in the current theoretic approach to nursing; results of the study are used to enhance understanding and analysis of nursing practice. Another choice is to use the findings as a direct model for action, to test the research findings in a new setting.[19]

For the CC-CNS and nursing staff the Stetler-Marram model is particularly useful, since it provides both a model and a tool for the actual eval-

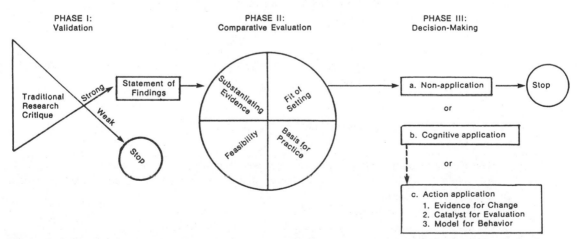

Figure 14–2 Model for utilization of research findings in nursing practice. (From Stetler C, Marram G: Evaluating research findings for applicability in practice, *Nurs Outlook* 24:559-563, 1976.)

uation of the applicability of the research. The tool is intended to guide the clinician in the process of RU (Table 14–5).[40] The model and tool help nurses improve critical care nursing practice through the utilization of nursing research.

Regardless of which model in Table 14-2 is used in clinical practice, there are four features of each of these models:

1. Each model represents a systematic and sequential process for creating change in clinical practice.
2. Each model identifies the research critique as an essential and first step in the utilization process.
3. Each model includes an evaluation component that provides the nurse clinician with ways to determine if the potential change should or should not become a permanent feature of nursing practice within a particular setting and a feedback mechanism for communicating concern and new areas of inquiry to nurse researchers.
4. Each model takes into account the structural issues involved in effecting change in the institutional setting.[17]

Research Utilization Among Critical Care Clinical Nurse Specialists

The RU process requires the collective input of nursing personnel who are knowledgeable about

---

TABLE 14–5 Stetler-Marram Tool for Evaluation of Applicability of Research Findings

I. Phase 1A: Validation

  A. What are the methodological strengths of this study?
  B. What are the methodological weaknesses and the limitations of this study?
  C. Given A and B above, to what degree are the findings acceptable for potential application in practice?

  Low degree   ____   ____   ____   ____   ____   High degree

          1   2   3   4   5

II. Phase IB: Statement of findings

In your own words, write a brief statement specifying the findings or conclusions of the study.

III. Phase II: Comparative evaluation

  A. Fit of setting:
    1. How similar are the characteristics of the sample to those of the population with which you work? (Briefly describe the two groups and then make a decision.)
    Study setting:
    Your setting:
    Level of similarity: _____ acceptable   _____ unacceptable
    2. How similar is the study's environment to the one in which you work? (Briefly describe both settings and then make a decision.)
    Study sample:
    Your clients:
    Level of similarity: _____ acceptable   _____ unacceptable

  B. Basis for practice:
    1. Do you have a theoretical or scientific basis for your current practice behavior?
    _____ No   _____ Yes (specify the theory and/or research findings that currently provide a rationale for your practice)
    2. How effective is your current method of practice in your area?
    Not at all effective ____ ____ ____ ____ ____ ____ Highly effective
    Source of evaluation data:

TABLE 14–5 Stetler-Marram Tool for Evaluation of Applicability of Research Findings *Continued*

   C. Feasibility (risk, resources, and readiness):

      1. What degree of potential **risk** could be associated with implementation of these findings? (Consider patients and staff.)

      No risk _____ _____ _____ _____ _____ High risk

      2. Readiness:

         a. What levels of organization would need to be involved in this change in practice? Check all that apply.

            _____ only you as an individual practitioner
            _____ other nurses on a single unit
            _____ upper nurses administration
            _____ other departments
            _____ others _____

         b. Given the levels involved, what is the degree of **readiness** for such a change in practice?

         (Specify level _____)
         Not at all ready _____ _____ _____ _____ _____ Highly ready
         (Specify level _____)
         Not at all ready _____ _____ _____ _____ _____ Highly ready
         (Specify level _____)
         Not at all ready _____ _____ _____ _____ _____ Highly ready
         (Specify level _____)
         Not at all ready _____ _____ _____ _____ _____ Highly ready

      3. What amount of **resources** would be needed to implement such a change?

      No resources _____ _____ _____ _____ _____ Great resources

   D. Substantiating evidence:

      1. What other **research** has been conducted that examined a similar question or hypothesis?
      2. Were the findings the same, similar or conflicting? (Specify)
      3. What other, **nonresearch information/knowledge** is available re this topic?
      4. Overall, to what degree are the findings substantiated?

      Low degree _____ _____ _____ _____ _____ High degree

IV. Phase III: Decision making:

   A. Given **all** of the above factors, do you believe these research findings are:

      _____ Not applicable at this time
      _____ Applicable, but only at the cognitive or conceptual level
      _____ Applicable at the action level

   Briefly explain your decision.

   B. If they are applicable at the action level, indicate the following:

      1. Exactly how would the findings be used? Who would be using them?
      2. Would any resources be needed to apply them? If yes, specify.
      3. Would "change" steps be needed to implement the findings? If yes, list and describe.
      4. Would informal or formal methods be needed to evaluate the effectiveness of this application of research findings? Explain.

From Stetler CB: A strategy for teaching research use, *Nurse Educator* 13(3): 17-20, 1989.

research critique and planned change theory and who have experience within the organizational structure and politics of the institution. The facilitator of the RU process must be effective in influencing and motivating others. Consequently the CC-CNS as content expert (i.e., has clinical and research expertise) and process expert (i.e., is knowledgeable about RU and change theory) has the major role in the RU process. The CC-CNS is responsible for establishing standards and maintaining quality care for a population of patients. Quality depends on research findings that validate practice. As a master clinician the CC-CNS is able to identify clinical problems that must be addressed to maintain quality care. In addressing these problems, the CC-CNS's goal is to develop and implement research-based protocols or innovations to alleviate problems and improve patient outcome.[13]

In addition, the CC-CNS acts as a magnet in bringing innovations into practice. The CC-CNS brings these innovations through the process of strategic scanning described by Rogers.[22] In this process the CC-CNS continually scans the environment, searching for new knowledge and innovations to apply to practice. The CC-CNS values such innovations, strategically scans for them, receives and recognizes them, and uses these innovations to solve practice problems and improve care.[41] Thus the CC-CNS has the potential to lead the nursing services organization in the process of improving patient care through RU.

Of the few investigations conducted examining RU in practice, most have found little evidence of use of research findings in nursing practice.[42] Where evidence was found it was unclear whether subjects were consciously using research.[43] Stetler and DiMaggio[44] explored utilization behavior of CNSs relative to research-based information. The specific research question addressed was as follows: what are the extent and nature of utilization of research-based information by CNSs in terms of (1) level and related frequency of use, (2) types of use, (3) sources of information, and (4) criteria for utilization? Twenty-four CNSs were interviewed in a field survey. Results indicated that subjects most frequently (75%) use findings conceptually (i.e., information was used to change one's understanding of something or the way one thinks about a situation). The remaining 21% in-

dicated they most frequently used the information instrumentally (i.e., utilization that is concrete, such as adoption of an explicit nursing intervention or other information that will help facilitate decision making). Only half of the subjects, however, could list one or more explicit criteria for evaluation of the applicability of findings to practice. No CNS was able to list a comprehensive set of criteria for determining the applicability of research findings for practice.

One explanation proposed by the investigators is that subjects had implicit criteria for evaluation of research into practice and were merely unable to articulate them. However, future research should test this hypothesis by critiquing case histories of utilization.[44] The potential hazards of misusing research are great.[45,46] CNSs and their educators must take the responsibility of applying research into practice seriously. Although most CNS programs have a course in research methodology, few programs emphasize RU to the same degree.[47] Critical analysis and synthesis of research knowledge may take a higher level of knowledge and skill than the conduct of research. In addition, in the RU process the CC-CNS is asked to examine not only the statistical significance but also the clinical significance of research results. Results may be statistically significant but may not be useful in clinical practice.[48] Only an expert in both research methodology and clinical practice can make these determinations accurately. Consequently equal attention needs to be given to both the utilization of research and the conduct of research.

RU is an integral component of the CC-CNS role. Mechanisms to provide CNSs with knowledge and skill regarding RU must begin with appropriate courses at the graduate level. Once a knowledge base is established, the CC-CNS can build on this through a variety of mechanisms such as RU conferences, networking with colleagues interested in RU, mentoring with doctorally prepared CNSs and faculty, subscribing to research journals, incorporating research into classes, clinical conferences, and staff meetings. As the CC-CNS develops in RU sophistication, the benefits are many: that is, nursing staff members become increasingly aware of the scientific basis of their practice, patient care improves, and the value for nursing practice becomes evident.

PRACTICE IMPLICATIONS

The success of the CC-CNS in RU requires a readiness by not only the staff and the institution, but also the CC-CNS. Once readiness is achieved, the CC-CNS can be instrumental in developing a working group (e.g., RU committee) to facilitate the RU process. An RU process approach or model provides the committee with a mechanism for conducting the RU program in an organized, systematic manner. This section offers practical advice to the CC-CNS on assessing and developing system and self-readiness and carrying out an RU program.

Assessing and Developing CNS Readiness

Each CNS brings to the role a unique set of values, education, and experiences. It is unrealistic to assume that every CNS possesses all of the qualities, knowledge, and skill necessary for incorporating research into practice. Before embarking on an RU project, the CC-CNS must assess personal capabilities for and attitudes toward implementing research in the clinical area. The CC-CNS's educational preparation, role development, and values will have a significant impact on ability to conduct a successful RU program.

Educational Preparation

Successful RU requires that the CC-CNS be familiar with the research process, be able to critique research literature, and be aware of the process for implementing research into practice. Many resources are available to the CC-CNS who needs to improve her or his RU knowledge base. The CC-CNS may opt to attend a refresher course on research, critiquing research or RU. Another means of increasing the CNS's expertise is to develop a mentoring relationship with doctorally prepared CNSs and faculty members from a nearby school of nursing. Research partnerships formed between the CC-CNS and nurses in academia are critical to narrowing the gap between the conduct and utilization of research findings. Attending research-oriented conferences and networking with other CNSs involved with RU are other ways the CC-CNS can develop the unique skills needed for implementing an RU program. Videos are also currently available as resources for institutions interested in conducting RU projects.[49]

Role Development

It is not unusual for research activities to be given a low priority compared to the other CC-CNS role components, namely, educator, practitioner, and consultant. This is especially true for the new CC-CNS, who is attempting to master and implement the various components of the role and to set priorities. Successful RU programs also demand that the CC-CNS have insight into the staff, unit, and institution's attitudes toward research and RU. The combined need for role clarity and knowledge of the "system" generally makes it difficult to conduct an RU program in the first (or even second) year as a CC-CNS.

Time spent developing the other role components is not wasted with regard to RU. In these roles the CC-CNS has the chance to observe staff, identify clinical problems, and test the "institutional waters." For example, as a practitioner the CC-CNS has the chance to interact with the staff and stimulate questions and discussions regarding clinical practice issues (e.g., what is the effect of lateral positioning on hemodynamics and cardiac output?).

Value of Innovative Thinking

Nothing is as important to the success of an RU project as the spirit of inquiry by those involved. The CC-CNS plays a pivotal role in promoting innovative thinking, creativity, and questioning by the staff. The word innovation is the essence of RU. Innovative thinking offers an alternative to the status quo. Therefore it means change for the CC-CNS and staff.

Successful RU demands that the CC-CNS be able to tolerate the uncertainty inherent in the change process. Expressing a spirit of inquiry is not as simple or straightforward as increasing one's knowledge base or developing one's role. A self-examination by the CC-CNS about personal attitudes toward and beliefs about research and research-based nursing practice often helps to identify whether a commitment to RU exists. Examples of questions the CNS may use for this assessment include the following:

- How many hours per week do you spend on research-related activities?

- Are standards of care (protocols or procedures) in your unit research based?
- Do you encourage staff members to question why nursing practice is delivered a certain way?
- Do you actively seek new innovations to bring into practice?
- Have you had discussions with your administrator about the benefits of research-based practice?
- Do your short- and long-term goals reflect utilizing research findings in practice?

Formal evaluation tools designed to measure research readiness are also available.[50]

Networking with other CC-CNSs involved in changing practice often helps to cultivate inquisitiveness. Exposure to RU through personal contact, newsletters (e.g., *American Association of Critical Care Nurses [AACN] News*), or nursing journals also may foster an interest in RU. A spirit of inquiry is contagious but only to susceptible individuals with an open mind. The following questions provide a self-assessment checklist that the CC-CNS can use to assess self-readiness for RU and to identify both strengths and areas of needed growth:

1. What educational preparation do I have regarding RU?
   a. RU content in master's program
   b. Research-critiquing skills
2. Where am I in my role development regarding research utilization?
   a. Stage of CC-CNS development
   b. RU as a priority for staff or administrator
3. How much do I value research innovation?
   a. Comfortable with change or ambiguity
   b. Spirit of inquiry

Assessing and Developing Staff Readiness

Many of the same factors that influence the CC-CNS's readiness for RU also apply to the staff nurse. Assessing staff readiness can be challenging in that each nurse's knowledge, role development, and values are different.

Depending on how long a CC-CNS has worked with a group of nurses, various types and amounts of assessment may be needed. For example, a CC-CNS who has worked with the same staff for 5 years may be acutely aware of the staff's attitudes toward and knowledge of RU. The CC-CNS new to an area may not have the same information and may want to use a formal tool to obtain these data.[50]

Developing staff readiness for RU may be a simple or complex process, depending on the staff's baseline knowledge. Strategies such as discussions at staff meetings, classes on critiquing research findings, and informal discussion of problems are all ways to prepare staff nurses for RU.

Successful RU usually has little to do with a staff's educational level or role development. Instead, it is a spirit of curiosity and creativity and value for research that ultimately allows scientific inquiry to thrive. The CC-CNS can begin to nurture this type of environment by asking questions such as the following: "Why do we do it this way? Is there a better way to do this? Has this been studied? Interesting idea, can I see the data?"

The CC-CNS can assist the staff in developing an appreciation for research even before a formal RU program is attempted by demonstrating to staff members the applicability of research to their setting and specifically addressing how research findings could improve patient care. Examples of critical care research ready to be implemented include the following:

- Chest tube stripping
- Cardiac output measurement and positioning
- Pulmonary artery measurement and positioning
- Hyperoxygenation before endotracheal suctioning
- Family visits in the ICU
- Epidural narcotics for pain control
- Weaning from ventilators[51]

In addition, the Agency for Health Care Policy and Research (AHCPR) has developed research-based guidelines for clinical practice.[52] Implementation of these guidelines in critical care is an excellent way the CC-CNS can begin working with staff members in the process of RU. Table 14–6 lists ways to introduce research to a unit and disseminate research findings.

TABLE 14-6 Suggestions for CC-CNS for Introducing and Disseminating Research Finding into Clinical Setting

- Base content of educational programs on research findings.
- Incorporate at least one nursing research finding into nursing rounds.
- Use research studies as the basis for nursing care plans and clinical conferences.
- Establish "research of the month" article. Topics should be timely and should relate directly to patient population. Save monthly articles in a three-ring binder kept on the unit.
- Subscribe to at least one research journal (e.g., *Nursing Research, Heart and Lung, American Journal of Critical Care, Critical Care Medicine*).
- Convey excitement and enthusiasm about recent discoveries in the research literature, and encourage staff to display the same type of enthusiasm to one another.
- Develop research-based standards of care. Include references at end of standard.
- Encourage staff to attend conferences such as the National Critical Care Nursing Research Conference at the AACN National Teaching Institute, where opportunities are available to network with nurse researchers.
- Develop a unit-based research journal club, where research is reviewed, critiqued, and evaluated for application to practice.
- Demonstrate evidence of having read and critiqued a wide range of clinical nursing research studies during bedside discussions and rounds with staff, physicians, and other health care disciplines.

Assessing and Developing Institutional Readiness

It has been suggested that the success of an RU program depends on an institutional philosophy that values and supports research.[19] Unless research and RU are valued, the CC-CNS will have a difficult time trying to implement an RU program. An assessment of institutional readiness is so critical that information about RU should be gathered as early as during the CC-CNS's job interview (Table 14-7).

The department of nursing's philosophy statement and the CC-CNS job description also offer a means of assessing institutional readiness. Performance expectations such as "The CC-CNS will participate in the interpretation, dissemination, and utilization of nursing research into clinical practice" indicate a value for research and RU in the clinical setting. The CC-CNS must investigate further, however, how these statements actually translate into practice. This requires a dialogue between nursing administrators and the CC-CNS regarding the specifics of what is expected in terms of research-related activities and the type of support available to the CC-CNS for carrying out these activities. Examples of organizational commitment include the provision of resources such as time, space, secretarial support, and money.[53]

A lack of administrative support creates a formidable but not insurmountable barrier to RU. The CC-CNS in this situation has two options. The first is to delay any RU activities until a more supportive climate is established. In this situation the final goal of carrying out a specific RU plan may be deferred, but in the long run this may be more beneficial to the organization and less stressful for the CC-CNS. Acquiring administrative support requires a concerted, deliberate effort by the CC-CNS. The most appealing RU project will be one that maintains an acceptable standard of care yet allows the institution to realize a savings (e.g., changing intravenous tubings every 72 vs. every 24 hours).

The second option is to initiate an RU activity without administrative support in an attempt to demonstrate its value to the organization. The CC-CNS can do this by (1) choosing a high-volume patient problem of concern to the nursing staff and administrators, (2) revising a policy or procedure based on research, or (3) turning a continuous quality improvement project into an RU project. The second option may be undertaken if the CC-CNS sees a specific RU activity as a priority and cannot wait for the institution to change its philosophy toward RU. This option demands that the CNS carefully plan an implementation strategy. A proposal for the RU project must be scrupulously outlined, with specific attention paid to the implications for the institution and all parties involved.[54] In particular, the CC-CNS must be able to project

TABLE 14–7 Suggested Questions Regarding RU for CC-CNS to Ask During Interview Process

---

Nursing administrators

1. Does the nursing philosophy include a statement supporting research?
2. Does your institution have an institutional review board? Does the board have nursing members?
3. Does the department of nursing have an active research committee? How is membership for that committee determined?
4. Are nursing standards of care and hospital policies and procedures research based? What are some examples?
5. How many nursing research projects are currently underway?
6. Is there a nursing school associated with the hospital or medical center? If so, what is the relationship between the school of nursing and university medical center? What are examples of collaborative projects between the two institutions?
7. Do nurses in the hospital/medical center know what nursing research is? Have they been involved in RU programs?
8. Is there a "housewide" mechanism for disseminating the results of nursing research studies (e.g., an in-house publication)?
9. Does the career ladder include criteria for the utilization of research?
10. Are there rewards or awards for research involvement?
11. Are there any personnel on staff who conduct nursing research as their primary responsibility?

Staff or nurse manager

1. Does the unit subscribe to a research journal?
2. Does the unit have a journal club?
3. Are there any mechanisms in place for sharing the results of research studies?
4. Is practice based on research findings?
5. Have any research studies been conducted in the unit?
6. Is anyone interested in conducting studies or implementing research-based findings into practice?

---

the potential cost impact of the program as well as the clinical impact.

Determining the Forum for RU and Developing Staff

Once the CC-CNS and the system have been assessed, developed, and determined to be ready, the CC-CNS's next task is to establish a forum for implementing RU. This necessitates recruiting a group of motivated and enthusiastic nurses interested in promoting research-based nursing practice. These groups may be formal, such as a hospital-based RU committee, or informal, such as a unit-based journal club. Some groups that choose to get involved in RU are part of a larger group such as a hospital research, policy and procedure, or continuous quality improvement committee. The committee should be open to all interested parties, and staff nurses must be represented. Once the group is established, the charge of the committee and ground rules should be determined. The CC-CNS

may initially assume the role of chairperson of the committee or may act as a consultant or member, depending on the group's needs.

Initially, the charge of the group will be to educate its members about the RU process. The CC-CNS may provide classes, handouts, and guest speakers based on the committee's needs. For many staff members, participation on the RU committee may represent their first exposure to research in any form. In-depth or specific learning needs of individual members can be met through reading materials and self-study packets. Examples of issues that should be addressed by the CC-CNS include (1) definition of RU; (2) differentiating among research utilization, research dissemination, and research conduct; (3) models of RU; and (4) research critique skills.

It is also important that the CC-CNS assist the RU committee in understanding the importance of the research critique process. This is not to say that members of the committee or even the CC-CNS has to be highly skilled in the critique process for RU to occur. Rather, they should understand the rationale for evaluating the clinical and scientific integrity of a study before implementing its findings into the clinical setting. Either the CC-CNS who is skilled in critiquing research or a consultant (such as a doctorally prepared CC-CNS or faculty member from a school of nursing) should spend time with the RU committee explaining the critiquing process. One teaching technique is to have a skilled individual critique an article from start to finish for the committee. This method requires that the members have read the research article beforehand and have an outline to follow as the critique is performed. The more choice the staff members have in choosing the article and the more the study relates to their patient care area, the more successful this strategy will be. Several tools are available to use as guides in the critique process.[20,55]

The ability to critique research requires a significant knowledge of the research process. It must be emphasized that not all staff members or even the CC-CNS needs to have a complete grasp of the critiquing process for RU to occur. However, it is imperative that the committee recognize the value of the critique process and have access to individuals who are skilled at the process.

Before an RU project can begin, the committee must decide on a model to use in guiding their decision making. The term "model" may have negative connotations for many staff members who consider models to be purely theoretic and associated with academia. Care must be taken by the CC-CNS to demonstrate how the selection of an appropriate model can serve to facilitate the process of RU. As previously discussed, a variety of models are available to the CC-CNS, each with various attributes including degree of user friendliness.

Implementing an RU Program

Once the committee is established, the CC-CNS is ready to begin the RU process. Regardless of the model used, the organization of an RU program follows similar steps. The following example of the RU process uses the seven phases described in the CURN Project (see Table 14-3) and highlights the role of the CC-CNS in implementing the steps in an RU program.

Problem Identification

Identifying clinical issues that require resolution is rarely difficult for either the CC-CNS or the staff. Questions such as "Why do we do this this way?" probably come up on a daily basis for many CNSs. This is especially true in units where staff members are encouraged to question the status quo and to be independent thinkers. Continuous quality improvement monitors, incident reports, and published research studies are sources of information that lead to problem identification. However, the CC-CNS must be aware from the onset that if the issue is not perceived as a problem by the staff, the chances of a successful RU program are severely diminished. Therefore choose a problem that is part of your day-to-day practice.

Once high-priority issues have been identified, the CC-CNS can help the staff to define the problems more clearly. It is common for the identified problem to be so broad or vague that it is not amenable to investigation or intervention. For example, the staff of an ICU in a large teaching medical center prioritized blood pressure measurement as the number one problem in the unit. The CC-CNS's knowledge of unit practices and continuous quality improvement data allowed the CC-CNS to guide the staff in further narrowing and defining the problem. After discussion with the staff, the problem was revealed to be a conflict between nurse and physicians over the use of arterial lines vs. cuff pressures for monitoring blood pressure. The nurses wanted to use the arterial line, but the physicians said they did not trust it. The decision was eventually made by the group to investigate the research on the validity and reliability of various methods of blood pressure monitoring in the critical care setting in order to develop a research-based protocol.

Assessment

The CC-CNS plays a major role in assisting the RU committee to obtain research articles for review and then facilitating the critique process. Technologic advances have made retrieval of literature possible even in areas without access to biomedical libraries. Sources of information about published reports include computer searches, citation indexes (e.g., *Cumulative Index to Nursing and Allied Health Literature*), and review articles (e.g., *American Journal of Critical Care, Heart and Lung,*

Applied Nursing Research, and *Critical Care Medicine*). When computer searches are used, the CC-CNS's knowledge of the literature can be very helpful in identifying the key words associated with a body of knowledge.

Critiquing the relevant literature on a topic is often one of the most interesting yet challenging components of the RU process.

The critique process is conducted to establish the scientific merit of the study. Establishing scientific merit is a part of the RU process that will benefit from the skills of a doctorally prepared nurse scientist. The purpose of this component of the critique process is to scrutinize the study's methodologic and data analysis techniques.

When undertaking an RU project, it is also important to establish the applicability of the study findings to the new setting and the feasibility of implementing the research-based innovation. It is this section of the RU process that depends on the knowledge, expertise, and experience of the staff and CC-CNS. For example, a study evaluating a family intervention program may be critiqued and determined to have high scientific merit. However, the staff and CC-CNS determine that the study is not applicable to their setting for a variety of reasons, such as differing patient populations or lack of similar resources. In addition, an assessment of the feasibility and cost benefit of an innovation is necessary.

Designing and Adopting the Research-based Innovation

Once the relevant research has been critiqued and the scientific merit and clinical applicability established, the next step is to design a research-based innovation. In some cases the practice change can be identical to the innovation used in the original study (or studies). In many cases, however, the innovation is altered in some way to meet the needs of a particular unit or patient population. Care must be taken when developing the protocol to avoid altering the intervention in such a way that it no longer achieves the intent of the original research from which it was derived. The CC-CNS's knowledge of the staff and the unit's resources (e.g., budget, support personnel) is invaluable in developing an innovation that meets the needs of the unit and is practical as well.

Implementation

Like any successful program, an RU program requires careful planning before a clinical trial is conducted. Overzealous attempts to implement changes in practice without having a well–thought out plan typically end in disaster. Before implementing any change, the CC-CNS must perform a complete evaluation of the driving and restraining forces that exist in the institution and unit.

The CC-CNS as a change agent can be instrumental in ensuring that the groundwork is properly laid before any changes in practice are begun (see Chapter 16). Steps in the implementation process include the following:

1. Writing the RU program proposal (including time frames)
2. Sharing the proposal with key personnel (e.g., staff nurses, nurse manager, unit medical director)
3. Revision of proposal as necessary
4. Education process of staff regarding practice change
5. Implementation of the practice change as a pilot program

When the program proposal is written, realistic time frames must be determined for each step of the process. The CC-CNS's insights into the unit's needs and priorities are invaluable in setting realistic goals. Not being able to meet time frames can be a significant source of frustration for the staff.

The CC-CNS is in a key position to disseminate the RU plan to various personnel involved in the change. Practice changes typically involve other disciplines beside nursing. Every effort therefore should be made to share the RU plan with the other disciplines involved with or affected by the change and to incorporate their suggestions into the plan. The CC-CNS's role as a consultant makes the CC-CNS the logical person to collaborate with other members of the health care team. A CC-CNS who is respected by colleagues will serve as an important facilitator to the change process.

Ensuring that staff are knowledgeable about the planned change is an important responsibility of the CC-CNS. An optimal situation would be one where the members of the RU committee are actively involved in educating their peers under the direction of the CNS. The CC-CNS can facilitate the education process by helping the committee members to determine learning objectives and creative ways to achieving those objectives. Educational programs may take on a variety of forms, including classes, information fairs, posters, videos, and self-study packets.

There are a variety of reasons for initially implementing the RU program on a small scale. A pilot study allows for the proposed change to be implemented and evaluated in a thorough yet less costly manner than a full-scale implementation. Perhaps even more important, it does not send a "fait accompli" message to the staff that can serve as a significant barrier to change. A pilot study suggests that the innovation and the method by which it is being implemented are being evaluated for effectiveness and that modifications and revisions will be performed as needed.

Evaluation

The RU process is not complete unless an evaluation is conducted to determine whether the desired outcomes were achieved. Although staff satisfaction with the change in practice is a desirable outcome, it should not be the only one. Other areas that may be affected by a change and require evaluation include patient and family satisfaction and patient outcome.

In addition to outcomes, the evaluation process also gives information about components of the RU process, such as the educational process and the methods used to implement the change. Data derived from the evaluation are initially used to revise the planned change and then later to maintain it.

The CC-CNS and staff are in a unique position to monitor outcomes of nursing care. Hence the CC-CNS can integrate the evaluation component of RU into ongoing data collection of patient outcomes. The RU committee and staff should also actively participate in the evaluative phase so that they understand when revisions to the plan are needed.

The CC-CNS must be prepared for situations in which the planned change process has improved patient care outcomes but is unpopular with the staff. Staff satisfaction is always a desirable outcome of an RU program but not a required one. If the effect on the staff is very negative, it is unlikely that the new innovation will ever be adopted. In most cases, however, the CC-CNS can often use the positive data from the evaluation program to justify the planned change's worth to the staff. It also may be possible to modify the intervention slightly to diminish the negative effects on the staff. An awareness of Roger's concept of rate of adoption of a new idea will help the CC-CNS to set realistic expectations for how quickly and enthusiastically a new idea will be accepted.[22]

At the end of the initial evaluation period a decision must be made to retain the change as introduced, to modify the change, or to abandon the change altogether. If major revisions to the initial plan are made, a continued evaluation period is necessary.

Extending and Diffusing Findings

Once an acceptable plan has been implemented and positively evaluated, it is appropriate to extend the findings on a larger scale or to other areas. The CC-CNS's role as a consultant to other units or divisions will facilitate this process.

Maintaining Innovation Over Time

The excitement of a new program is typically short lived, especially in an ICU setting where new innovations are common. Ensuring that a new research-based practice is maintained over time depends on the continuous evaluation of its effects on patient outcome (by the CNS, nurse manager, and staff). Integration of the new protocol into the unit standards and continuous quality improvement monitoring will assist in maintaining continuity of the practice innovation.

CASE STUDY

The RU committee of a surgical intensive care unit (SICU) was interested in using the results of AACN's[56] Thunder Project to determine if their practice of routinely using heparin in arterial line flush solutions should be changed. The CC-CNS consulted with the RU committee and guided the group through the following steps of the RU process.

1. Determining the problem: Is heparin required to maintain patency of arterial line catheters?
2. Critiquing research-based literature on the use of heparin versus no heparin to maintain arterial catheter patency.
3. Designing a research-based innovation. This in-

novation included an education and practice component for all staff nurses that presented the following:

a. Research findings of the variables affecting patency.

b. Three clinical scenarios of critically ill patients so that nurses could apply the research findings and determine which patients needed heparin.

c. A new unit policy based on the research that stated, "the critical care nurse applies research knowledge of the variables affecting patency and makes the decision to add or not to add heparin in the arterial line flush solution." This policy was signed by the unit medical director of the SICU.

4. A clinical trial of the new research-based policy was conducted and evaluated. The evaluation indicated that these nurses were successfully making a **research-based** decision on whether or not to add heparin to arterial line flush solutions. There were no negative patient incidents, and the innovation was adopted by the unit.

SUMMARY

The CC-CNS acts as a link between nursing practice and research. Through clinical expertise and knowledge of research methodology, the CC-CNS can identify clinical problems that can be addressed through RU. However, for RU to occur, commitment to support and encourage research-based practices must exist from agencies and academic settings. This chapter provides the CC-CNS with a theoretic perspective of RU, concrete examples of how to involve staff in the RU process, and sample tools to use when evaluating research ready for practice.

References

1. McClure ML: Promoting practice-based research: a critical need, *J Nurs Admin* 9(11):66-70, 1981.
2. Wabschall JM: The CNS as researcher. In Menard SW, editor: *The clinical nurse specialist: perspectives on practice,* New York, 1987, John Wiley & Sons.
3. American Nurses' Association, Commission on Nursing Research: *Guidelines for the investigative function of nurses,* Kansas City, Mo, 1981, The Association.
4. Fuhs MF, Moore K: Research program development in a tertiary care setting, *Nurs Res* 30:24-27, 1981.
5. Davis MZ: Promoting nursing research in the clinical setting, *J Nurs Admin* 11:22-27, 1981.
6. Diers D: Preparation of practitioners, clinical specialists, and clinicians, *J Prof Nurs* 1:41-47, 1985.
7. Hefferin EA, Horsely J, Ventura M: Promoting research-based nursing: the nurse administrator's role, *J Nurs Admin* 12:34-41, 1982.
8. King O, Barnard K, Hoehn R: Disseminating the results of nursing research, *Nurs Outlook* 29:164-169, 1981.
9. Engstrom JL: University, agency, and collaborative models for nursing research: an overview, *Image* 16:76-80, 1974.
10. Felton G: The dean's research support function in minimizing performance gaps, *J Prof Nurs* 1:125, 1985.
11. Haller KB, Reynolds MA, Horsley JA: Developing research-based innovative protocols: process, criteria, and issues, *Res Nurs Health* 2:45-51, 1979.
12. Fawcett J: A topology of nursing res
h activities according to educational preparation, *J Prof Nurs,* pp 75-78, March/April 1985.
13. Hickey M: The role of the clinical nurse specialist in the research utilization process, *Clin Nurse Specialist* 4(2):93-96, 1990.
14. Horsley J: Using research in practice: the current context, *West J Nurs Res* 7:135-139, 1985.
15. Stetler CB: Research utilization: defining the concept, *Image* 17:40-44, 1985.
16. Krueger J: Utilization of nursing research: the planning process, *J Nurs Admin* 8(1):6-9, 1978.
17. Rempusheski VF: Using art and science to change practice, *Appl Nurs Res* 4(2):96-98, 1991.
18. Stetler C, Marram G: Evaluating research findings for applicability in practice, *Nurs Outlook* 24:559-563, 1976.
19. Phillips LRF: A clinicians guide to the critique and utilization of nursing research, Norwalk, Conn, 1986, Appleton-Century-Crofts.
20. Burns N, Grove SK: Utilization of research in practice. In *The practice of nursing research conduct, critique and utilization,* ed 2, Philadelphia, 1993, WB Saunders Co.
21. Glasser EM, Abelson HH, Garrison KN: Putting knowledge to use facilitating the diffusion of knowledge and the implementation of planned change, San Francisco, 1983, Jossey-Bass.
22. Rogers EM: *Diffusion of innovations,* New York, 1983, Free Press.
23. Rogers EM: *Diffusion of innovations,* New York, 1983, Free Press.
24. Havelock RG: *A guide to innovation in education,* Ann Arbor, Mich, 1970, Center for Research on Utilization of Scientific Knowledge, Institute for Social Research, The University of Michigan.
25. Havelock RG: *The change agent's guide to innovation in education,* Engelwood Cliffs, NJ, 1973, Educational Technology Publication.

26. Havelock RG: *Ideal systems for research utilization: four alternatives.* Contract 22893/5-01, Social and Rehabilitation Service, Washington, DC, 1974, US Department of Health, Education and Welfare.

27. Havelock RG, Lingwood DA: *R & D utilization strategies and functions: an analytical comparison of four systems,* Ann Arbor, Mich, 1973, Center for Research on Utilization of Scientific Knowledge, Institute for Social Research, University of Michigan.

28. Lewin K: Group decision and social change. In Newcomb T, Hartlet E, editors: *Readings in social psychology,* New York, 1947, Holt, Rinehart & Winston.

29. Lewin K: Field theory in social sciences. In Cartwright D, editor: New York, 1951, Harper Brothers.

30. Horsley JA et al: *Using research to improve nursing practice: a guide,* New York, 1983, Grune & Stratton.

31. King D, Barnard K, Hoehn R: Disseminating the results of nursing research, *Nurs Outlook* 24:164-169, 1981.

32. Donaldson N: *Improving nursing practice through research utilization* Washington, DC, US Department of Health and Human Services, 1988.

33. Dracup K, Breu C: Strengthening practice through research utilization, In M. Batey, editor: Communicating nursing research, Boulder Colo, 1977, Western Interstate Commission for Higher Education, vol 10, p 341.

34. Krueger J: Research utilization, Western J Nurs 1:148-152, 1979.

35. Goode C, et al: Use of research based knowledge in clinical practice, J Nurs Admin 12:11-18, 1987.

36. MacLachlar LW: General considerations about the utilization of research by clinicians. In Phillips LRF, editor: A clinician's guide to the critique and utilization of nursing research, Norwalk, Conn, 1986, Appleton-Century-Crofts.

37. Horsley JA, Crane J, Bing JD: Research utilization as an organizational process, *J Nurs Admin* 8(7):4-6, 1978.

38. Horsley JA, Crane J, Reynolds N: *Pain: deliberate nursing interventions: CURN project,* New York, 1982, Grune & Stratton.

39. Barnard KE: Proceedings of the 1982 Conference of the Western Society for Research in Nursing. The research cycle: nursing, the profession, the discipline, West J Nurs Res 4(3):1-12, 1982.

40. Stetler C: A strategy for teaching research utilization, *Nurse Educator* 13:17-20, 1989.

41. Donaldson N: Personal communication, 1993.

42. Kirchhoff K: A diffusion survey of coronary precautions, *Nurs Res* 31:196-201, 1982.

43. Brett J: Use of nursing practice research findings, *Nurs Res* 36:344-349, 1987.

44. Stetler C, DiMaggio G: Research utilization among clinical nurse specialists, *Clin Nurse Specialist* 5(3):151-155, 1991.

45. Cook T, Levinson-Rose J, Pollard W: The misutilization of evaluation research, *Knowledge Creation Diffusion Utilization* 1:477-498, 1980.

46. Gerber R, Van Ort S: Topical application of insulin to pressure sores: a questionable therapy, *Am J Nurs* 81:1169, 1981.

47. Mallick M: A constant comparative method for teaching research critiquing to baccalaureate nursing students, *Image* 15:120-123, 1983.

48. LeFort SM. The statistical versus clinical significance debate *Image* 25:57-62, 1993.

49. *Research utilization: a process of institutional change,* Ida Grove, Iowa, 1988, Horn Video Productions.

50. Rempusheski VF: Incorporating research role and practice role, *Appl Nurs Res* 4:46-48, 1991.

51. Dracup K: *Research utilization in practice.* Sigma Theta Tau, Gamma Tau Chapter, presentation, Los Angeles, 1993.

52. Institute of Medicine, Committee to Advise the Public Health Service on Clinical Practice Guidelines: *Clinical practice guidelines—directions for a new program,* Washington, DC, 1990, National Academy Press.

53. Cronenwett LR: The research role of the clinical nurse specialist, J Nurs Admin 16:10-12, 1986.

54. Rempusheski VF: Nursing administrators: What are their research needs? How can they support critical care research? *Heart Lung* 17:456-457, 1988.

55. Downs FA: *Source book of nursing research,* Philadelphia, 1984, FA Davis Co.

56. American Association of Critical-Care Nurses: Evaluation of the effects of heparinized and non-heparinized solutions on patency of arterial pressure monitoring lines: The Thunder Project. Am J Crit Care 2:3-15, 1993.

The Critical Care Clinical Nurse Specialist as Leader / Manager

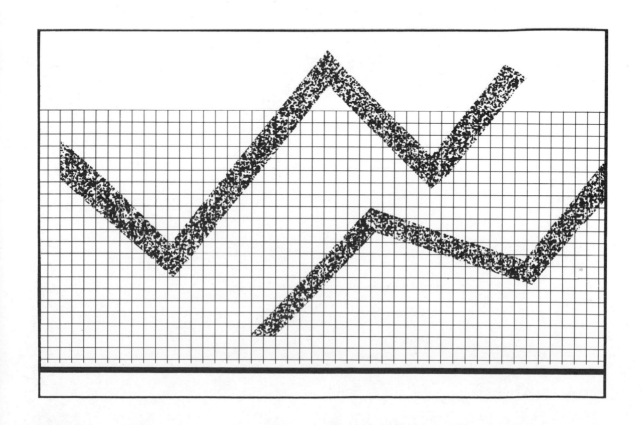

The Critical Care Clinical Nurse Specialist as Leader

Janet C. Howard, RN, MSN, CEN, CCRN

The leadership role is predominantly demonstrated by the critical care clinical nurse specialist (CC-CNS) in working with staff and in consultation with other professionals. In each of the traditional roles, the CC-CNS's primary objective is to advance the delivery of effective care to critically ill patients and their families. Except as a direct care provider, however, the CC-CNS affects the quality of patient care only by influencing the behavior of others. The CC-CNS's success depends as much on ability to work with staff as on expertise. Additional skills for working with staff supplement the traditional roles. At times the CC-CNS serves as a salesperson in selling an idea, a cheerleader in providing positive feedback, and a spring trainer in developing a team.[1] Positive working relationships with staff members are crucial not only to the CC-CNS's success but also to the quality of patient care and the success of the organization as a whole. Health care organizations that strive to provide cost-effective, quality care value the CC-CNS who is able to influence the work of staff toward this end, especially in critical care, where the cost of care is high and where complications become life threatening.

In the process of improving patient care, the CC-CNS strives to achieve a secondary goal: empowering staff nurses by assisting them to gain the knowledge, skills, and self-confidence that will assure their success. As important as the CC-CNS's ability to produce quality care are the ability and commitment to empower staff members through enabling their professional development.

THEORETIC PERSPECTIVES

Appreciating the CC-CNS's ability to influence the quality of care through working with staff requires an understanding of the fundamentals of *power, leadership,* and *empowerment.* Nurses frequently avoid thinking or talking about power because they negatively equate power with dominance and control. Wynd, however, warns of the consequences of viewing power only as a negative force: "Avoidance of power in nursing contributes to a lack of progress in achieving professional, occupational goals, the greatest of which is promotion of excellence in patient care."[2] It is therefore crucial that nurses begin to differentiate the positive (or constructive) from the negative (or controlling) aspects of power in order to exert positive and useful energy in promoting quality patient care.

Power and leadership have been described as reciprocal forces. If power is "the basic energy needed to initiate and sustain action" then leadership is the "wise use of power."[3] Effective leaders use power when they direct resources and empower employees to achieve a desired result.[3] Leadership, of course, is not confined to those with formal positions of power.

As a resource, power can be created, accrued, and shared. Empowerment is commonly defined as the sharing of formal power or authority. This definition focuses on empowerment as a process of passing legitimate power from one person to another and is contingent on the leadership style of the person in a formal position of power.[4] This relational view of empowerment is limited, because it emphasizes power as dependence of one person on another. As a result, it often encourages participative management and delegation as "empowering" strategies.[4] Unfortunately, discussions of empowerment are frequently restricted to this view alone.

Power also arises from a person's view of self and the ability to make things happen. Therefore a more balanced view of empowerment encompasses a personal or internal perspective. In this context, empowerment is also the enabling of people by assisting them in gaining the knowledge, resources, information, and support to be successful.[4] This view of empowerment is broader and less restrictive, because it does not depend on those in formal positions of power but is applicable to any leader, including clinical nurse specialists (CNSs).

Consistent with this internal perspective, strategies that enhance the staff's understanding and ability to act in situations that confront them are empowering. Four specific strategies that are fundamental to empowerment are (1) strengthening collegiality, (2) engaging staff in change activities, (3) assisting staff in gaining the necessary skills to resolve interpersonal and organizational problems, and (4) extending sponsorship to guide staff in resolution of difficult practice problems.[5]

RELATED RESEARCH AND LITERATURE

Specific literature detailing use of power by CNSs is scarce. This may be due in part to the persistent understanding of power as control, not from an empowerment perspective. However, the question of how a leader influences the behavior of others is the basis of various leadership theories. One popular theory is situational leadership.[6] Although frequently applied to management functions, situational leadership applies equally well to any person in a leadership role.

The concept of situational leadership is based on the belief that effective leaders use a repertoire of leadership styles that are adapted to a unique combination of variables present in each situation.[7] Leadership styles are "consistent behavior patterns that leaders [demonstrate] when they are working with and through other people as perceived by those people."[6]

Communication between leaders and followers is thought to be an important determinant of leadership; people can be motivated to achieve goals through the influence of words matched by action. Accordingly, four patterns of communication (directing, coaching, supporting, and delegating) are recognized in situational leadership.[7] The four styles differ in the combination of two basic leader behaviors: directive behavior and supportive behavior. Directive behavior is the extent to which a leader provides instructions, whereas supportive behavior is defined as the extent to which the leader encourages followers to take responsibility for their own work.[7]

In the directing leadership style, the leader provides specific instructions and closely supervises performance; supportive behavior is low. Coaching is a second highly directive behavior; the leader explains directions and provides opportunity for clarification and suggestions. The leader is also highly supportive of the follower, however, in providing opportunity for clarification. A third pattern, supporting, scores high in supportive behavior but low in directive behavior. The leader is less directive by sharing ideas and encouraging participation in decision making. The final style, delegating, involves both little direction and little support.[7]

The situational leader also considers the developmental level of the learner, defined by the elements of competence (knowledge and skills) and commitment (motivation and confidence).[7] There are four levels of development. The first developmental level encompasses the beginner who lacks competence but usually exhibits high commitment. Competence increases at the second level, but confidence and motivation often drop. The employee at the third developmental level demonstrates moderate to high competence but variable commitment. Finally, the top level is characterized by a "peak performer" who demonstrates both high competency and high commitment.[7]

The effective leader chooses a leadership style that matches the development level of the staff. For instance, as the level of staff competence increases, the effective leader decreases direction; with a highly committed employee, the leader offers less support.[7]

The potential for misuse of power exists, especially when the leader does not learn a leadership style that is consistent with the development needs of staff members. Abuse can result if the CC-CNS fails to recognize staff competence and commitment and fosters staff's dependence on the specialist.[8] Two common manifestations of abuse are rescuing and pleasing behaviors.

Rescuing often results from the CC-CNS's need to reaffirm expertise and skills. It is commonly displayed when staff members are struggling to provide care to a patient. As an expert the CC-CNS is called on to lend assistance in solving a patient care problem. If, however, the CC-CNS takes over and corrects the problem without considering the staff nurses' need to be part of the problem solving, rescuing has occurred. The CC-CNS emerges from the situation having reaffirmed her or his expert skills and knowledge as a means of reinforcing confidence and pride. At the same time and often without the CC-CNS's realization, however, the staff members emerge from the situation confused about the solution and how the CC-CNS arrived at the solution. In addition, the staff members are frustrated and less confident about their ability to handle similar situations and therefore depend on the CC-CNS when future problems arise.

A variant of rescuing occurs if the CC-CNS retains exclusive reponsibility for a certain aspect of care, not because it is in the patient's best interest or is even the most appropriate way to deliver care, but because of an underlying need to maintain control and demonstrate expertise. Keeping information from staff is abusive and subordinates the staff to a dependent position. If the CC-CNS does not share knowledge and skills, staff members remain unprepared to assume responsibility when the CC-CNS is unavailable.

Another abuse of power occurs if the CC-CNS falls into pleasing behaviors. In this situation the CC-CNS has difficulty recognizing the limitations of expertise and offers less than adequate advice in an attempt to please others. Sneed[8] refers to this misrepresentation of qualifications as the halo effect. The CC-CNS may also slip into pleasing behaviors in an attempt to maintain the status quo and avoid difficult change.

PRACTICE IMPLICATIONS
Working with Staff

Effective and rewarding working relationships begin with the recognition and acknowledgement of the staff's intrapersonal needs. These include the need for a positive self-esteem and a sense of self-efficacy. Low self-esteem is frequently diag-

nosed as a problem of nurses. One author[9] suggests, in reference to nurses, that Maslow's pyramid be redrawn as an hourglass with a bottleneck at the level of self-esteem. Further, nurses need to feel a part of meaningful work and to see meaningful outcomes of their work.[10]

They need to use the four strategies fundamental to empowerment[5] discussed earlier.

The CC-CNS becomes a member of a recognizable work group, whether a single unit, division, or department. Devoting time and energy to strengthening collegiality within the work group influences the success of future strategies. The CC-CNS who is new to the role or the practice setting needs to gather data about the staff, standards of practice, and the practice setting. Many practitioners recommend a brief 15- to 30-minute conversation with each staff member as a useful assessment technique. This initial assessment serves several important functions. Primarily, it provides an opportunity to assess each nurse's skills, particularly clinical and interpersonal skills. At the same time, however, the CC-CNS gains insight into the staff's level of self-esteem and self-efficacy. For instance, the CC-CNS may explore aspects of patient care that a nurse finds rewarding or challenging. At the same time, staff members are able to judge the CC-CNS's knowledge and clinical objectives.

A second highly recommended assessment technique is dedicated clinical time. The opportunity to work with staff in a purely clinical role may not be appreciated by the CC-CNS unless viewed as an opportunity to observe the staff's knowledge, skills, and commitment. Given clinical time, many CC-CNSs choose to practice alone by providing direct care to patients. When working in isolation, however, the CC-CNS is unable to directly interact with staff. In contrast, working with staff members allows firsthand observation of staff and more direct role modeling by the CC-CNS. It also avoids misleading the staff who may otherwise view the CC-CNS primarily as a direct care provider.

On a daily basis the CC-CNS can use various strategies to strengthen a working relationship with the staff. The CC-CNS is consistently linked with the staff through clinical involvement as practitioner and consultant. The practitioner role is traditionally recognized as the basis of clinical specialization.[11] For the CC-CNS this requires demonstrating advanced cognitive and psychomotor skills in diagnosing, treating, and evaluating human responses to actual or potential life-threatening health problems.[12]

The patient is the primary benefactor of CC-CNS interventions as a practitioner. The CC-CNS's influence is further extended, however, when the staff is able to observe skilled practice. Specifically, staff members witness assessment techniques that demonstrate in-depth knowledge of the population, negotiation of care with patients, and care based on future thinking.[13] Staff members also learn by watching the CC-CNS discard ritualistic practice and provide care based on research findings. Finally, watching how the CC-CNS behaves under stress can be very supportive to staff.[14]

The CC-CNS may practice in a setting surrounded by very experienced and accomplished staff practitioners. Instead of feeling threatened by an experienced staff, the empowering CC-CNS recognizes, incorporates, and supports the staff's knowledge and skills.

In addition to technical expertise, the specialist models caring practices. This is especially crucial in critical care, where humanism is easily blurred by technology. The CC-CNS challenges the staff members to expand their understanding of responses to critical illness by guiding the staff to consider other interpretations of the patient's needs or behaviors. For example, the CC-CNS may coach the intensive care unit (ICU) staff to see that the manipulative behavior of a spinal cord–injured patient is a manifestation of powerlessness.

Beyond the role as practitioner, the CC-CNS must also effectively implement the indirect role of consultant to broadly influence the quality of care.[15] Generally, the consultation role arises from earlier interactions of the staff with the CC-CNS as practitioner or educator. Because the CC-CNS is not immersed in direct care on a daily basis, she or he is often in a position to identify needs and suggest approaches not apparent to the direct caregivers.[16]

Clinical rounds are recommended as an unstructured way to be available as a consultant. Because of the rapidity of changes in critically ill patients, frequent, regular rounds are required. One recommendation is to do rounds early in the shift to elicit patient care problems and to problem solve; later rounds can be used to evaluate progress.[17]

In consulting the CC-CNS uses critical care expertise to support the staff's ability and desire to manage care. For example, the CC-CNS may discuss an idea or assessment finding with a staff nurse. The CC-CNS makes a valuable contribution by encouraging and validating staff members' clinical observations that might otherwise go unnoticed.[14]

At the same time the CC-CNS protects against rescuing behavior that is disempowering to the staff nurse. Rescuing can be a problem for expert nurses whose practice is so highly refined by past practical experiences and theoretic knowledge that they have difficulty seeing a patient care situation from the same perspective as a beginning nurse.[13] In other situations, anxiety about the patient's condition makes it difficult to "let go" and allow the less experienced nurse to make independent decisions. However, the CC-CNS can guide the staff nurse in addressing the problem appropriately. The CC-CNS assesses the problem and determines what approaches the nurse has already attempted and what further interventions are needed. Prompts such as "How has Mr. X's cardiac index responded to the nitroprusside?" work well for a more experienced nurse who quickly realizes the significance of the problem. Advanced beginners often require more direct communication, such as "Mr. X's cardiac index is too low. Which drug can you titrate to improve the parameter?" Of course, if a situation is harmful for the patient, the CC-CNS must step in to correct the immediate problem, but she or he should make time later to discuss the situation with the nurse so that learning occurs.

As a consultant the CC-CNS is primarily concerned with facilitating the staff's ability to manage an immediate problem. By providing recommendations to solve a patient care problem, the CC-CNS simultaneously ensures appropriate care and reduces the staff's anxiety. However, the empowering consultant also considers how to ensure the staff's ability to handle similar problems in the future.[18] "The goal of consultation should be one of 'empowering' others by helping them to [work] through a problem, identify resources to meet goals, and become more confident in carrying out their tasks and nursing responsibilities."[19]

From these daily interactions with the staff, the CC-CNS comes to know the staff's practices intimately and is thus able to provide opportunities for recognition. The CC-CNS can assist staff nurses to examine their own practice to recognize overlooked expertise and the resulting outcomes. While doing rounds the specialist can encourage nurses to share their contributions to patient care. By asking probing questions such as "How did you know what this patient needed?" or "How did this patient challenge you?" the CC-CNS exposes the staff's significant work to the nurses themselves and to others.

Additional opportunities for recognition are available with limited planning. For example, the vice president for nursing at one hospital asks the CNSs each year to provide exemplars from clinical practice to present as part of her yearly report to the board of trustees. Formal awards, scholarships, and grants, such as those offered by the American Association of Critical Care Nurses (AACN), are also available. Such opportunities highlight the work of nurses and the outcomes they achieve. In particular, critical care nurses need to be prompted to see the extraordinary in what they perceive to be ordinary, everyday work.[13]

A second strategy for empowering staff is to involve them in meaningful change activities. The CC-CNS must stay informed about the staff's current issues and goals. Staff meetings offer one setting in which the CC-CNS can gain information about the unit's agendas and offer support. Many units also gather on a regular basis (e.g., a retreat day) to formulate goals. As topics are discussed, the CC-CNS can identify a role in achieving the goals and making a public commitment to supporting the goals.

The specialist can often assist the group in writing patient-centered goals with measurable outcomes. For example, a problem with excessive cost of suction in canisters may result in a goal "to decrease the cost of suction canisters." As an alternative, the CC-CNS can guide the group to explore factors increasing the supply use, such as an increased incidence of pulmonary complications. This direction may result in a very different goal, "to decrease the incidence of pulmonary complications." The CC-CNS's guidance assists the group to address both patient needs and unit financial goals.

Conflict Management

While present in the clinical area, the CC-CNS often encounters conflicts that disrupt patient care. Although conflict is uncomfortable and is frequently avoided, the CC-CNS recognizes that conflict must be resolved completely in order that it not reappear. Further, the CC-CNS appreciates that conflict can be positive; new solutions and channels of communication are often uncovered when issues leading to conflict are explored, confronted, and resolved.[20]

Fenton[16] found that the CNS plays an important role in conflict management by encouraging staff to see the positive side of conflict, by actively listening to staff, and by facilitating the development of problem-solving skills. The CC-CNS makes a particularly suitable conflict manager because of the organizational placement within a work group and because of interpersonal skills.

The CC-CNS makes a significant contribution by identifying sources of and traditional methods of dealing with conflict. The labor intensity and complex nature of critical care frequently give rise to conflicts among staff members. Pressure from patients, ancillary personnel, physicians, administrators, and accrediting agencies all contribute to conflict.[21] However, overt conflict erupts when crucial resources, such as time, money, or personnel, are limited relative to perceived need.

Traditionally used approaches to conflict management include avoidance, competition, accommodation, compromise, and collaboration.[20] Avoidance is evident when neither party confronts the issue. Although peace and harmony are perceived when conflict is avoided, the approach is rarely satisfactory, because the situation remains unresolved and tensions remain high. When competition is the chosen mode, the two parties assume assertive but uncooperative positions from which personal interests are argued. Accommodation is the opposite approach in which one party defers its interests to satisfy the other's concerns. When nurses choose compromise as the conflict management method, they attempt to find a solution that represents a middle ground. However, in many cases of compromise, neither party is satisfied. Collaboration is the most satisfying but tedious solution in that it is an attempt to come to a fully mutually agreeable solution.[20]

In managing conflict the CC-CNS benefits from a broad vantage point not only of the parties involved but also of the larger organization. The CC-CNS often suggests other factors that might influence the issue and conflict management mode. As an objective third person the CC-CNS is able to independently gather data and listen to staff members' interpretations of the situation.[22] The CC-CNS also uses active listening skills to assist both parties to identify the underlying problem and to determine each party's driving interest. A CC-CNS can also serve as a formal conflict manager in a nursing staff support group; the formal group provides a forum in which staff members recognize and correct behaviors, such as ineffective communication skills, contributing to conflict.[23]

The CC-CNS may coach the staff in using a particular conflict management method. For example, the CC-CNS may suggest that the involved parties negotiate a solution through a structured problem-solving technique. Although negotiation skills are not frequently taught in graduate curriculums, many CC-CNSs necessarily acquire these skills through practice in a variety of situations.[24]

Mentorship of Staff Members

The CC-CNS's commitment to the professional growth of staff naturally leads at times to formal mentorship of a staff member. Mentorship is an engaged, caring relationship between two persons: a mentor who provides gentle guidance to a less experienced nurse to promote personal and professional growth. Thus mentoring fulfills the fundamental need to believe in oneself and one's ability.[25] Mentoring is an ultimately empowering relationship that leads the staff member to realize the potential of personal power.

Although infrequently mentioned in the literature, the CC-CNS serves as an ideal mentor for staff members who choose to remain in clinical practice. The CC-CNS has accomplished a professional goal and continues to find challenge and fulfillment in a clinical nursing role.[25] Further, the CC-CNS often demonstrates the professional qualities of expertise, accountability, and commitment combined with the personal qualities of authenticity, responsiveness, and availability.[25]

Characteristics of the inexperienced staff member are equally important to the relationship. Mentoring may be more effective for the staff nurse who responds positively to authority figures, functions well with consistent direction, and is in the early stages of a career.[26]

Throughout all interactions with staff, communication is often best and most efficiently handled verbally. Verbal communication has the benefits of informality and collegiality. Nevertheless, some situations require a written note, such as when the CC-CNS wants to give positive feedback to a staff member who has provided skillful nursing care. A handwritten note by the CC-CNS to the staff nurse with a copy to the manager can be very effective.

As a result of close working relationships with staff, the CC-CNS may be approached or offer to provide input into staff evaluation. The clinical manager can take advantage of the clinical viewpoint offered by the CC-CNS to validate staff members' clinical skills, strengths, and developmental needs, as well as interpersonal skills such as communication with patients, families, and other health care providers.[27] However, delivery of performance appraisal is usually reserved for the manager.

Indicators of CC-CNS Effectiveness in Working with Staff

Successful implementation of the CC-CNS role must consider not only the impact on the CC-CNS, but also the growth and development of recipients of the CC-CNS's service, namely, staff nurses. Regardless of individual activities, the driving goal for the CC-CNS must be the empowerment of staff for the purpose of advancing clinical practice and patient care. As the CC-CNS plans utilization of time, a major concern should be, "How will this contribute to the knowledge, skills, and abilities necessary for staff success?"

An evaluation system that uses structure, process, and outcome measures is useful in documenting the CC-CNS's effectiveness in working with staff. Structural measures form a foundation for the evaluation by focusing on the CC-CNS's attributes and the setting in which the specialist functions.[28] Structural components often include numbers or frequencies, for example, the number of consultations requested of the CC-CNS or staff turnover rates. Another popular strategy is to document the percentage of time the CC-CNS spends in different activities using time studies.[29] Structural measures can be helpful and useful for a new CC-CNS. However, in evaluating the CC-CNS's impact on staff, structural measures are indirect and insensitive at best.

Including process measures provides an additional measure of reliability to the evaluation method. The CC-CNS's effect on staff practice is considered a process measure, because it focuses on activities of the CC-CNS and the resulting changes in practice. Because the staff nurse is the recipient of service, process evaluation is a useful and valid approach. Several research studies have explored changes in staff behavior as a result of CC-CNS involvement. One of the earliest studies compared information recorded by nurses on Kardexes on units with and without CNSs. The researchers found that clinical nurse specialization resulted in fewer errors; better use of assessment data; and better reflection of independent, interdependent, and dependent aspects of practice.[30] Preoperative teaching and documentation by staff nurses were the dependent variables of interest in another process study.[31]

The CC-CNS or supervisor may also evaluate the CC-CNS in relation to some staff outcome. For example, in appraising the CC-CNS's skill as a conflict manager, a peer or supervisor may observe actual interactions with staff and then measure the outcomes of the conflict management or changes in staff behavior.

A highly desirable method of evaluation involves measuring both the process (CC-CNS's effect on staff) and the staff's impact on patient outcome; such a strategy is known as process-outcome.[32] However, many methodologic problems make process-outcome measurement difficult and therefore underused.

Qualitative methods overcome some of the difficulties posed by these quantitative methods. Whereas qualitative methods have been used to describe the clinical competencies and skilled performance of CNSs in working with patients and staff,[33,34] they have been less commonly used for evaluation purposes. Nevertheless, CC-CNSs are encouraged to use anecdotal records to provide evidence of their success in working with staff.[35] Commonly encountered indices of success include staff members emulating the CC-CNS's behavior or incorporating the CC-CNS's recommendations into the care they provide. Descriptions of specialist actions paired with staff outcome within clinical contexts provide powerful evidence of the CC-CNS's value to the organization.

CASE EXAMPLES

The ongoing relationship the CC-CNS shares with members of the nursing staff must be flexible

to respond to different staff needs, as illustrated in the following case study.

CASE STUDY 1

Chris, a CC-CNS, is working with three nurses with varied experience who are being oriented to the coronary care unit (CCU). Specifically, Chris is working with each nurse to establish competence in hemodynamic monitoring.

The first nurse is a highly experienced nurse who possesses the requisite cognitive and psychomotor skills and confidence in those skills. Chris acknowledges this nurse's expertise and suggests that she demonstrate competence in actual clinical situations. The CC-CNS also encourages the nurse to share her expertise as a staff resource.

The second nurse has limited experience with hemodynamic monitoring through a previous job. Although this nurse possesses some of the pertinent theoretic knowledge, she lacks skill in accurately interpreting parameters and making treatment decisions based on her interpretation. She doubts she will ever be as knowledgeable as the more senior nurses in the unit. In this situation Chris chooses to use techniques, such as paper and pencil tests, to validate the nurse's formal knowledge. The CC-CNS then uses walking rounds or case studies to allow the nurse to practice interpretation in a safe environment. Chris also helps identify staff experts to serve as resources for this orientee.

The final orientee is a newly graduated nurse who has no practical experience with hemodynamic monitoring. As an advanced beginner, this nurse possesses very little competence but is very eager to learn. In this instance Chris works alongside the orientee to provide careful direction and close supervision as the beginner builds skills. In both verbal and nonverbal communication the CC-CNS conveys the message that learning is supported.

An important step to foster self-development of staff is to promote a positive self-esteem and sense of self-efficacy. In this example the CC-CNS acknowledges each staff nurse as a fellow professional. Further, the CC-CNS recognizes the nurse's skill and desire to perform sucessfully. The CNS demonstrates situational leadership by altering the teaching style to match each learner's needs.

An important strategy for empowerment is to provide staff with the skills necessary to resolve interpersonal and organizational problems. In critical care settings the staff nurse's experience in resolving conflict is often limited. However, most staff members are open to CC-CNS intervention and coaching. The following case study illustrates the negotiator role of a CC-CNS.

CASE STUDY 2

Susan, a veteran CC-CNS, often seizes opportunities to coach staff in the development of important conflict resolution skills. One such opportunity arose when the emergency department (ED) and the intravenous (IV) team were arguing about who should be primarily responsible for IV starts in the ED. The IV team was concerned about an increased incidence of phlebitic complications and patient complaints. The ED nurses were concerned about maintaining their IV skills.

Susan encouraged the two parties to negotiate a solution to this problem. She chose not to be directly involved, but rather to serve as a neutral facilitator. In this capacity she was available to coach the staff in the negotiation process.

As a facilitator, Susan guided the discussion so that the involved individuals viewed the conflict as a problem to be solved. At the outset she clarified the topic and purpose of the discussion to establish a common understanding. She asked questions such as "What is the problem as you see it?" and "What factors are creating the problem?" Once the issue was clearly identified, Susan encouraged each party to state their interests. For the ED this translated into maintaining the ability to deliver timely IV therapy based on patient age and status. The IV team's interest was to reduce the rate of complications and improve patient satisfaction.

The next step was to generate alternative solutions. The question "How can we efficiently start IVs and prevent complications and patient complaints?" was used to prompt a list of ideas. Once the list of alternatives was generated, each suggestion was considered by both parties. Acceptable solutions included doing in-service programs for the ED staff on newer techniques and increasing patient teaching. The parties than decided on a timetable for implementing the solution. Finally, Susan ensured that the staffs met to evaluate progress.

SUMMARY

Effective CC-CNS leaders use their position to accomplish two objectives: to advance the delivery of skilled nursing care to patients and their families and to empower staff members by assisting them in gaining the knowledge, skills, and confidence to ensure their success. Fulfilling both objectives requires a fundamental understanding of power as a positive force that can be created, accrued, and shared. Conversely, misunderstanding leads to misuses and abuses of power, exhibited by rescuing or pleasing behaviors.

Four specific leadership strategies were discussed and illustrated through case studies. Through each strategy the CNS role models effective behavior, provides resources to staff, and coaches the professional development of staff members.

References

1. McCaffery D: Unspoken subroles of the clinical nurse specialist, *Clin Nurse Specialist* 5(2):71-72, 1991.
2. Wynd CA: Packing a punch: female nurses and the effective use of power, *Nurs Success Today* 2(9):15-20, 1985.
3. Bennis W, Nanus B: *Leaders: the strategies for taking charge,* New York, 1985, Harper & Row Publishers.
4. Conger JA, Kanungo RN: The empowerment process: integrating theory and practice, *Academy Management Review* 13(3):471-482, 1988.
5. Gorman S, Clark N: Power and effective nursing practice, *Nurs Outlook* 34(3):129-134, 1986.
6. Hershey P, Blanchard K: *Management of organizational behavior: utilizing human resources,* Englewood Cliffs, NJ, 1988, Prentice-Hall.
7. Blanchard K, Zigarmi P, Zigarmi D: *Leadership and the one minute manager,* New York, 1985, William Morrow & Co.

8. Sneed NV: Power: its use and potential misuse by nurse consultants, *Clin Nurse Specialist* 5(1):58-62, 1991.
9. Chenevert M: *STAT: special techniques in assertiveness training,* St. Louis, 1983, Mosby–Year Book, Inc.
10. Bandura A: Self-efficacy: towards a unifying theory of behavioral change, *Psychol Rev* 84(2):191-215, 1977.
11. American Nurses' Association: *Nursing: a social policy statement,* Kansas City, Mo, 1980, The Association.
12. American Association of Critical Care Nurses: *Competency statements for critical-care clinical nurse specialists,* Aliso Viejo, Calif, 1989, The Association.
13. Benner P: *From novice to expert: excellence and power in clinical nursing practice,* Menlo Park, Calif, 1984, Addison-Wesley Publishing.
14. Koetters TL: Clinical practice and direct patient care. In Hamric AB, Spross JA, editors: *The clinical nurse specialist in theory and practice,* ed 2, Philadelphia, 1989, WB Saunders Co.
15. Holt FM: A theoretical model for clinical nurse specialist practice, *Nurs Health Care* 5(8):445-449, 1984.
16. Fenton MV: Identifying competencies of clinical nurse specialists, *J Nurs Admin* 15(12):31-37, 1985.
17. American Association of Critical Care Nurses: Letter by clinical nurse specialist special interest group, 1987.
18. Barron A: The CNS as consultant. In Hamric AB, Spross JA, editors: *The clinical nurse specialist in theory and practice,* ed 2, Philadelphia, 1989, WB Saunders Co.
19. Chisolm M: Use and abuse of power, *Clin Nurse Specialist* 5(1):57-58, 1991.
20. Bray KA: Managing conflict, *Critical Care Nurse* 3(2):77-78, 1983.
21. Levenstein A: Negotiation vs. confrontation, *Nurs Management* 15(1):52-54, 1984.
22. Walker ML: The clinical nurse specialist as a consultant, *Nurs Management* 17(5):61, 1986.
23. Guillory BA, Riggin OZ: Developing a nursing staff support group model, *Clin Nurse Specialist* 5(3):170-173, 1991.
24. Beare PG: The essentials of win-win negotiation for the clinical nurse specialist, *Clin Nurse Specialist* 3(3):138-141, 1989.
25. Pilette PC: Mentoring: an encounter of the leadership kind, *Nurs Leadership* 3(2):22-26, 1980.
26. Darling LAW: Mentor matching, *J Nurs Admin* 15(1):45-46, 1985.
27. Barden RM: Evaluating critical care staff personnel. In Cardin S, Ward CR, editors: *Management in critical care nursing,* Baltimore, 1989, Williams & Wilkins Co.
28. Hamric AB: A model for CNS evaluation. In Hamric AB, Spross JA, editors: *The clinical nurse specialist in theory and practice,* ed 2, Philadelphia, 1989, WB Saunders Co.
29. Robichaud AM, Hamric AB: Time documentation of clinical nurse specialist activities, *J Nurs Admin* 16(1):31-36, 1986.
30. Georgopoulos BS, Jackson MM: Nursing Kardex behavior in an experimental study of patient units with and without clinical nurse specialists, *Nurs Res* 19(3):196-218, 1970.
31. Girouard S: The role of the clinical nurse specialist as change agent: an experiment in preoperative teaching, *Int J Nurs Studies* 15(2):57-65, 1978.
32. Oleske DM, Otte DM, Heinze S: Development and evaluation of a system for monitoring the quality of oncology nursing care in the home setting, *Cancer Nurs* 10(4):190-198, 1987.
33. Steele S, Fenton MV: Expert practice of clinical nurse specialists, *Clin Nurse Specialist* 2(1):45-51, 1988.
34. Schaefer KM, Lucke KT: Caring—the work of the clinical nurse specialist, *Clin Nurse Specialist* 4(2):87-92, 1990.
35. McCaffery D: Indices of success, *Clin Nurse Specialist* 4(4):200, 1990.

Chapter 16

The CNS as Change Agent in Today's Political Health Care Environment

Debbie Tribett, RN, MS, CCRN

Question any critical care clinical nurse specialist (CC-CNS) about the responsibilities of the CNS, and without a doubt, change agent will be included in the answer. This particular activity of the role is difficult to actualize for many CC-CNSs. Although change theory is included in the CNS curriculum, graduate nursing programs allow little time to practice the strategies and techniques used to implement change theory. Once the CC-CNS is employed, organizational expectations include the change agent role in the CNS job description and incorporate evaluation criteria in the annual performance review. In addition, the critical care environment poses constant challenges for change such as incorporation of new technologies into practice. This places the burden of implementing change on the CC-CNS, and the CC-CNS must perform at a level to meet this expectation.

To be effective in implementing change, a CC-CNS must evaluate the organization in which she or he is employed to analyze the factors impeding and enhancing implementation of this role and other aspects of the position. Within the existing situation the CNS must devise plans to implement behavior changes that lead to nursing practice changes in harmony with organizational needs and goals. Leadership and power must be developed by the CC-CNS to be successful in the change agent role. Often the CC-CNS feels overwhelmed or powerless in an organization to influence positive outcomes. This chapter will assist the CC-CNS to identify ways to become more influential and

powerful within the political environment of the critical care unit and in the hospital to contribute to successful implementation of change.

THEORETIC PERSPECTIVES

Like it or not, the influences of today's health care system on institutions are demanding that change occur more rapidly at all levels within the organization to meet the health care needs of the customers. The professional goal of improving nursing practice that exists for the CC-CNS fits perfectly with the current health care climate. The CC-CNS can implement the change agent component of the role, but the changes must be congruent with the needs for change within the organization. The CC-CNS leads the process of change and manages the process to minimize resistance and maximize the results.

Change can be defined as the difference between what is now and what will be at some time in the future.[1] Change is a process, not an event or a destination, because it never ends.[2] For a CC-CNS, change becomes a lifetime endeavor. When the CC-CNS is an effective agent managing the process of change it can be an enjoyable and rewarding professional journey.

Lewin's theory of change[3] is a helpful tool for CC-CNSs in implementing the role of change agent within their practice. Lewin's theory looks at the tendency of systems to maintain the status quo. Forces or factors affecting the system may tend to move or restrain the system. With the forces at equilibrium the system is frozen. Altering the relative strength of certain forces causes a disequilibrium or an unfreezing. Movement or a change can then take place. When new forces reach an equilibrium the system is once again frozen, until any further shift in forces causes another disequilibrium or change to occur.[3]

The CC-CNS can facilitate the change process by unfreezing the staff. Building a sense of urgency and developing a positive attitude can help the staff to see the need to change. The CC-CNS can help staff members see where they can be as a result of changing and anticipate obstacles along the path. As a role model, the CC-CNS must consistently demonstrate the behavior of the desired change to demonstrate the path for the staff to follow. The CC-CNS needs to be able to provide resources to staff members to assist them in changing their practice. This may be in the form of providing new information, teaching a new skill, or providing them with opportunities to practice or for role-playing sessions. Then the CC-CNS will help to refreeze the staff by positively rewarding and reinforcing the new behavior when it is demonstrated.

The process of change is unique within each nursing unit, service, and hospital because of the responses of the individuals affected by the change, but common characteristics of change can be predicted to occur. Change produces anxiety in most people. Anxious people can create a resistance that is difficult to overcome. Obstacles to change can be overcome, with anticipation and planning of strategies to deal with each one. Change always takes longer than anticipated. The larger the change, the longer it will take. People will have exaggerated expectations of the results. Problems must be anticipated. Skeptics and critics can be helpful by identifying potential problems that might occur or areas of weakness in the planned change. Procrastination in the implementation process will be inevitable. The bigger the change, the more it will be postponed by those who must make it. Small steps toward a large change are better tolerated by most people than large steps. The change will not be a perfect process. The CC-CNS must turn imperfection into an opportunity for learning along the way. Striving for constant improvement vs. perfection can make the change more realistic.

To be effective in implementing change within the political environment, the CC-CNS must be able to use power to influence the behavior of others. Therefore an understanding of the concepts of power is essential for the CC-CNS as change agent. The concepts of power politics and leadership were discussed in Chapter 15.

RELATED LITERATURE AND RESEARCH

Successful implemenation of change in critical care nursing practice is well documented in the literature. Whether it is documentation,[4] change of shift report,[5] or visiting policy,[6] the specific change implemented was a planned, systematic, managed process in which collaboration of CC-CNS with nurse managers, nursing staff, and other disciplines was founded on change theory.

The CC-CNS has a vantage point to view the practice and outcomes of the critical care unit or service as a whole and can identify problems or deficient areas common to the practice of the nursing staff. With advanced knowledge and expertise in clinical practice, the CC-CNS is aware of alternatives to the status quo of critical care nursing practice in the organization. Therefore the CC-CNS may identify a need for change to occur. To successfully implement change the CC-CNS uses knowledge of the principles of change theory to accomplish the goal of improving nursing practice.

Although the CC-CNS may be intensely aware of the need to make a change, the change must be embraced by the staff for the change to be made and sustained. The CC-CNS must also consult with the nurse manager of the unit regarding the change. As the nursing leadership of a unit, it is important to work together in implementing change and to ensure the change is consistent with the goals of the unit, department, or organization. The nurse manager's support of the change can assist the staff in making a change, whereas a mandate by the "boss" is not always met with staff support.

The CC-CNS plays an important role in unfreezing the staff by weakening or breaking the bonds that support the present system. Raising the consciousness of the staff, gaining interest in a new idea, and ultimately generating some acceptance for the idea can be accomplished using a variety of strategies.

When making daily rounds the CC-CNS can make comments to the staff or ask questions to get them thinking about an area targeted for change by the CC-CNS. This gets key staff members talking and asking questions about the same topic and fosters interest in the change.[5] At a staff meeting the CC-CNS may ask an evaluative question specific to the targeted area for change. For example, if the form of nursing documentation is targeted for change, the CNS might ask, "What is the purpose of nurses' notes?"[4] Based on the staff response, the CC-CNS would follow with a question to probe the staff's perceptions of whether their present practice was meeting that purpose.[4] The CC-CNS may conduct a specific attitude survey of the staff to determine staff satisfaction with the current practice or policy.[6] One difficulty in using these methods is that the preparation time and idea-planting time are lengthy.[5] Ultimately, if staff members become involved early in the process, resistance to the change can be minimized, because it will be viewed as "theirs" and not dictated to them from above.

Once staff members have gotten interested in a topic, the CC-CNS can provide reference materials for them to read on the area targeted for change. This information should include both the positive and negative aspects of the subject. The CC-CNS can also provide examples of how the change could be implemented within the existing critical care environment.

Forming a committee of staff members to investigate a potential change allows staff truly to own the change in practice. Depending on the nature of the potential change, other disciplines affected by the change should be involved. This may also include the input of the patients or family members in the critical care unit.[6] The CC-CNS should not chair the committee but should be the expert consultant to the group. This again prevents the perception of imposed change vs. a voluntary participation in the process. The CC-CNS can act as a mentor to the committee chairperson to assist the staff member in performing in the role of chairperson, to teach group process, and to introduce the concepts of change theory into practical actions to be taken by the group.

One technique that has proven effective for staff groups implementing change is the Claus-Bailey model for problem solving[5] (Table 16–1). The CC-CNS can assist the staff in using this problem-solving approach for the implementation of a change. This is yet another example of how the CC-CNS can manage change through the application of an advanced theoretic knowledge base.

TABLE 16–1 Steps of Claus-Bailey Systems Model for Problem Solving

1. Define overall needs, purposes, goals.
2. Define the problem.
3. Specify constraints, capabilities, resources, claimant groups.
4. Specify approach to problem solution.
5. State behavioral objectives and performance criteria.
6. List alternative solutions.
7. Analyze options.
8. Choose the best solution.
9. Control and implement decisions.
10. Evaluate effectiveness of action.

Data from Bailey J, Claus K: *Decision making in nursing: tools for change,* St Louis, 1975, Mosby–Year Book, Inc.

The examples presented are some suggested strategies to assist in the unfreezing phase of the change process. To begin the moving phase of change, a process for the old system to convert to a new system must be developed. The implementation of planned change requires its own strategies.

Once a change has been decided on, an educational process is often needed by the staff involved with the change. This may include the dissemination of information, demonstrations, or practice sessions. The CC-CNS can function in the educator component of the CNS role by actually teaching or being a mentor for staff members in the preparation and presentation of educational offerings related to the desired change. Gathering or creating resource materials for the staff to use during the implementation phase is another example of a CNS activity to support the process. Frequent rounds or increasing time available to the staff to answer questions or provide moral support is another tactic the CC-CNS may use to assist with the implementation of change. The CC-CNS and the nurse manager can also be influential by role modeling the desired change in practice or behavior being implemented.

Because change is easier to accept if it is introduced gradually, implementation may include a pilot project or a trial period.[6] An evaluation of the situation following the pilot project can determine pitfalls that may have been overlooked or not anticipated by the CC-CNS and the staff. Positive and negative feedback on the change can be collected and evaluated by the CC-CNS and those involved in the implementation process. A trial period allows for the stumbling blocks to be smoothed out and gradual adjustment by those resisting the process.

Refreezing is necessary for the perpetuation of the change. This process integrates and stabilizes the change. The CC-CNS plays an integral part in the refreezing phase and may use a variety of approaches to ensure the successful integration of the change in the critical care environment.

Positive reinforcement of a change in behavior or practice can go a long way to strengthen the commitment of staff to accept the desired change. The CC-CNS has the opportunity to be on the unit and observe the staff in action. Words of praise and encouragement to a staff member struggling with the new or unfamiliar rewards effort and will likely influence future behavior.

Recognition of successful changes in nursing practice can be in the form of articles in hospital or nursing newsletters. The CC-CNS can write articles or supply information to the editor to publicize the results of the change process. If staff members are interested in publishing in nursing journals, the CC-CNS can also act as a mentor in helping them prepare an article on their change project for submission to a journal. Additional routes for acknowledging successful implementation of change are preparing a poster or a proposal for a presentation at local or national American Association of Critical Care Nurses (AACN) programs. This can be done by the CC-CNS alone, or interested staff members can be included in the process.

The CC-CNS can help with making the change official by assisting with the writing of policy, procedure, guidelines, or other documents used by the organization to specify expectations or responsibilities of staff. The CC-CNS can also see that unit-based changes are integrated into larger ongoing programs such as orientation of new staff members.

Integration of change into continuous quality improvement (CQI) activities of the critical care unit must also be accomplished. Sometimes a change is initiated as a result of CQI activities, but if it was initiated from other routes, monitoring of that change can provide documentation of efforts to improve the quality of patient care. The CC-CNS can be instrumental in linking quality improvement activities with the change process.

Formal evaluation of the change as a final step of the process is again an area for CC-CNS involvement. Not only will this provide feedback to the staff on their accomplishments, but also it will provide documentation of CC-CNS involvement as a change agent. This visibility is essential for the CC-CNS in meeting the expectations of her or his role as a change agent within the organization.

PRACTICE IMPLICATIONS
Assessment of Political Environment

To be effective as a change agent, the CC-CNS must possess a clear understanding of the politics of the organizational setting. Analysis of the formal and informal organization is essential to determine where the scheming factions for power and status are within an organization and to determine the methods for dealing with them.

The CC-CNS must acquire a knowledge base of the organization before assuming a leadership role in effecting change. To obtain this knowledge the CC-CNS must analyze the unit or units for which she or he is responsible, the nursing service within the organization, as well as the hospital and corporate structure. The CC-CNS must be aware of the channels of authority, power, influence, and information in order to navigate through the system. Table 16–2 presents the areas to include in this analysis.

The organizational chart is the source of the formal structure that exists. The hierarchy, chain of command, position authority, and areas of responsibility can be identified from this document. Job descriptions and evaluation tools for the CC-CNS and other nursing positions help to delineate the official expectations of the different roles within the nursing structure. The philosophy, values, and objectives of the hospital and critical care area should be examined for compatibility.[7] The CC-CNS should examine personal nursing philosophy to determine the fit between the organization and the CC-CNS. An initial impression can be formulated from a review of these items. However, it takes observational time or a reliable mentor in the organization to act as historian to validate if those

TABLE 16–2 Assessment of Political Environment

Areas	Questions or Actions
Formal structure	Review organizational charts
	Read job descriptions
	Compare evaluation tools with job descriptions
	Review philosophy, values, and objectives of hospital, nursing service, critical care department
Power bases	Determine position of CNS in organization
	Question administrators, nurse manager, and other CNSs on perceived support for role
	Determine key persons with control of resources (budgets and allocation of supplies and equipment)
Decision or policy making	Identify committees, councils, and groups that determine policy and procedure
	Review bylaws of these gruops
	Find out if a formal decision-making process exists
	Attend meetings as an observer or read meeting minutes
	Determine group membership
	Differentiate administrative and clinical practice groups
	Determine how unit-based decisions are made
	Identify issues that may be political landmines
Leadership	Assess leadership styles:
	Hospital administrator
	Nursing service leaders
	Critical care nursing manager
	Critical care medical director
	Key physicians using critical care services
	Compare with your style for compatibility
Communication systems	Identify formal methods for information distribution
	Determine flow of information
	Assess amount of communication
	Identify informal sources of information (grapevine)
Organizational climate	Review organizational survey (if available)
	Determine if union or nonunion
	Talk to staff members about their perceptions of workplace
	Compare staff perceptions with the following:
	Existing programs for staff development
	Schedules and patient care assignments
	Patient classification data
	Educational attendance records

in authority act in congruence with the official documents.

Visible nursing executive support for the role of the CC-CNS further strengthens the CNS position. Referent power from management can reinforce the expert power held by the CC-CNS by virtue of clinical skill and knowledge.[8] If the CC-CNS is working in a union environment, the po-

sition must clearly be identified as management or nonmanagement. If the CNS position is management, then the CC-CNS must be aware of the manager's role in union drives; if a contract exists, the CC-CNS must know the terms of the contract to help administer it correctly.[9] However even if the CNS is not part of management, knowledge of these restrictions is essential to being able to implement change within the union environment. In a joint appointment the CC-CNS may overlap two distinct organizational charts. Reporting to more than one boss with different expectations can be challenging. Percentages of time spent in each organization may be defined. The CC-CNS in this setting may be more difficult to analyze, because analysis would involve looking at the clinical practice and the academic organizations for their impact on the role. Once the CC-CNS knows where the position lies within the existing structure, then the CC-CNS can work to maximize its strengths.

The organizational chart describes only part of the power base of the CC-CNS and other positions. Control over resources is a major power base in the organization. Money for travel and education, patient care equipment and supplies, audiovisual equipment, classroom space, secretarial services, or work schedules may all be sources of power. This power may be wielded by persons located at lower levels within an organizational structure. The CC-CNS must clearly identify the power derived from interpersonal relationships and personal power bases within the organization. Tapping into the informal power network can be more productive for the CC-CNS than using the legitimate structure. Observation and individual conversations are methods to determine key power bases within the unit, nursing service, and hospital. Reading meeting minutes or attending a variety of nursing or interdisciplinary committee meetings can reveal true power players. In addition, issues that are political landmines can be identified by the CC-CNS. Once sources of power are clear, then strategies to cultivate relationships with those individuals in powerful positions can be planned.

Assessment of decision and policy making is only partially liked to the formal organizational structure. Often it cuts across hierarchic channels. Key questions to answer are who makes decisions, when, and how. Look for the key committees, councils, or meetings in the organization and within the nursing service. If bylaws exist for groups, review these documents. Also, identify which major decision-making groups have nursing representation. If other CNSs are in the nursing department determine their involvement with committees or councils and with decision making of these groups. Look for involvement of nursing staff within their untis and in the nursing service. How

do they participate, and what types of issues are addressed?

The actual decision-making process reflects the leadership style prevailing within a group or organization. Determine if important decisions are made in groups, with or without input of those affected by the decision, or exclusively by management. Try to attend a variety of meetings to observe the process of decision making. If this is not possible within an organization, read meeting minutes to obtain an indication of participatory or autocratic decision making. After attending meetings or reading minutes, follow up on the method used to communicate the decision to those it affects.

An important area for the CC-CNS to focus on is the decision-making process related to clinical practice issues. Determine who makes decisions related to standards, procedures, supplies, and equipment. Find out if there is a nursing department or critical care service procedure committee or standards group. Look at the representation at meetings. Find out if the committees are nursing or multidisciplinary groups and if they involve staff or management representatives.

Meeting with the director of procurement or central supply can provide a wealth of knowledge about decision making regarding supplies and equipment in the organization. Within the critical care unit, the relationship of nurses, physicians, ancillary staff, patients, and families in making patient care decisions must also be scrutinized.

The style of leadership used by those in formal and informal leadership positions within the organization should be determined. Many people are consistent in the way in which they lead, using a style that is comfortable for them. It may not be effective in influencing others' behaviors. The style used by the leader may not be perceived as the same by others in the organization.[10]

Individuals with whom the CC-CNS has the most interactions are important to observe. Through observation of interactions and interviews the CC-CNS should determine the leadership style of the nurse managers she or he will be working with and the response of the staff to this style. Knowing the style of the immediate supervisor of the CC-CNS will also help the CC-CNS. Key physicians in the critical care unit must also be included in this assessment.

The CC-CNS must be aware of the predominant style of leadership she or he most often practices. The style of the CC-CNS and those in management may be in direct conflict. Conflicting styles between the CC-CNS and those with whom she or he works most intimately may contribute to an unsatisfactory work environment for the CC-CNS.

The communications system within the unit, nursing service, and hospital must be examined during the organizational analysis. The key to success in most interactions is the ability to communicate effectively. To do this the CC-CNS must find out how to get information within the system and how to use it to accomplish the desired effects. Look for the direction of flow of information. Is it always unidirectional, or is it a two-way flow? Determine if communications are direct and open or vague or distorted. The amount of communication should be quantified. Is there minimal opportunity for communication or too much information bombarding the staff? The methods used for communication should be identified. Are there staff meetings at different levels within the nursing service, circulation of memos or documents, newsletters, computerized electronic mail, communication books, or other formal means for information sharing? The pathways for communication between disciplines must also be identified. Determine if the communication system follows the chain of command or if it is controlled by interpersonal relationships. The informal or "grapevine" system is also important to identify. Cultivating the grapevine can be an important source of information about the entire organization for the CC-CNS. It is easy to identify individuals with inside information on the organization. These people may not be peers or members of the nursing staff. Sharing what they know enhances their perceived power base. Invite your source to have coffee or lunch regularly, and use good listening skills.

The final area included in the organizational analysis is the general climate of the organization. This can be thought of as the overall feeling of the people working in the organization. The feelings of the staff may differ among disciplines or a more global positive or negative attitude may be perceived in the organization. Organizational climate issues are often the determining factor affecting unionization of an organization.[9] While looking at the general climate, the CC-CNS should identify the factors that facilitate and inhibit patient care management and the functioning of the CNS.

Some organizations have conducted formal organizational climate surveys that may be reviewed. If such a survey has not been conducted, things that affect the organizational climate such as compensation, working conditions, work loads or assignments, staffing, scheduling, and opportunities for personal and professional growth must be examined individually. Census records, patient classification data, and staffing and scheduling records are sources of factual, objective documents that can be reviewed and compared to the perceptions of the staff on these subjects. Clinical ladders or professional practice models may be reviewed; however, what exists on paper vs. actual participation in such programs must be compared. Lip service to the support of staff development may be observed. The CC-CNS should assess the mechanism for staff members to attend unit in-service programs. When programs are presented but lack attendance because staffing is minimal, prohibiting staff participation, or when budgets lack funds earmarked for continuing education for staff, there is no evidence of true support.

From this thorough examination of the organization, the CC-CNS can adequately diagnose the system. This paves the way for the process of planning change. It can also help the CC-CNS to set reasonable goals, so as to be successful in her or his individual setting. Understanding the complexities of the system allows the CC-CNS to be a more effective leader and to work collaboratively with other nursing leaders such as the nurse manager in effecting change.

Conflict and Change

Even when practicing ideal management strategies, conflicts will arise as part of the change process. Anticipation of the potential conflicts and planning strategies for handling them must be included in the planned change process. However, almost daily in the complex environment of the critical care unit unanticipated conflicts arise. The CC-CNS must deal with conflict in a positive way. Ignoring the situation will inevitably make a bad situation worse. The CC-CNS must use the problem-solving process intertwined with effective negotiation techniques to gain power and influence in the organization.

Negotiation is defined as a process for reaching satisfactory settlement of differences between parties in a conflict situation.[8] The goal of a negotiation is to change a conflict into a manageable situation for the parties involved.[8] Table 16–3 lists the steps of negotiation.

First, the CC-CNS must get the facts before negotiating a conflict. There are at least two sides to every issue (and sometimes more) that must be determined before the real probelm or issue can be identified. It is important to separate people from the problem at hand. Depersonalize a situation by asking who, what, where, when, and why types of questions. Collect facts. Avoid trying to link a cause or a solution to the issue at this point.

Once the issue or problem is defined more knowledge or information may be needed. Policies, standards, procedures, or regulations that apply to the situation may need to be researched. Resources such as time, money, or materials may be involved. A description of the situation should result from this step.

Analysis of each party's interests or motives must occur. As the negotiator, the CC-CNS must decide what she or he wants to accomplish as the absolute bottom line from the negotiation. A third party may need to be consulted to clearly understand the other side's position and motivation. It is usually wise to start with higher expectations, so that during the process you can make concessions or compromises that the opposition feels are valuable to their position.

It is important to brainstorm options, or possible ways of getting what you want. In negotiation you want to have multiple options or possibilities that will be agreeable to all involved. Entering into negotiation with only one position, you have assumed there is a single answer to the problem.

TABLE 16–3 Steps of Negotiation Process

1. Identify issue or problem.
2. Collect facts of situation.
3. Analyze situation from each party's perspective.
4. Identify best alternative or possibility for action.
5. Develop a strategy.
6. Use negotiation tactics to reach a consensus.
7. Document outcome in writing for confirmation by participants and future reference.

In developing your strategy, you must decide if you want to win the battle (the short-term situation) or win the war (the long-term result of letting the other side feel that they have won also). Each CC-CNS must make a choice. Generally the win-win strategy where both parties feel they have won the negotiation has benefits when future conflict and negotiation are anticipated.

The CC-CNS can use a variety of tactics in preparation for and during the actual negotiation. Role playing the negotiation process builds confidence and allows one to practice anticipated reactions by the other side. It may also help to identify alternatives. Try to schedule the meeting in a neutral territory so neither side has the power advantage. Sit opposite one another at a table or in a circular chair arrangement to avoid the leadership or power position at the head of the table. Keep language objective, and avoid placing blame or making accusations. Try to listen nonjudgmentally. Check frequently for understanding, and restate or summarize what you think you heard. Ask the other person if you heard correctly. Try to keep the other side talking and get as much information as possible. In bringing up issues, bring up one issue at a time and raise less controversial topics first. If the opposition tries to evoke your emotions, maintain your composure verbally and in your body language. Uncontrolled emotion can lose a negotiation.

Deciding on a mutually agreeable outcome or reaching a consensus may not be possible. If a permanent solution cannot be reached, an interim plan may be agreed on. This allows for people to adjust gradually to new proposals. The outcome of the negotiation should be written and confirmed by the participants so that both sides are clear about the details and responsibilities and the documentation can be used for future reference.[11]

Extending Your Political Power Base

The CC-CNS can develop an extensive political power base within an organization. The CC-CNS must use the power to accomplish goals or create changes that are valuable to the organization. Evidence of one's contribution must be visible at a variety of levels.

On a larger scale within the organization the experienced CC-CNS can enhance perceived power and leadership ability by participating in and volunteering to lead key committees within the nursing department. As the committee chairperson, it is important to use strategies for improving the efficiency and productivity of committee meetings.

Another avenue for expanding the CC-CNS's leadership role is through activities outside the organization. For the CC-CNS, involvement in local chapters of AACN, regional special interest groups, or national AACN activities provides a wealth of opportunities for networking (see Chapter 19), increasing one's knowledge base, and accessing resources to assist in the implementation of changes in critical care nursing practice. Volunteering for leadership positions within the professional organization enables the CC-CNS to practice and develop leadership skills. Likewise, participation in local and state nursing associations provides opportunity to broaden the focus beyond critical care to more general nursing issues.

Both AACN and the American Nurses' Association have legislative committees that provide the CNS with opportunities for participation in local community political forums related to health care issues. Politics in its positive definition (participation in political affairs) can be practiced by the interested and motivated CC-CNS.

The following case study is provided to demonstrate application of the techniques discussed in this chapter. It provides a basis for discussion and suggestions of other means of dealing with these and similar situations facing the CC-CNS on a daily basis.

CASE STUDY

You are the CNS of an intensive care unit (ICU) that has just been assigned to work with a nurse manager of a medical-surgical unit on a project. This project involves planning and implementation of long-term ventilator support as a specialty on the unit.

After 2 weeks you feel very frustrated. Every meeting you have attempted to have with the nurse manager has been started late, interrupted by staff, or cancelled because she has been to busy. Today you hear from your boss that she has complained to her that you have not done anything. She has questioned your competence and expressed concerns

about working with you. Your boss wants an update and a plan for how you will address the situation.

Your immediate reaction might well be anger and hostility. Although you recognize the importance of meeting with the nurse manager immediately, you decide to first gain more information. Working in a new unit environment you need to complete an analysis of the unit, including the implementation of the nurse manager role by this individual. You tap into your informal network as well as reviewing formal records available. You find a large, busy unit, with a mixture of new graduates and experienced staff members and a few vacancies. A modified form of primary nursing is their model for care delivery.

The unit has been selected for the pilot project because of its relative stability. The patient population is predominantly pulmonary and postoperative surgical cases. The length of stay of the patients is long, and many of the patients are elderly and receiving Medicare. The unit is physically located near the respiratory therapy department.

The nurse manager has been in her position for 10 years. She has her BSN but is being pushed to go to graduate school by her director. She has never had a clinical specialist assigned to her unit before. She is perceived by her staff and her peers as being a controlling manager. She sets high expectations for the staff and is often critical of their performance. However, the unit operates efficiently and seems well organized.

Your initial impression is that the nurse manager is feeling out of control and resisting the changes imposed on her and the unit. You think she may be intimidated by you because of your knowledge base and educational preparation. In addition, you remember an incident during a code on her unit last year when you snapped at her during the emergency when a piece of necessary equipment could not be found.

The next step you take is to validate your perceptions and get more information from the nurse manager. You arrange to meet her for coffee, off the unit, to prevent interruptions. She comes, and you begin to explore how she feels about this project that the two of you have been assigned. This exploration reveals the nurse manager is experiencing anger and powerlessness. You find out that she does not want to have ventilators on her unit. She does not have the knowledge base concerning ventilators. She lacks direction on how to proceed to help her staff gain expertise to care for ventilator patients. She is feeling overwhelmed and that too many changes are happening in the hospital at the present time.

With much of your analysis confirmed, you express that you can understand how she feels. You let her know that you are there to help her and the staff and ask her what you can do for her that would be most helpful. She rattles off a list of several minor activities but expresses that she does not really know what to expect in terms of the patients.

As a starting point to build your working relationship and increase her knowledge, you suggest that the two of you spend a day together in the ICU taking care of a typical ventilator-dependent patient. You will perform the necessary care, and she can identify the knowledge or skills that her staff may need to learn and develop to feel comfortable with the situation. She likes the idea, and you compare calendars to schedule a date.

Looking at the list of things to do that she identified, you can determine which may be able to be contracted to be done by you as the CC-CNS, such as acquiring educational resource materials on mechanical ventilation and developing and presenting an in-service program on tracheostomy care for the staff. When dealing with an organized, controlling person the contracting method can be a very agreeable way to delineate responsibility.

You suggest that together you schedule a meeting with the director. This will provide an opportunity for the nurse manager to discuss her concerns and for more effective problem-solving strategies to be developed. Additionally, this will provide you with the opportunity to demonstrate your abilities to the director and to clarify your efforts thus far with this project.

Commentary In this situation, if the CC-CNS had approached it from a wounded ego perspective and tried to immediately clear up the perception that she is incompetent, little would have been accomplished. Eliciting information and feelings, she found the reason for the behavior of the nurse manager. By allowing the nurse manager to maintain control, she can avoid a battle of wills. Working together clinically, the CNS can demonstrate her knowledge and competence to the nurse manager, allow the nurse manager to identify the needs of her staff, and allow the nurse manager to increase her knowledge base and feel more comfortable and in control over the imposed change.

SUMMARY

The CC-CNS is embroiled in the change process on a daily basis. To be effective the CC-CNS must be flexible and utilize a variety of techniques and strategies. The information presented in this chapter was selected to assist the CC-CNS in identifying ways to increase power, influence, and leadership abilities to effect change in the practice of critical care nursing.

References

1. Walker D: Future directions in administrative utilization of the CNS. In Hamric AB, Spross J editors: *The clinical nurse specialist in theory and practice*, Orlando, Fla, 1983, Grune & Stratton.
2. Belasco JA: *Teaching the elephant to dance*, New York, 1990, Crown Publishers, Inc.
3. Lewin K: *Field theory in social change*, New York, 1951, Harper & Row.
4. Gawlinski A, Rasmussen S: Improving documentation through use of change theory, *Focus Crit Care* 11:12-17, 1984.
5. Young PY, Maguire M, Ovitt E: Implementing changes in critical care shift report, *Dimen Crit Care Nurs* 7:374-380, 1988.
6. Owen J et al: Changing visiting policy, *Dimen Crit Care Nurs* 7:369-373, 1988.
7. Reddcliff M, Smith EL, Ryan-Merritt M: Organizational analysis: tool for the clinical nurse specialist, *Clin Nurse Specialist* 3(3):133-136, 1989.

8. Harrell JS, McCulloch SD: The role of the clinical nurse specialist: problems and solutions, *J Nurs Admin* 16:44-48, 1986.

9. Cardin S: Applying labor relations in critical care nursing. In Cardin S, Ward CR, editors: *Personal management in critical care nursing*, Baltimore, 1989, Williams & Wilkins Co.

10. Kotter JP: *The leadership factor*, New York, 1988, The Free Press.

11. Beare PG: The essentials of win-win negotiation for the clinical nurse specialist, *Clin Nurse Specialist* 3(3):138-141, 1989.

Chapter 17

Working in an Era of Cost Containment

Thomas S. Ahrens, RN, DNS, CCRN

We are living in a dynamically changing health care environment. As hospitals adapt to changing reimbursement patterns they are downsizing inpatient populations and expanding outpatient services. The downsizing of inpatient populations and changing reimbursement patterns have reduced hospitals' profit margins. As profit margins have decreased, most hospitals have reduced expenses that do not directly affect the "essential services" of the hospital. What exactly are essential services still varies from hospital to hospital.

In nursing the attempt to reduce resources has frequently centered on the reduction in personnel. The focus on personnel reduction has created concern among many nurses, but particularly nurses in indirect patient care positions. These nurses do not actually assume responsibility for direct patient care during a given period. Therefore indirect positions, such as the critical care clinical nurse specialist (CC-CNS), may not be viewed as an essential part of the nursing organizational structure. They are vulnerable when downsizing occurs.

Although the value of the CC-CNS position has been difficult to quantify, it is not without value. The CC-CNS must overcome the perceived value of the position by demonstrating how the CC-CNS position is an essential component of the critical care nursing environment. This chapter explores the theoretic foundations of the value of the CC-CNS as well as demonstrates the value of the CC-CNS. From this foundation the CC-CNS should be able to articulate her or his value to administrators facing difficult budget constraints.

Perhaps the most important aspect of the CC-CNS role and economics is identified in the actual concept of the clinical specialist. The CNS, by definition, is a relative expert in the practice of nursing within a given specialty.[1] To truly be a CNS a nurse must have a knowledge and experience base that separates her or him from other nurses in the organization. Because of this greater knowledge base, the CNS can impact the outcome of patients in a manner few other clinicians can. This unique nature of the CNS position is essential to make the position valuable to the organization.

THEORETIC PERSPECTIVES
Health Care Economics

It is important for the CC-CNS to understand health care economics and concepts. Health care economics is a broad topic that has many concepts. The CC-CNS should develop a working knowledge of (1) direct and indirect hospital costs, (2) cost vs. charges, (3) CC-CNS salary determinations, (4) product acquisition costs, (5) payer mix, (6) cost per registered nurse (RN) workload, (7) hospital reimbursement processes, and (8) physician/hospital relationships. In addition, an understanding of how clinical practice can impact these economic variables through changes in patient outcome, length of stay, and improved organizational efficiency is essential.

Unfortunately, few of these concepts are routinely taught in CNS graduate curriculums.[2] The lack of formal education in these topics leaves the CC-CNS ill prepared to discuss their role relative to hospital economics. The CC-CNS is left to learn these concepts alone. Because of the broad range of topics involved in health care economics, many

CC-CNSs never fully acquire the requisite knowledge involved in health care economics. A CC-CNS who cannot articulate the value of the CNS position in terms of health care economics to an administrator may fear losing the position as it comes under scrutiny.

The CC-CNS can increase understanding of health care economics in several ways, such as by taking graduate courses in health care financing or by arranging for hospital administrators to hold a series of classes or attend courses at national conferences, such as the National Teaching Institute (NTI). Whatever method is chosen, the CC-CNS must supplement formal education in health care economics.

Intensive Care Unit Costs and Charges

Understanding the direct and indirect costs incurred during the care of a patient provides a perspective for developing a standard of value. Measuring *direct costs* in an intensive care unit (ICU) is essentially an objective task that examines such factors as nursing salaries and equipment and supply acquisition. Terms such as cost per work load index may be applied to quantitate how much it costs to take care of a patient with a given nursing assignment. However, the only personnel typically factored into the direct costs of the ICU are the personnel actually giving direct patient care. This level is considered to be the minimum staffing requirement to perform care. The quality or sophistication of care is not assessed by measuring direct costs.

Indirect costs do not directly factor into the care of a patient but are necessary to provide management and support of the direct care costs (Table 17–1). In addition, building costs and utility and maintenance expenses are considered examples of indirect costs. Indirect costs are difficult to quantitate and even more difficult to measure in terms of affecting quality patient care. If the value of the indirect positions were clear, hospitals would be able to consistently determine the number and type of indirect personnel needed. Some hospitals have more management, dietary, housekeeping, or security personnel than others, with no clear evidence of the impact of these positions on patient outcomes, satisfaction, or hospital success in the marketplace.

TABLE 17–1 Examples of Direct and Indirect Costs

	Nursing	Ancillary
Direct cost positions	Bedside nurses	Respiratory therapists
Indirect cost positions	CNS Educators Nurse managers	Chief executive officer Security personnel Housekeeping personnel

Charge vs. Costs

The manner in which a hospital can recoup its costs varies from patient billing to the stock market. The primary method, however, should be from patient revenue. One method of patient revenue is through charging the customer or patient a rate higher than the actual costs to make up for the indirect costs. For example, a hospital may have a ventilator charge of $400/day when the actual costs directly associated with the ventilator are only $150. The indirect costs faced by the hospital can be partially offset if the difference between the charge and cost is actually paid by the customer, since this difference represents a profit margin.

CC-CNS Salary Determination

The major charge in an ICU setting is the room charge. Generally the nursing salaries are built into this charge. The ICU room charge is frequently near the actual cost. If an ICU costs $800/day, the direct costs will be near this figure. This is important since the CC-CNS salary must come from the profit margin of the hospital. The profit margin in an ICU is often relatively small to nonexistent. The profit margin difference between costs and charges is usually determined by hospital administration and finance departments rather than nursing, although it is generated from a nursing division. This leaves nursing administrators little leverage when attempting to justify actual or additional indirect positions such as the CC-CNS.

Reimbursement Methods

It is unfortunate that the hospital charges are not necessarily going to be paid by the consumer. Hospitals may be reimbursed for costs by government programs, through self-pay, or by third-party private insurers (Table 17–2).

Governmental reimbursement includes federal (Medicare, Medicaid), state, and local programs. Most of these programs are prospective payment systems where the government provides the hospital with a set amount of money to care for a patient with a specific diagnosis. For example, if a patient is in the ICU for acute respiratory failure, becomes ventilator dependent, and requires a tracheostomy, the reimbursement pattern allows about $48,000 to care for this patient. Most hospitals will care for these patients for months with the net cost exceeding $48,000. As a rule, the hospital can expect to get a return of about 50 to 60 cents for every dollar spent. This figure varies by state and locale, but government reimbursement is limited relative to the actual cost incurred by the hospital. The significance of this for the CC-CNS is to demonstrate the ability to decrease hospital cost in high-risk or high-volume areas of care.

Self-pay reimbursement includes patients or customers without insurance and those failing to qualify for governmental assistance who are expected to pay for their care. With an average ICU day costing a minimum of $1000, a typical hospitalization requiring ICU care can easily cost in excess of $10,000. Many patients are unable to pay their entire bill, resulting in a decrease in money to the hospital. The hospital loses money in providing care for customers in this category.

Private insurers are companies paid by the customer to provide financial coverage for hospitalization. Private insurers are more likely to pay for the majority of charges requested by the hospital. The hospital can receive more money from this group than it actually expended in the care of the customer, thereby creating a positive profit margin.

Private insurers can be insurance companies or preventive health organizations, but their reimbursement patterns are more favorable than the self-pay and governmental reimbursement methods.

One important concern for hospitals is their payer mix, or the percentage of customers in each reimbursement group. The more patients in the private insurer group, the higher the profit margin of that hospital. Hospitals with a higher private payer mix are able to fund indirect positions simply because they can absorb the costs. Despite this, the most important parameter in determining available funding for CC-CNS positions is the understanding of the hospital administration of the value of advanced clinicians. The CNS can help to educate the administrator as to CNSs' value through monthly reports, CNS evaluations, joint CNS/administrator projects, and literature updates.

Administrators' Understanding of Advanced-Practice Roles

Nursing and hospital administrators are not routinely educated about the value of advanced clinicians for patient outcomes and organizational efficiency. Few programs in administration address the value of advanced clinicians in an organization. In addition, if the administrator does not have a graduate degree, his or her understanding of the value of the advanced clinician is generally limited to individual learning or exposure to advanced clinicians.

The administrator who does not understand the value of advanced clinicians may not see the benefit of placing clinicians in positions of importance in the organization or may fail to hire advanced clinicians at all. Most U.S. hospitals do not routinely hire persons for CNS-level positions, primarily because of the perception that the cost of the CNS position is excessive or unnecessary to achieve similar patient outcomes.[2] Those hospitals that do have CNS positions frequently have only a small number of these positions. The inconsistency in number of CNS positions in hospitals across the United States points out the importance of being able to describe the value of the role to hospital administrators. Hospital administrators who understand the role of the CC-CNS in managing hospital costs, facilitating effective discharge planning, and providing clear direction and support to nursing staff caring for high-risk patients are more likely to fund CC-CNS positions.

TABLE 17–2 Reimbursement Methods

Method	Payer
Governmental	Medicare/Medicaid
Self-pay	Patient pays own bill
Third party	Blue Cross/Blue Shield

RELATED RESEARCH AND LITERATURE
CC-CNS and Hospital Expenses

The CC-CNS position is usually paid for by the hospital from the profit margin covering indirect personnel. A unit-based CC-CNS is often a part of the unit budget for the area she or he is assigned to cover. In this system the unit manager expects the CC-CNS to demonstrate a positive impact on the unit budget. Activities beyond the unit or those that negatively impact the unit budget do not benefit the unit manager. Therefore CC-CNS activity that does not directly aid the unit could be viewed negatively by the nurse manager. Helping an ancillary department or another area of the hospital would conflict with unit priorities.

Hospital-based CNSs may be part of the general nursing service budget. In this system the CNS often performs more system nursing activity than direct unit activity. Regardless of the system used, the CC-CNS should be aware of how the position is perceived to understand how to demonstrate role value.

CC-CNS's Impact on Hospital Economics

The ability of the CC-CNS to positively impact the hospital financial situation is determined by the specific skills of the CC-CNS. Every CC-CNS has the potential to positively impact the economic situation in an institution, primarily through the five major role components of the CC-CNS (practitioner, educator, researcher, consultant, and leader or manager). The ability of the CC-CNS to positively impact the hospital economic situation is a function of individual CC-CNS strengths in each of these role components. The significance of the impact is a combination of the CC-CNS's capabilities and the hospital's needs.

PRACTICE IMPLICATIONS
Methods of Affecting Economics Through Clinical Expertise

The clinical knowledge base of the CC-CNS has a positive impact on patient care and therefore the economics of the institution. Assessing and therapeutically intervening at strategic points in the hospitalization can accelerate patient discharge. Through advanced assessments the CC-CNS offers the potential for appropriate use of resources as well as reducing the length of stay. The key point to reducing the length of stay and conserving re-

sources is tied to the ability of CC-CNSs to make assessments of clinical situations that normally would not be made or would not be made in a timely manner.

Many examples of the CC-CNS's ability to impact patient outcome can be demonstrated. For example, in patients with acute respiratory failure, therapies designed to improve ventilation/perfusion (V/Q) ratios are frequently assessed through blood gases. However, blood gases are only a small part of the assessment of V/Q ratios. The CC-CNS is able to assess more specific aspects of the V/Q concept such as measurements of intrapulmonary shunts or dead space to more clearly define the impact of a specific therapy.

Understanding the impact to a therapy results in more appropriate use of resources. For example, unnecessary blood gases can be avoided or more blood gases required to accelerate the assessment process. The CC-CNS may recommend placement of an SvO_2 line to continuously assess critical care patients more appropriately. The goal is appropriate resource utilization to improve patient condition and outcomes as quickly as possible. If the CC-CNS is not available, the advanced assessment of V/Q may not take place or may be delayed until another clinician, such as physician specialist, arrives. In this case the length of stay may be increased since the physician generally would not arrive immediately and is not available to make frequent assessments.

It is important for the CC-CNS to understand how to figure the cost of a particular service. Each hospital has a method for identifying a particular service charge. Ancillary service departments as well as nursing service can provide the CC-CNS with service cost information. Using this information, the CC-CNS can compute cost savings for a change in practice. For example, a blood gas may be charged to the patient at a cost of $75. However, the actual cost may be only about $5. If an assessment of a CC-CNS saves 50 blood gases, the actual hospital savings is not 50 × $75 ($3750) but rather 50 × $5 ($250).

A reduction in hospital services is usually financially advantageous; however, a paradox exists in regard to resource reduction. If a patient has third-party reimbursement, then it is not necessarily advantageous for the CC-CNS to reduce hospital services since the hospital profit margin is good for this type of patient. However, with the increase in fixed reimbursement patterns, it generally is useful to avoid using any unnecessary resources.

The advanced assessment capability of the CC-CNS has the potential to decrease the length of stay of many critically ill patients. Assuming the majority of care given to patients is adequate, the CC-CNS may not impact every patient. However, a high-risk and complex patient exists in every hospital who can be affected by a CC-CNS. The percentage of this population varies with the clinical competence of the staff in each hospital.

If the CC-CNS makes recommendations that could impact the length of stay of 1 or 2 patients per week, it would more than justify the salary. Specific examples of how the CNS can impact economics are described in many different ways.[3-9] Over a 15-month period, assessments were made by a CC-CNS of the nursing-medical care plan of patients in a 15-bed critical care unit (CCU). Following the nursing-medical staff assessment, the plan was reviewed by the CC-CNS for appropriateness. In over 200 instances the care plan was thought to have inadequate development or potential areas for improvement. Recommendations were provided to both nursing and medical staff based on these reviews. Most of the recommendations resulted in a reassessment and adjustments in the care plan. Documentation of the specific impact on economics was difficult in many instances. It was difficult to determine if length of stay or resources employed were altered by changing medication or initiating a new treatment or another assessment. However, in 27 cases it was clear that the length of stay was affected, since the patient was discharged from the unit following the recommendation to alter the proposed therapy. Based on this impact, ICU costs were reduced by approximately $27,000. Unfortunately, the net impact on hospital costs was not calculated. In a similar study in the same institution, hospital costs did not change, reflecting a net improvement in the efficiency of care and reduced cost.[10]

The ability of a CC-CNS to routinely impact care and hospital economics is at the heart of the CC-CNS position. Improved documentation of this impact is essential to demonstrate the value of the CC-CNS position to nursing and hospital administration.

CC-CNS as Educator

The CC-CNS has the potential to change clinical practice in nursing through the education of nursing staff and other health care clinicians. The impact of education can be translated into improved patient assessment and therefore into reduced length of stay. Two relevant issues in assessing the impact of the CC-CNS through education are the control of the CC-CNS over the education process and who the CC-CNS is teaching.

In theory it is relatively easy to make an impact on clinical practice through teaching. In reality it is very difficult because of the difference between classroom education and transfer of learning. For the CC-CNS to change practice, two educational components are necessary, namely state of the art classroom education and practical application in the clinical setting. Last, the motivation of the nurse must be present for a behavioral change to occur. All components must be present for actual practice changes to occur. Classroom education alone will not provide enough time or opportunity to change behavior.[11] The CC-CNS must help the learner actually apply concepts in the practice setting, or retention of the new information will be minimal and the benefit to the organization will be reduced.

The CC-CNS does not have to teach all of the nurses after the class in order to generate the retention of knowledge but rather is better used in educating the educators. The CNS is unlikely to be able to spend time with each nurse after a class and is more likely to achieve success through the education and empowerment of other advanced staff nurses such as preceptors and unit educators.

The CC-CNS who is able to provide for both the classroom education and clinical follow-up is more likely to be successful in demonstrating that specific educational efforts are significantly contributing to improving patient care.

Improvements in patient care reduce resource utilization and length of stay. In one example a weaning protocol was considered for a cardiothoracic ICU for nurses to make more consistent and advanced assessments of the patient's spontaneous breathing capability. After review with the medical director and nurse manager, classes were offered to the staff regarding implementation of the protocol. To be successful, however, the education concept had to go beyond a class setting. One graduate-prepared staff nurse and several volunteer staff nurses were targeted as unit advisors. These nurses acted as key unit resources and catalysts to implement the protocol and help other nurses in this practice change. Use of the unit advisors in this educational endeavor increased the likelihood of a successful change.

Based on the implementation of this protocol, the ICU length of stay was reduced in this patient population by 33%. The use of resources such as blood gases and sedation was decreased by 75%. The resultant saving to the hospital was in excess of $30,000 from the ancillary resources alone.[12] Cost of length of stay was not specifically figured. The key point is that the CC-CNS can change economics with education, provided the education is applied in the practice setting beyond the classroom.

Research Effects of CC-CNS Practice

One of the key elements in demonstrating the value of a CC-CNS rests in the capability for the CC-CNS to provide the institution with a service that is unavailable or difficult to achieve within the system. Because of the limited number of people in hospital organizations with research skills the role of the CC-CNS in research is valued.

Research principles can be applied to health care economics. Understanding research principles is at the heart of safely introducing new practice concepts, evaluating new methods of delivering nursing care, or introducing new technology. Without an adequate knowledge of research concepts, errors in evaluation techniques are common. Confusing associations and causal relationships in reported research result in jumping to conclusions between events that are clinically significant and those that are spurious. A simple example will help illustrate this point.

A different intravenous catheter was brought to the attention of the materials manager by a local sales representative. This catheter was commonly used in other hospitals, according to the salesperson, and would save the hospital about $10,000 per year. An evaluation of the catheter was proposed by the nursing product committee to take place in a medical ICU. A sample of 50 catheters was left in the unit with all nurses asked to participate in evaluating the catheter. During the evaluation, complaints were made by the nursing staff

that the new catheter seemed to cause more pain. To test the potential for pain by the new catheter, two volunteers were obtained to compare the new catheter with the current catheter. The participants were blindfolded to avoid seeing the catheter being inserted. Both volunteers picked the new catheter as causing more pain than the current product. The issue was referred back to the nursing product committee. At this time the CC-CNS raised the issue of lack of basic research evaluation techniques, including failure of randomization, lack of interrater reliability, biased sampling, inadequate sample size, and several other limitations. Because of these limitations, a research study was proposed to evaluate the issue of pain induction from the new catheter. With funding from one of the involved companies a formal study was developed to evaluate all major catheters in the marketplace relative to pain. In this study of seven catheters the results demonstrated the new catheter actually as superior to the current catheter regarding pain.[14] The hospital was able to negotiate a better price with the catheter vendor, with the net result of saving several thousand dollars.

This example is easy to replicate in many situations, ranging from products to practice techniques. The need for a clinician with an understanding of sound research principles in an advisory position to nursing is crucial. The CC-CNS can fill the research need faced by the hospital because of the number of issues, ideas, and concepts that need to be tested. The issues are too numerous for a single person to address, but the CC-CNS can chair a nursing research committee to address nurses' own problems and changes that need evaluation; multiple CNS positions are required within any institution.

Through understanding research concepts, the CC-CNS offers the organization an opportunity of advancing practice in a safe manner and allows the organization to practice state-of-the-art techniques. Without research guidance an organization is likely to make the many errors associated with inadequate evaluation techniques.

Consultative Effects on Economics

Clinical practice, education, and research are all areas that have a clear impact on economics. Consultation effects are frequently based on the capabilities of the CC-CNS in these three areas.

Depending on the expertise and level of development of the CC-CNS, the impact of the CNS is seen in various degrees.[14] The CC-CNS serves as an advisor to nursing administrators regarding changes and the potential impact on practice. The changes are evaluated using the principles of research. Education of staff and others regarding proposed changes is facilitated by the CC-CNS. Subsequently, the CC-CNS uses the skills acquired in practice, education, and research to serve as the consultant to the organization. The CC-CNS consultant role is helpful as a nursing representative to medical staff, allied health professionals, and community organizations. Legal matters and cooperative interhospital arrangements are often facilitated by the CC-CNS as consultant for clinical practitioners. The direct economic impact results from the changes or decisions the organization takes based on the CC-CNS consultation. For example, if the CC-CNS is routinely consulted on new products the CC-CNS can bring advanced clinical skills and research understanding to properly evaluate the product. Evaluating whether a new product is clinically acceptable allows the hospital a stronger bargaining position in dealing with manufacturers. In this area alone, savings can be in excess of the yearly salary of the CNS.[15]

Some administrators advocate the use of the CC-CNS in a consultative role to generate income for the hospital. The clinical skills of the CC-CNS can be provided in a consultation to aid those hospitals without the CC-CNS's expertise. However, it is important to keep in mind that the primary value of the CC-CNS is in clinical practice in their own clinical areas. For the CC-CNS to be free to consult outside her or his organization, an assumption must be made that the practice within the organization is at a level where the CC-CNS is not routinely needed. Although this situation is ideal, it is unlikely that an organization has a level of practice that does not need further development. Once the CC-CNS is removed, influence is reduced and there is a tendency to revert to the level of practice present before the CC-CNS was available. Although there are always exceptions to this rule, particularly with significant staff empowerment and development, the tendency to revert back to a less sophisticated level is powerful and should be viewed with caution.

Manner in Which Impact is Seen

The ability to reduce length of stay and improve patient outcomes can be accomplished through clinical, educator, and research roles. The CC-CNS can also reduce the length of stay through consultation to the system. The CC-CNS is able to direct the development and implementation of a clinical program used by the system. The CC-CNS must continually help educate both nursing and hospital administrators regarding the value and impact of the CC-CNS on clinical practice through these roles. Advanced practice that impacts quality is by itself cost effective. This concept is currently advocated throughout the business sector.[16]

The clinical specialist often views methods that impact health care from a clinical perspective. The CC-CNS focuses on changing clinical issues. This perspective allows the CC-CNS to identify problems no one else can see, particularly an administrator who does not have an advanced clinical practice background. Although this perspective is the source of the CC-CNS's value, it also is a source of frustration. Others may not see the problems identified by the CC-CNS as important.

Nursing administrators may have a different perspective that allows identification of problems unrecognized by the CC-CNS. Because of this potential for divergence in perspectives, the CC-CNS benefits from a collaborative relationship with nurse managers regarding the best methods to change practice, maintaining quality patient care, and doing so in the most cost-effective manner. Both perspectives are needed in order to achieve these goals.

Plan of Action to Support CC-CNS's Value

Several articles in the literature have been cited that address the value of the CNS. However, it is important to keep in mind these articles can be viewed as somewhat self-serving, since they are generally written to demonstrate the value of the CNS position. More research is needed in institutions with and without CC-CNS positions in the areas of length of stay, patient outcomes, resource utilizations, staff capabilities, patient satisfaction, nursing satisfaction and turnover, and cost per work load or index. Studies need to be multihospital in scope with expertise in research methodology at an advanced level. Without more objective research into the area of CC-CNSs' value, CC-CNS posi-

TABLE 17-3 Effect of Implementing Oximetry Protocol

	Before Protocol	After Protocol	Protocol Impact
Number of ABGs (average)	3/pt/day	1/pt/day	−2 ABGs/pt/day
Charge/cost per ABG	$60/$10	$60/$10	$120/$20/pt/day
Number of ABGs (average)	1326/yr	434/yr	$53520/$8,920

ABGs, arterial blood gases; pt, patients.

tions will continue to be viewed more as important but expendable indirect positions in the health care organization.

In addition, education of administrators at the graduate level is essential. Unless administrators are well schooled in the capabilities of all their staff, including advanced clinicians such as the CC-CNS, the potential exists for ineffective nursing structures. In an attempt to address this concern, CC-CNSs should attempt to offer classes for local universities during the graduate administration course work, offer presentations at administrative seminars (such as the national meeting of the American Organization of Nurse Executives [AONE]), and publish in administrative journals. It is essential to educate administrators relative to the value of the advanced clinician.

CASE STUDY 1

Pulse oximetry is a common technology in clinical practice but one that has not yet necessarily been applied to its proper extent. For example, the technology for using oximeters is accurate enough to allow a close correlation with actual oxyhemoglobin values.[17,18] Because of this close correlation, arterial blood gas sampling for oxygen tension values (Pao_2) has become almost unnecessary. However, many units still continue to do blood gases despite pulse oximetry.

In one medical unit where oximetry was standard, the CC-CNS developed a protocol in conjunction with the medical director that allowed nursing staff to manipulate oxygen and positive pressure therapy in specific patients based on pulse oximeter values rather than blood gas values. The net result was a substantial savings in blood gas utilization (Table 17-3). This

result is common, and other citings in the literature support this concept.[19,20] This intervention is important because of the CNS's assessment that technology was being used improperly. No other clinician in the institution had raised this concern.

CASE STUDY 2

A wound care CNS noted the potential value of placing high-risk patients on beds that reduced the risk for skin breakdown. The CNS assessed the types of beds on the market and decided a research study was necessary to fully evaluate the effect of any of the beds. In conjunction with a manufacturer, who funded the study, the CNS was able to demonstrate a major economic benefit by having nursing staff members identify high-risk patients and placing these patients on a special bed (Advance 2000 by Hill Rom). The savings to the hospital, as demonstrated over a 3-year period, far exceeded the cost of purchasing new beds (Table 17-4).[21] The importance of the CNS in this project was the requirement to make an advanced clinical assessment. Without the CNS's role, this hospital would have continued to incur high costs secondary to unnecessary skin breakdown.

TABLE 17-4 Length of Stay Differences Between Two Types of Beds in Population at High Risk for Pressure Wounds

	Number of Cases	Average Length of Stay (days)	Average Total Charges
Experimental bed	43	12	$1483
Rental beds	24	23	$1641

SUMMARY

Overt empiric evidence supports the value of the CC-CNS position in the five role components. Literature is available that supports the CC-CNS position from an economic perspective in several nursing specialties. In becoming knowledgeable about health care economics; by educating hospital and nursing administrators about the CC-CNS role; and through the implementation of clinical, education, research, and consultation role strategies; the CC-CNS will continue to be increasingly viewed as essential to the organization.

References

1. American Association of Critical Care Nurses: *Competence statements for the critical care clinical nurse specialist,* Aliso Viejo, Calif, 1989, The Association.
2. Radke K et al: Administrative preparation of the clinical nurse specialists, *J Prof Nurs* 6:221-228, 1990.
3. Gurka AM: Process and outcome components of clinical nurse specialist consultation, *Dimen Crit Care Nurs* 10:169-175, 1991.
4. Field J: A specialist role in patient nutrition, *Nurs Stand* 6:38-39, 1992.
5. Gardner D: The CNS as a cost manager, *Clin Nurse Specialist* 6:112-116, 1992.
6. Boyd NJ et al: The merit and significance of clinical nurse specialists, *J Nurs Admin* 21:35-43, 1991.
7. Brunk QA: The clinical nurse specialist as an external consultant: a framework for practice, *Clin Nurse Specialist* 6:2-4, 1992.
8. Shawler C, Stepler H, Kinnaird S: Model for integration of CNS with nursing management and staff development, *Clin Nurse Specialist* 4:98-102, 1990.
9. Harrison EA: Product evaluation and the clinical nurse specialist: an opportunity for role development, *Clin Nurse Specialist* 3:85-89, 1989.
10. Ahrens TS, Padwojski A: Economic effectiveness of an advanced nurse clinician model, *Nurs Management* 21:72J-72P, 1990.
11. Ahrens TS: Recruitment, retention and education of critical care nurses. In Heater B, editor, *Controversies in critical care,* Rockville, Md, Aspen Publishers, 1988.
12. Bommarito J: Weaning protocol—establishing standardized parameters for withdrawing cardiothoracic surgical patients from mechanical ventilation, *PRN News—Barnes Hospital* 5:3, 1990.
13. Ahrens T, Wiersema L, Weilitz PB: Differences in pain perception with intravenous catheter insertion, *J Intraven Nurs* 14:85-89, 1991.
14. Wolf GA: Clinical nurse specialists: the second generation, *J Nurs Admin* 20:7-8, 1990.
15. Ahrens TS, Padwojski A: Economic impact of advanced clinicians, *Nurs Management* 19:64D-64F, 1988.
16. Iacocca L: *Talking straight,* New York, Bantam Books.
17. Barker SJ, Tremper KK: Pulse oximetry: applications and limitations, *Int Anesthesiol Clin* 25:155-175, 1987.
18. Szaflarski NL, Coene NH: Use of pulse oximetry in critically ill adults, *Heart Lung* 18:444-453, 1989.
19. Rotello LC et al: A nurse directed protocol using pulse oximetry to wean mechanically ventilated patients from toxic oxygen concentrations, *Chest* 102:1833-1835, 1992.
20. Bierman MI, Stein KL, Snyder JV: Pulse oximetry in the postoperative care of cardiac surgical patients: a randomized controlled trial, *Chest* 102:1367-1370, 1992.
21. Wiersema LA: Impact of advance care 2000 bed on length of stay and resource utilization, *PRN News—Barnes Hospital*. (In press.)

Chapter 18

The Critical Care Clinical Nurse Specialist and Delivery Systems and Practice Models in Transition

Denise M. Lawrence, RN, MS, CS

Issues facing the health care system of today are markedly different from those that shaped the health care environment of the past. Escalating health care costs, the aging of America, and the explosion of technology are driving forces mandating an overhaul in health care in the United States.

It is predicted that by the year 2000, 15.5% of the gross national product will be spent on health care, which translates to greater than 13 trillion dollars for health care services alone.[1] At the beginning of this decade, 31 million Americans (1 in 8) were 65 years or older, and it is predicted that the number of elderly persons will more than double at the end of the decade.[2] Major advances in medical technology and therapeutic interventions have transformed our ability to obtain and interpret clinical data, to manage critical illness, and ultimately to extend life. These advances have created enormous ethical and financial dilemmas within health care. We are being challenged to design a health care system for the future that will provide the highest quality services and interventions for patients within a fiscally manageable framework. Meeting these challenges will require flexible, creative, and innovative clinical leadership.

The critical care clinical nurse specialist (CC-CNS) will influence and be influenced by this evolving health care system. The CC-CNS, as practitioner, educator, consultant, researcher, and leader or manager, is both positioned and suited to direct and lead changes to meet health care needs of the future. In addition, new CC-CNS practice models will be developed to meet the demands for advanced nursing care within this changing environment.

This chapter describes selected nursing delivery systems and practice models designed to meet these evolutionary and revolutionary changes in health care. The chapter further discussed strategies of how the CC-CNS can facilitate changes in delivery systems and nursing practice models and provides direction for CC-CNS practice within this evolving health care system.

THEORETIC PERSPECTIVE

The words "delivery system" and "practice model" appear repeatedly in the literature but often lack clarity, discrimination, and consistency. Although they are interrelated concepts, they are not synonymous. For this discussion, delivery system will refer to the *framework* in which care is provided to patients; practice model will refer to the *process* used to deliver care. The delivery system defines the structure for providing care. It delineates how care is organized and provided to groups of patients within an organizational system. How the system is organized, how parts of the system relate to one another, and how the work (tasks) of delivering care is allocated and assigned are all components of a delivery system. Primary nursing, team nursing, and managed care are examples of delivery sytems.

Practice model, on the other hand, refers more

directly to the process of giving care. A practice model describes the manner in which the caregiver role is executed. Inherent in any professional practice model is the philosophy of the professional role, role definition, and role components. The model defines and operationalizes a scope of practice. Practice models exist within a delivery system, and several different practice models may occur within the same delivery system. Collaborative practice and differentiated practice are examples of practice models.

The CC-CNS is in a key position to assist organizations, groups, and individuals to create, test, implement, and evaluate care delivery systems and nursing practice models. The CC-CNS is a pivotal resource in a changing health care delivery system. Since the changes that need to be made center around patient care (clinical expertise) and the ability to structure a system to provide this care (process expertise) the CC-CNS becomes a major force in the evolving health care system.

RELATED RESEARCH AND LITERATURE
Nursing Delivery Systems and Practice Models

Health care costs, a changing population, decreased length of stay, technologic advances, and the changing work force are influencing the way in which we deliver care today and are mandating the changes of tomorrow. Consequently health care providers are examining ways to achieve high quality care at the lowest possible cost. Because nursing service is a high cost item in health care organizations, great emphasis is placed on delivering quality nursing care at a decreased cost. This has resulted in a surge of new nursing delivery systems and practice models.

A recent compendium of innovative nursing practice models includes the selected examples in Table 18–1.[3,4] These models, which have been evaluated to varying degrees, represent a wide variety of structural approaches to reorganizing nursing practice. Some have been motivated primarily by the need to address nurse staffing shortages, whereas others have been motivated primarily by the need to contain costs. Cost savings might be achieved through better coordinated care, through the use of non–registered nurse (RN) providers, or through reductions in turnover and replacement costs. In addition to the models already described in the published literature,

there are some ongoing evaluations on innovative models.[4]

Twenty projects have been funded by The Robert Wood Johnson Foundation and The Pew Charitable Trusts in their program entitled "Strengthening Hospital Nursing: A Program to Improve Patient Care." The implementation phase of these projects began in the fall of 1990, and results of implementing these practice models have not yet been published. According to the projects' proposals, the models range from system-wide interventions to unit-based practice models. Most of the models have a patient-centered focus. Further, 14 of the 20 proposals indicated that patient outcomes would be measured to assess the impact of the models.[5] These projects are likely to produce some interesting findings with regard to patient outcomes by 1994.[4]

Two research demonstration projects funded by the National Institute of Nursing Research (NINR) and the Division of Nursing are underway in New York and Arizona. The University of Rochester (New York) School of Nursing is implementing and evaluating an Enhanced Professional Practice Model for Nursing, designed to increase nurses' control over practice at the unit level and to provide professional compensation. The University of Arizona College of Nursing is implementing and evaluating a unit-based Differentiated Group Professional Practice Model that has three components: group governance—including participative management, staff bylaws, peer review, and professional salary structure; differentiated care delivery—including differentiated RN practice, use of nurse extenders, and primary care management; and shared values—including a culture-building process that values quality of care, entrepreneurship, and recognition for excellence in practice.[4]

NINR is also funding the evaluation of The Johns Hopkins Professional Practice Model. That model consists of a contract between a unit's RNs and the hospital in which the nurses agree to provide 24-hour patient care on the unit for 1 year in exchange for unit self-management (including peer review, self-scheduling, and quality assurance), salaried compensation, and shared savings if the unit contains its costs.[4,6]

Another project with plans to collect patient outcome data is the New Jersey Nursing Incentive Reimbursement Awards (NIRA) program.[7] This

TABLE 18–1 Nursing Practice Models: Selected Cases*

Model	Location	Key Attributes
ProACT (Professionally Advanced Care Team Model)	Robert Wood Johnson University Hospital, New Brunswick, N.J.	Case management; multidisciplinary teams
Professional Nursing Practice Model	Beth Israel Hospital, Boston, Mass.	Primary nursing; case management
NEMCH Case Management Model	New England Medical Center Hospitals, Boston, Mass.	Primary nursing; case management
Johns Hopkins Professional Practice Model	Johns Hopkins Hospital, Baltimore, Md.	Self-managed units; salaries
VUMC Cooperative Care Model	Vanderbilt University Medical Center, Nashville, Tenn.	Primary nursing; multidisciplinary teams
CSMC Cost Containment Model	Cedars-Sinai Medical Center, Los Angeles, Calif.	Primary nursing
IVH Model	Iowa Veterans Home, Iowa City, Iowa	24-hour accountability; self-governance
Professional Nursing Network	Carondelet St. Mary's Hospital and Health Center, Tucson, Ariz.	Case management across service continuum
Patient Care Technician (PCT) Model	New England Deaconess Hospital, Boston, Mass.	Nurse extenders supervised by RN; multidisciplinary teams
Primary Case Management Practice	Hermann Hospital Houston, Texas	Case management; differentiated

*This is not intended as an exhaustive list. The models listed here are described in Mayer et al.[3]
From Weisman CS: Nursing practice models: research on patient outcomes. In U.S. Department of Health and Human Services, editor: *Patient outcomes research: examining the effectiveness of nursing practice* (proceedings of a conference sponsored by the National Center for Nursing Research) 1991.

project is evaluating nursing innovations in 23 New Jersey hospitals. The innovations include redesigned work environments, including case management models; shared governance structures; computerized nursing process; and educational programs to address nurse satisfaction.[4]

Current projects in critical care include studies of nursing practice models in specialty units, such as special care units for chronically critically ill patients,[8] pediatric critical care units,[9] and intensive care units.[10]

Clinical Nurse Specialist's Role in Changing Health Care Delivery Systems and Nursing Practice Model

Little literature exists on the specific role of the CC-CNS in changing health care delivery systems and nursing practice models. However, the literature does reflect essential components of the CNS's

role in today's health care delivery system. These essential components are advanced nursing practice, clinical expert judgment, and leadership. Advanced nursing practice is described as the broad range and depth of specialized clinical knowledge, the ability to anticipate problems and issues that affect patient and system outcomes, the ability to analyze information, and the ability to assess nonclinical variables that influence patient outcomes.[11] Although different health care delivery systems and nursing practice models emphasize various competencies and functions of the CNS role, the essential components of advanced nursing practice, clinical judgment, and leadership prevail.

The CNS model of practice described by Holt[12] identifies the goal of CNSs and advanced practitioners to improve patient care and patient outcomes through *direct* and *indirect* care activities. An example of a direct care activity is the CC-

CNS's experienced assessment of patients on mechanical ventilation. The CC-CNS's assessment can lead to early removal from mechanical support and earlier discharge from the ICU. Considering that the cost of an ICU stay and ventilator use exceeds $1,000 per day, the advanced clinician only need to perform such an assessment once a week to more than justify his or her entire salary.[13] An example of an indirect care activity is a CC-CNS's input on administrative decisions in the acquisition of appropriate technology and products. The CC-CNS is better able to understand the potential effect of new products and to evaluate their suitability for clinical application. The CC-CNS can also identify key features required of a product and is able to identify less expensive alternatives to currently used products.[13] Thus the CC-CNS improves patient care through advanced clinical judgment and leadership. Holt states: "A clinical nurse specialist must influence the quality of nursing care in a larger group of patients than she can personally attend."[12] The CC-CNS does this specifically through the roles of educator and researcher. As educator, the CC-CNS uses educational material to demonstrate how to prioritize and put knowledge to use. If the CC-CNS does not follow classroom teaching, much of what is learned in that setting is forgotten, and there will be little improvement in patient care.[13] Thus the CC-CNS influences the quality of care rendered by other nurses. As researcher, the CC-CNS assesses new trends in practice that need evaluation from a scientific perspective before they are implemented in routine practice. Institutions that implement practice changes without this kind of evaluation run the risk of introducing changes that do not advance patient care. Thus the ability of the CC-CNS to critique and implement research-based practice will safely advance nursing practice at an institution.[13]

Calkin[14] emphasized the analytic skills of the CNS in executing the various role components that are based on deliberate reasoning. Calkin states that the CNS role includes the abilities "to be articulate about the nature of nursing practice, to use reasoning to deal with practice innovations, and to develop or contribute to newer forms of practice."[14]

Brown[15] described a model called multidisciplinary partnership, in which the CNS (attending nurse) and physician manage the care of a specific patient population. The CC-CNS relates to the staff nurse much as the attending physician relates to residents and interns. The CC-CNS enters into joint practice with a physician and has clinical practice privileges. Effective interpersonal and interprofessional communication skills are at the core of successful implementation. Brown states that CNSs should "be able to define nursing practice creatively and soundly; they are on the frontier of interprofessional relationships."[15]

One example of the role of the CC-CNS found in the literature is in the development of a special care unit for chronic critically ill patients.[15] The CC-CNS in this setting has a major role as project leader. The CC-CNS functions within the five role components as practitioner, educator, consultant, researcher, and leader/manager. For example, clinical teaching and overall clinical management of the patients are the responsibilities of the CC-CNS. In addition, the CC-CNS facilitates a case management delivery system and shared governance management model. Case management delivery system holds the nurse accountable clinically and financially for the patient outcomes throughout the whole spectrum of care. Shared governance gives the nurse authority and responsibility for managing the environment through collaboration and joint decision making.

Successful implementation requires strong nursing leadership by the CC-CNS. In addition, equally important are consensus among the nurses regarding commitment to the patient and professional practice and support from administrators and nurses assuming accountability for their decisions.[16] Inherent in the expanded scope of practice are the increased autonomy and self-regulation of nursing practice.

The nurse-managed special care unit is composed of a physical design that is limited in technology. Care is aimed at family involvement and rehabilitation. Success is determined by continually looking at length of stay, cost, and patient outcomes. Beside the clinical and educational activities, the CC-CNS functions as a liaison for the unit to the hospital and coordinates the operational details.

In addition to nurse-managed units, other nursing practice models that are emerging in critical care include case management, managed care, patient care extenders, and multiskilled workers. However, regardless of the health care delivery system or nursing practice model instituted, advanced nursing practice is essential in providing cost-effective quality care. As Styles[17] stated:

The future of all nursing is linked to the development of advanced nursing practice today. Advanced practitioners are crucial to rational, systematic restructuring of the occupation; recruitment into nursing; generation of knowledge for practice; the approach to ethical issues which are at the heart of truly professional behavior.[17]

Advanced assessment, planning, decision making, and management of care by protocols occur through the entire spectrum of care. It is the CC-CNS who functions as coordinator, director, and evaluator of clinical care. The CC-CNS in today's health care delivery system and practice model has more direct care activities, independent interventions, autonomy, and accountability than ever before.

PRACTICE IMPLICATIONS

The importance of the CC-CNS's role in the implementation of a new delivery system in critical care cannot be overemphasized. The successful implementation of a delivery system that reassigns patient care responsibilities among critical care nurses and support personnel requires skillful attention to the care requirements of critically ill patients and the values and charactertistics of critical care nurses. The CC-CNS today must deal effectively with the dual challenge of facilitating a high degree of staff involvement in the changes and giving time and attention to the emotional and relationship aspects of nurses' role changes.[18]

Successful CC-CNSs in the changing health care delivery environment are those who will do the following:

• Be energized by changes in nurses's clinical roles
• Coordinate activities of all areas of practice
• Provide links to the organization and its resources[19]

A key concept of the CC-CNS's role in implementation of new practice models is supporting, guiding, and developing staff. The new workers of today want to be active participants rather than passive recipients of change. Consequently, the CC-CNS must facilitate a high degree of staff involvement in planning a change in health care de-

livery system and nursing practice model. The American Association of Critical Care Nurses (AACN) supports collaborative approaches to developing new delivery systems.[20] In high-intensity, high-stress areas such as critical care units, staff participation and ownership of the work redesign are of the utmost importance.

Another role of the CC-CNS in the changing health care delivery system and practice model environment is facilitating physician collaboration. Physicians and medical directors of critical care units are key stakeholders in the patient care delivery system and must be closely involved in its redesign. As Knaus et al.[21] reported: "The highest quality of care appears to require a high degree of involvement by both dedicated physicians and nurses in ongoing clinical care." It is the CC-CNS who facilitates collaborative relationships between physician and nurses while developing, implementing, and expanding the new practice model. This is achieved by the following:

• Physicians, nurses, and CC-CNSs working together to develop clinical care protocols, critical paths, and standing admitting orders
• Combined nurse-physician advisory committees that review clinical practice issues
• Incorporating feedback from physicians regarding changes noted when new health care delivery systems or practice models are implemented
• Combined nurse and physician meetings for joint analysis of patient variances from critical paths or clinical protocols

CASE STUDY

The following case study demonstrates the role of the CC-CNS in facilitating a change to a new nursing practice model. The shortage of RNs created a continuously high work load level for the nurses in a critical care pediatric unit of a large, mid Atlantic, private, nonprofit, teaching hospital. The nurse manager of the unit consulted with the pediatric CC-CNS because of his concern about the negative consequences of the consistently high workload in an understaffed situation. Both the nurse manager and CC-CNS were aware of the decrease in quality of care in the pediatric intensive care unit (ICU) and the dissatisfaction among the nursing staff. Together they brainstormed creative strategies to support the nursing staff and help meet the demands of the critically ill children. Both agreed that the solution had to be budget neutral and that ideas they generated would have to be brought to the staff meeting for consideration, further brainstorming, and discussion.

Together the nurse manager and CC-CNS brought to the staff meeting several ideas from their meeting. The staff expressed much interest in the idea of using support personnel to assist in performing selected activities usually done by the nurse. The nurse manager discussed this as a strategy being implemented in a growing number of institutions.

The CC-CNS used supportive literature which documented that as much as 40% of nursing time is spent performing tasks that unlicensed persons could perform.[22] The CC-CNS shared examples of non-nursing tasks from the AACN publication "Delegation of Nursing and Non-Nursing Activities in Critical Care Nursing."[23] In addition, the CC-CNS shared the position statement "Use of Nursing Support Personnel in Critical Care Units" developed jointly by the AACN and the Society of Critical Care Medicine.[24] The CC-CNS discussed those activities that constitute professional nursing practice and therefore should not be delegated. These include the initial patient assessment or intervention, establishing nursing diagnosis, establishing nursing care goals, developing a nursing care plan, and evaluating patient progress or lack of progress toward achieving goals.[25]

The nursing staff agreed to support a change to a nursing practice model that used support personnel who would be called patient care technicians. The group decided their new model of nursing practice would be called the RN/technician model. In this model each RN would pair with a nursing technician who acted as a helper in delivering nursing care. The RN would delegate specific direct and indirect patient care tasks.

The CC-CNS and nurse manager outlined a plan for implementation that would incorporate staff input at all levels. The plan was divided into four phases.

The nurse manager was primarily responsible for phase 1. In phase 1 the nurse manager brainstormed feasible staffing patterns. Each vacant RN position would be changed to create two technician positions. This proposal was represented and accepted by the staff.

Phase 2 was primarily the pediatric CC-CNS's responsibility. This was the development and implementation of an educational program for the RN/technician partners. The content of the educational program included sessions for RNs on delegation, conflict resolution, and mutually valuing the RN and technician roles. The content for the technicians included a review of their responsibilities in the pediatric ICU, basic aspects of pediatric nursing care, and care of the pediatric critical care environment and equipment.

Phase 3 was the responsibility of both the nurse manager and CC-CNS. This was the actual implementation phase. During this time the nurse manager and CC-CNS made rounds in the unit to assess the progress and problems as the change was occurring. In addition, the CC-CNS spent extra time in the unit, answering questions, reassuring the nurses they could delegate tasks to the technicians, educating the technicians and staff when necessary, and role modeling clinical practice.

Phase 4 was the evaluation phase and was a shared responsibility of the nurse manager and CC-CNS. The nurse manager evaluated cost savings to the unit. The CC-CNS evaluated aspects of clinical practice and patient satisfaction. Together the nurse manager and CC-CNS developed a staff satisfaction survey. Because of the CC-CNS's knowledge of research, the CC-CNS was responsible for data analysis of the evaluation instruments. The results of the evaluations were positive and were reported at subsequent staff meetings. Everyone agreed that using this model of patient care delivery enabled the pediatric unit to increase the standards of nursing practice, decrease cost of care, and provide improved satisfaction among the nursing staff.

SUMMARY

The CC-CNS has the knowledge, commitment, values, and beliefs to help move organizations through changes in health care delivery systems and practice models. As health care technology increases and the environment becomes more complex, the CC-CNS will continue to have an important role as content expert (clinical practice) and process expert (organizational change). The CC-CNS has a major role in assisting with the successful redesign of the critical care practice environment to enhance the quality of care, and increase the nurse's, patient's and family's satisfaction cost effectively.

References

1. U.S. Department of Commerce: *Economics and Administration Bureau of Census,* Washington, DC, 1991, The Department.
2. U.S. Senate Special Committee on Aging, American Association of Retired Persons, Federal Council on the Aging, U.S. Administration on Aging: *Aging America: trends and projections,* Washington, DC, 1991.
3. Mayer GG, Madden MJ, Lawrenz E, editors: *Patient care delivery models,* Rockville, Md, 1990, Aspen Systems, Publisher.
4. Weisman CS: Nursign practice models: research on patient outcomes. In U.S. Department of Health and Human Services, editor: *Patient outcomes research: examining the effectiveness of nursing practice* (proceedings of a conference sponsored by the National Center for Nursing Research), 1991.
5. Information provided by Sue Taft, Associate Professor of Nursing, Kent State University, in her role as evaluator of the Robert Wood Johnson/Pew Charitable Trusts' "Strengthening Hospital Nursing: a Program to Improve Patient Care."
6. Mamon J et al: Impact of hospital discharge planning on meeting patient needs after returning home, *Health Services Res.*
7. Knickman J et al: *An evaluation of the New Jersey nursing incentive reimbursement awards program: an interim report,* New York, 1991, Health Research Program of New York University.
8. Daley J et al: Predicting hospital-associated mortality for Medicare patients: a method for patients with stroke, pneu-

monia, acute myocardial infarction, and congestive heart failure, *JAMA* 260:3617-3624, 1988.
9. Murphy CA, Walts L, Cavouras CA: The PRN plan: professional reimbursement for nurses, *Nurs Management* 20:64Q-64X, 1989.
10. Phillips RS et al: Decision making in SUPPORT: the role of the nurse, J *Clin Epidemiol* 43(suppl):555-585, 1990.
11. Sproxx JA, Baggerly J: Models of advanced nursing practice. In Hamric AB, Sproxx JA, editors: *The clinical nurse specialist in theory and practice,* ed 2, Philadelphia, 1989, WB Saunders Co.
12. Holt FM: A theoretical model for clinical specialist practice, *Nursing Healthcare* 5(8):445-449, 1984.
13. Ahrens T: Advanced clinicians can positively affect patient care, *AACN News,* Sept 1988.
14. Calkin JD: A model for advanced nursing practice, *J Nurs Admin* 14(1):24-30, 1984.
15. Brown SJ: The clinical nurse specialist in a multidisciplinary partnership, *Nurs Admin Q* 1:34-46, 1983.
16. Daly BJ et al: Development of a SCU for chronically critically ill patients, *Heart Lung* 20(1):45-51, 1991.
17. Styles MM: Clinical nurse specialist and the future of nursing. In Sparacino PS, Cooper DM, Minarik PA, editors: *The clinical nurse specialist: implementation and impact,* Norwalk, Conn, 1990, Appleton & Lange.
18. Curtin LL: Designing new roles: nursing in the 90's and beyond, *Nurs Management* 21(2):7-9, 1990.
19. Ritter J, Tonges MC: Work redesign in high-intensity environments, *J Nurs Admin* 21(12):26-35, 1991.
20. Searle DL: Efficient allocation of resources: support services, systems and personnel, *Heart Lung* 18(2):27A-28A, 1989.
21. Knaus WA et al: An evaluation of outcome from intensive care in major medical centers, *Ann Intern Med* 104(3):410-418, 1986.
22. American Hospital Association: *Proceedings of the Invitational Conference on the Nursing Shortages: Issues and Strategies,* Chicago, Oct 7, 1988, Chicago, 1988, American Hospital Association, Center for Nursing.
23. American Association of Critical-Care Nurses: *Delegation of nursing and nonnursing activities in critical care: a framework for decision making,* Laguna Niguel, Calif, 1990, The Association.
24. American Association of Critical-Care Nurses, Society of Critical Care Medicine: *Use of nursing support personnel in critical care units,* Newport Beach, Calif, 1986, The Association and the Society.
25. Cardin S, Kane S, Koch K: Use of patient care extenders in critical care nursing, *AACN Clin Issues* 3(4):789-796, 1992.

Part VII

Professional Development of the Critical Care Clinical Nurse Specialist

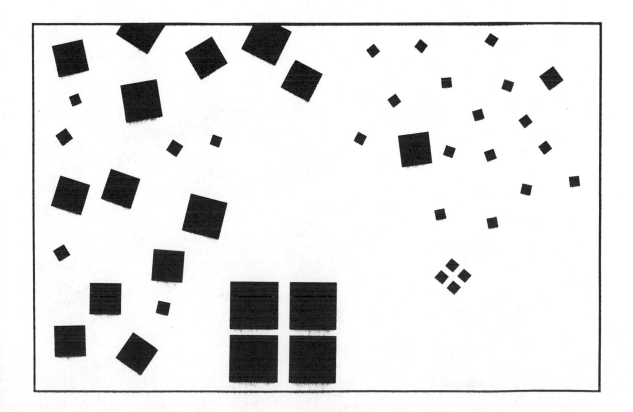

Networking: Making It Successful for the Critical Care Clinical Nurse Specialist

Joan M. Vitello-Cicciu, RN, MSN, CS, CCRN

We are what we repeatedly do. Excellence, then, is not an act, but a habit.

Aristotle

One of the most integral components of a critical care clinical nurse specialist's (CC-CNS's) career is the networks that she or he develops. The benefits of establishing networks can lead to a higher level of practice, greater career advancements, productivity, and empowerment of an individual. Additionally, advanced clinicians may learn best from joint problem solving with other experts. Networking can also develop the CC-CNS's practice and the practice specialty. This chapter describes the process and strategies to develop one's network as a CC-CNS.

REVIEW OF LITERATURE

Just what is a network and networking? Luebbert[1] describes a network as "an informal group of contacts who share advice, facts, techniques, job leads, plans and dreams, and lend each other moral support." Wake and Vogel[2] define networking as "the process by which groups share ideas, information, strengths, problems and resources." Along a similar tenet, Welch[3] states that networking is a "process of developing and using your contacts for information, advice, and moral support as you pursue your career." Networking as a CC-CNS may occur at conferences, symposia, journal clubs, and professional associations and in one's own facility. A word of caution is needed in that networking does not imply maintaining contact with everyone that you meet. One needs to remain focused on developing specific contacts that will most influence professional career. Davidson[4] refers to this as "focused networking," whereby you seek out 10 to 20 key people who will be most helpful to you in your career.

Making just one contact can be an extremely important step because of the rule of threes.[5] This rule implies that one contact knows three contacts, each of whom have three other contacts. Thus whenever you make one contact you have actually made 13 possible contacts, all of whom may be called for advice, information, and possible career opportunities. Further, the importance of establishing a network is emphasized in this revised adage by Murphy[6] as "It's what you know, who you know, and who knows you that really counts!"

A network also needs to be distinguished from a coalition. Harkavy[7] describes a coalition as a temporary alliance of persons or groups with a common shared cause who have their sights set on the achievement of one or more common goals. Networks tend to be more permanent, more information sharing, and more supportive in nature in contrast to coalitions, which are more temporary, influential, and goal directed. Further, in a coalition each member or group maintains its own identity and shares an equal partnership in the governing, planning, and decision-making processes of the coalition.

FUNCTIONS OF NETWORKS

Networks function in many important ways for a CC-CNS. They can serve as (1) channels for information about clinical issues impacting practice; (2) conduits for generating possible clinical or professional solutions for problems; (3) sources of support for the CNS; and (4) resources to share clinical expertise and to gain insight about new practice patterns or techniques in one's clinical specialty practice. Another important function of a network centers around the ability to gain a collective force that can affect decision making or policy making or implement necessary changes locally, regionally, or nationally. For example, several years ago the American Association of Critical Care Nurses (AACN) Research Committee asked the AACN Clinical Nurse Specialist Special Interest Group (CNS-SIG) to select a specific clinical topic for a multicenter national study. The clinical issue identified was to investigate the effect of heparinized and nonheparinized solutions on the patency of arterial pressure lines. This research investigation came to be known as the Thunder Project. The Thunder Project Task Force consisted of members of both the research committee and the CNS-SIG. Thus two networks came together to embark on a landmark research endeavor that answered an important clinical question.

TYPES OF NETWORKS

The type of network a person begins to develop should depend on the objectives one hopes or needs to accomplish. There are many types to pursue. These consist of social/personal, business, support, and professional networks.

In addition to those types of networks, a CC-CNS can develop horizontal, vertical, internal, external, organizational, or mixed professional networks. When a CC-CNS enlarges contacts chiefly to other critical care specialists then that CNS is developing a horizontal network involving only those persons holding similar positions. Conversely, if this same CC-CNS expands a network to include nursing educators, nursing administrators, and researchers, this is a vertical network involving people from various levels. An internal network mainly consists of individuals from one institution. External networks contain people from outside the CNS's institution. Occupational networks are developed with other nurses regardless of background or specialty. A mixed network is a group of contacts made by a CNS from other professions or disciplines such as physicians, respiratory therapists, social workers, dietitians, or clinical pharmacists. Development of all of these types of networks is valuable to the CC-CNS in order to derive the most personal and professional success. For example, a CC-CNS should belong to the American Nurses' Association as the professional organization (vertical, occupational), American Association of Critical Care Nurses (AACN) as the specialty organization (horizontal, occupational), and perhaps a nonnursing organization such as the American Heart Association or the American Cancer Society (vertical, mixed). These would all be external networks. The CC-CNS should also have internal networks consisting of horizontal (other specialists if employed), occupational (nurse managers, clinicians, educators), and mixed (physicians, pharmacists) groups. Investing in developing certain networks initially depends on the level of experience of the CC-CNS and the most pressing needs or issues confronting that individual. Regardless of the type of network one wishes to develop, the process of creating such a network is similar.

PRACTICE IMPLICATIONS

Developing certain networks depends on the level of experience as a CNS. A neophyte CC-CNS or an experienced CC-CNS who wants to initiate the networking process should ask two questions: (1) What internal and external contacts do I need in my role as a CNS? and (2) Where do I begin? As a beginning level specialist or networker, one can start exploring potential internal and external professional networks. Strategies to get started with internal networks consist of the following:

- Volunteer for membership on nursing and hospital-wide committees.
- Keep a notebook initially of all the contacts you have made within the hospital.
- Have an appointment book or pocket calendar for all scheduled meetings, lunch dates, and other potential networking opportunities.
- Choose a veteran CNS as a mentor to provide guidance and counsel.
- Offer to write a short piece for your hospital

newsletter or magazine to increase your visibility.

- Volunteer to talk to other disciplines in the hospital about a topic in your area of expertise.
- Project a successful, knowledgeable, and energetic image.

In addition to establishing internal networks it is equally important to expand one's external networks. One should decide as a CC-CNS what type of network to develop, that is, clinical specialty or role component (education, research, consultation). It is also essential to determine what outcomes one wishes to achieve. Decide how many contacts to make within a certain time frame. For example, I plan on making 10 new contacts next month. The following strategies are recommended to develop external networks:

- Have personal business cards available to distribute.
- Join professional organizations such as the American Nurses' Association, American Heart Association, American Thoracic Society, and Sigma Theta Tau.
- Join specialty organizations such as AACN, the Society of Critical Care Medicine (SCCM), and the American Neuroscience Association. Information on other nursing organizations is available in the *Encyclopedia of Associations* found in public libraries.
- Attend conferences, professional meetings, or seminars that are specialty based and global in nature. A premier conference for networking as a CC-CNS is AACN's National Teaching Institute (NTI), which meets annually in May. In anticipation of attending such a conference, set your own network objectives. Decide who you want to meet and what questions you want answered. Use the time before sessions or during exhibit hours or social events to meet your planned objectives. Table 19-1 gives an example of a possible networking agenda.
- Attend civic and community groups to broaden your professional contacts outside nursing.
- At any of the aforementioned meetings act like a host or hostess instead of a guest.[8] A host or hostess will introduce himself or herself; a guest waits to be introduced. It is important

TABLE 19-1 NTI Networking Agenda

1. Find speaker for local chapter's spring symposium.
2. Talk to hospital exhibitors regarding clinical ladders.
3. Ask about critical care nurse practitioners in ICUs.
4. Gain more information about left ventricular assist devices.
5. Talk to member of NTI task force about submitting proposal to speak at next year's NTI.

to take the initiative and invite people to meet for a beverage or a meal to get to know them and begin the network process. Attempt to meet as many people as you can at these gatherings.

- After these encounters maintain a file of the contacts you made. This can be accomplished by compiling business cards either alphabetically or by professional standings or by keeping an index-card file with names, addresses, and telephone numbers of all the contacts you made. I have found it useful to write some pertinent information such as where I met the person and some significant details of our conversation on the back of the business card or index card. A loose-leaf notebook or computerized list can also be helpful in keeping your contacts organized.
- Maintain your contact with an individual after meeting them either by telephoning or writing a note.
- Promote yourself through writing an article for publication or a letter to an editor in response to an article. Consider doing some professional speaking, because this is one means of expanding your visibility and credibility in nursing. Volunteer for task forces or committees in your local, state, regional, or national nurses' associations.
- Share with other professional colleagues the latest nursing or medical advances at your institution.
- Write letters of congratulations to professional colleagues who have recently published an article or received an award or professional advancement.

• Consider expanding your network in the political arena. Volunteer to support a particular candidate in any way that your schedule would permit. Such political contacts have proved invaluable to a number of clinical specialists, especially in gaining third-party reimbursement.

A CC-CNS should be selective about the number of contacts that are converted to an ongoing relationship. Davidson[4] offers the following questions for deciding which people you want to contact on a continuous basis:

1. Do I like that person?
2. Do I feel challenged and excited by my conversation with that person?
3. Does that person have a high energy level?
4. Does that person have knowledge I need or want?
5. Does that person have contacts in my field?
6. Could that person advance my career at some time?
7. Could I help that person with his or her career?

An effective network has been described by Lee Gardenswartz and Anita Rowe, partners in Training and Consulting Associates, as containing two kinds of supporters: maintainers and propellers. Maintainers are people who assist you in accomplishing your job more competently and effectively. Propellers push you into new areas to promote your advancement. A combination of both types of people is important in your professional network. In addition, effective networking requires time and perseverance. It takes time to nurture relationships and perseverance in maintaining these relationships. The important consideration is to maintain these networking relationships not only when you need information, advice, or support but on a continuous basis.

MAXIMIZING NETWORKING ACTIVITIES

The art of networking can assist critical care specialists in realizing their full potential in their current position as well as open new doors for career mobility. However, some caveats about networking will enable a CC-CNS to attain the greatest benefits from this process.

After one begins to make contacts, it is imperative that certain ground rules prevail. Networking is a two-way process. This means that one must give as well as receive from these professional contacts. It is crucial to help those who have helped you so as to maintain an active network. Moreover, it is critical to treat others exactly as you wish to be treated. It is very interesting to note how small our professional circles have become. A person's outrageous or unacceptable behavior can spread through a grapevine faster than anyone can imagine. Careers have literally been destroyed in this manner.

Another caveat is to provide timely feedback to others. Learn to listen and not always to speak. A CC-CNS should consistently project an optimistic attitude, especially to casual acquaintances. Avoid others with hidden agendas. If you do not like someone you have met, graciously excuse yourself, leave, and move on to meet other new people. On the other hand, you do not have to like everyone in your network. You just need to derive a mutual benefit from that association. Along this line is the important adage about not burning bridges or you may find yourself needing those bridges another day! Moreover, you do not necessarily need to become close friends with your professional contacts. In fact, one of the most skilled female networkers according to Novak[9] is the storybook character Cinderella. Novak describes Cinderella's skill as a networker in the following way:

Cinderella used her stepsisters to give her information about a key event. Then she plugged into her mentor, the fairy godmother, who had resources that were utilized on her behalf. When she got to the ball, she was imaged appropriately and knew how to dance. And then she knew when to leave.

Skillful networking also involves making a conscious effort not to become so overwhelmed with establishing one's contacts that a CC-CNS neglects work responsibilities. A careful balance should be achieved.

It may be noteworthy to examine how others go about the networking process. I surveyed 20 CC-CNSs from 12 states and the District of Columbia to assess their networking strategies. Demographics on the respondents were as follows:

• Age: range of 29 to 46 years; mean of 39 years
• Gender: all females

- Years as CC-CNS: range of 4 months to 14 years; mean of 7.6 years
- Type of facility: university affiliated (8), federal (3), community-teaching affiliated (2), community (2), teaching (1), nonprofit teaching (1), community for profit (1), community nonprofit (1), and military (1)

Five questions were asked of these CC-CNSs practicing throughout the United States, who were part of my professional network:

1. How did you get started networking as a CNS?
2. What types of networks did you develop first?
3. What strategies did you find especially helpful to networking?
4. How do you maintain or plan to maintain your networks?
5. What benefits have you gained from your networks?

In response to the first question, the majority of the respondents (70%) replied that they began networking through AACN, that is, through their local chapter, national committees, or task forces. Others (15%) began by using their contacts made through graduate school or through city-wide consortia with other clinical specialists. Additional responses by individuals included starting their networks through the following: Sigma Theta Tau (1), state council of CNS (1), CNS orientation in hospital (1), attending conferences (3), public speaking (1), and city-wide CNS support group (1).

Responses to the second question (What types of networks did you develop first?) yielded very interesting results. External networks were developed initially by 55% of the sample. Internal networks were first created by 35%. The remaining 10% stated that they began both internal and external networks at the same time. The major determinant voiced by those who began their external network first was that there were no other clinical specialists in their institution to network with so they had to explore others outside the facility. All (95%) but one respondent began with expanding their horizontal networks. One individual actually began developing a mixed internal network by sharing her office with a nurse manager and by attending multidiscipline discharge rounds where she ex-

panded her network to include social workers, secretaries, chaplains, and physicians.

The third question (What strategies did you find especially helpful to networking?) yielded multiple responses from each CC-CNS surveyed. The specific strategies and percentages are as follows: (1) involvement in group projects or working on committees (50%); (2) initiating phone contact with others (40%); (3) attending meetings, conferences, or other educational gatherings (55%); (4) reading journals and then contacting the authors (20%); (5) conducting informal surveys (5%); (6) clinical visits with students (CNS had joint appointment) (5%); and (7) sharing information with others (15%). One CC-CNS stated that she made a list of things she needed information about and brought that list to conferences. She would then seek out specific people to assist her in gaining the information. She also felt that it was important to have something you can bargain with (an area of expertise or information that you can share with others). Interestingly two other respondents made reference to the need to share information with others as a very important strategy.

Another respondent stated that when she is attending a conference she will often meet people by going up to a specific individual and introducing herself (acting like a hostess instead of a guest). Two other specialists responded that they had to overcome their reluctance and just introduce themselves to others in order to meet specific people.

Similar strategies were articulated by these respondents to question 4 (How do you maintain or plan to maintain your networks?) These included (1) continually attending conferences and seeking out people I have networked with previously (50%); (2) keeping active in my professional organizations (40%); (3) seeking people out when I have a need for information, advice, or support (40%); (4) gathering at social events (10%); (5) engaging in public speaking (10%); and (6) periodically calling people and seeing how they are doing (50%). Individual responses also included sending Christmas cards, frequently dropping a postcard to say hello, writing a note to someone to acknowledge an article that the person has written, and congratulating people on specific accomplishments. All the participants in this survey acknowledged that maintaining networks was extremely important.

BENEFITS OF NETWORKING

The literature is replete with the benefits of networking (Table 19–2). In addition to those listed in Table 19–2 the 20 respondents of the informal survey I conducted articulated the following specific benefits:

- "Making new friends"
- "New ideas about how to use a piece of equipment"
- "Principal expansion of my knowledge base"
- "Gaining new opportunities to publish"
- "Having someone to bounce ideas off!"
- "Incredible peer support during my first year as a CC-CNS"
- "Maintaining a pulse on what's going on in your area"
- "Staying current and competitive"
- "Feeling not so isolated"
- "People are calling me now because I've published and I do not have to seek out my networks—they are seeking me out now"
- "Asking to speak at meetings as a result of referrals by others"
- "Gaining more confidence in my practice"
- "Broader exposure to other people's experience"
- "Expanding my own horizons"
- "Facilitating the mentoring of my staff to also provide them with a network"
- "Invaluable—I can't imagine working in isolation"
- "Have opportunity to get into so many different people's mind"
- "Tremendous support for I'm OK, you're OK!"
- "Don't have to reinvent the wheel"

TABLE 19–2 Benefits of Networking

- Gaining valuable information
- Learning new ways of doing things
- Getting important feedback
- Psychologic support
- Expanding career opportunities
- Establishing a list of resources
- Mentorship
- Opening doors to publishing and speaking
- Impacting policy changes

- "Driven me to become more involved with research"

The following case studies exemplify successful networking strategies.

CASE STUDY 1

KI is a new cardiac surgical CC-CNS who is attending the NTI for the first time. She wants to begin building her external networks. Over the last several months, she developed three objectives as part of her networking strategy: (1) to meet two cardiac surgical CNSs with whom she might start building her horizontal network, (2) to gain insight into case management, and (3) to learn more about the local chapter of AACN.

To achieve the first objective, KI highlighted those talks given by cardiac surgical CNSs and attended them. After each presentation she went up to the speaker, introduced herself, and exchanged business cards. After the NTI she contacted each person by telephone and continued to correspond with those individuals, sharing at times new technologies at her institution as well as gaining new information and other contacts. KI was also able to seek valuable information about case management from the NTI by attending the two presentations on case management given by CNSs currently operationalizing the role. After both lectures KI remained behind to talk to other participants as well as the presenter. In addition, she noted that on Monday night there would be a networking event whereby she could meet other CC-CNSs. She did attend that evening activity and made wonderful contacts with whom she exchanged business cards and gained valuable information regarding case management.

In meeting her third objective, KI noted that there was a chapter resource center at the NTI where participants could find information regarding chapters. KI made a point on Tuesday to go to this room in the convention hall where she was greeted by a national AACN office staff member from the chapters department. She introduced herself and told Peggy (the AACN staff member) that she wanted to join her local chapter but did not know where to begin. Peggy gave her a list of the chapters in her state along with the names and telephone numbers of people to contact. Peggy also told KI that she knew that several chapter presidents were attending this NTI and suggested that KI leave them a message at the message center and perhaps arrange to meet them briefly. KI followed through on this suggestion and met a chapter president at lunch the next day and later joined the chapter nearest her home instead of the one near work. In attending the NTI KI was able to successfully begin her networking activities, which should influence the development of her professional career.

CASE STUDY 2

JS has been a CC-CNS for 10 years and is relocating to a different state for a new position as the coronary care CNS at a large medical center. In anticipation of this move, JS sent 15 letters to key people in his network informing them of his new position and enclosing his new business cards. Moreover, JS joined the local chapter of AACN in his new location and started attending meetings and conferences to expand his network. Once JS was in his new position he made a point of setting up individual lunch meetings with the nurse managers and other CC-CNSs in his department with whom he would be interacting on a regular basis. He also made a point of requesting to join several interdisciplinary committees in his institution to pursue a mixed network of contacts. In being proactive about developing both external and internal networks, JS was able to transition into his new position with relative ease.

SUMMARY

Networking is a dynamic process to be nurtured and maintained. It is the vehicle by which the CC-CNS's career can be advanced and numerous doors may be opened. More importantly, networking has the potential of accessing valuable information that the CC-CNS may use to impact patient care delivery. This outcome is crucial in light of the increasing technologic and scientific advances impacting our practice and the need to keep current.

References

1. Luebbert PP: Networking for survival and success, *Med Lab Observer* 19(6):39-42, 1987.
2. Wake M, Vogel G: Networking: reducing competition while increasing collegiality, *Dimen Crit Care Nurs* 4(3):132-134, 1985.
3. Welch M: *Networking,* New York, 1981, Warner Books.
4. Davidson JP: *Blow your own horn,* New York, 1987, Berkeley Books.
5. O'Connor PB: Ingredients for successful networking, *J Nurs Admin* 12(12):36-40, 1982.
6. Murphy JK: Networking across professional lines, *Pediatr Nurs* 14(2):133-134, 1988.
7. Harkavy LM: Coalition building and networking, *Am J Infect Control* 75(3):23A-25A, 1987.
8. Dossey B: Networking made easy, *Nurs 1987* 17(5):161-162, 1987.
9. Novak A: *Keynote address. Annual Conference on Continuing Education in Nursing,* Washington, DC, 1981, American Nurses' Association Council on Continuing Education.

Chapter 20

Career Opportunities for the Critical Care Clinical Nurse Specialist

Tess L. Briones, RN, MS, CCRN
J. Keith Hampton, RN, MSN, CS

The clinical nurse specialist (CNS) role has been described by Stevens[1] as the movement in nursing that "has contributed so much, so rapidly, to attempt to professionalize nursing and to substantiate its existence as an independent profession." The CNS role has existed for almost 50 years now. The primary purpose of this "nurse clinician," described by Reitner[2] in 1943, was to be the use of discriminative judgment and intellectual capabilities to bring about the highest quality of nursing care. Forces that led to the development of CNS roles were the knowledge explosion, technologic advancements, and an increasingly complex health care system.

Many experienced CNSs within nursing, and specifically within critical care nursing, have achieved the level of discriminate judgment envisioned by Reitner and are perhaps ready for a change or ready to move beyond an advanced-practice clinician role. What are the characteristics of the mature critical care CNS (CC-CNS)? What are the stepping-stones to self-actualization for the CC-CNS? What career options are CC-CNSs considering once they have achieved their goals as advanced clinicians? These are some of the questions this chapter will address.

THEORETIC FRAMEWORK
CNS Role Maturity

According to Mayo[3] CNSs are expert practitioners, because they have a broader knowledge base,

deeper insights and appreciations, and greater skills than those that can be acquired in a basic nursing course. By virtue of these characteristics, CNSs are then better able to analyze, explore, and cope with nursing situations for a specific clinical field and contribute to the improvement of service to patients.

The concepts essential to a model of advanced practice are *clinical judgement* and *leadership*. Although clinical judgment is exercised by all nurses when they make decisions about patient care, CNSs are expected to demonstrate an advanced level of clinical judgment.[4] Spross and Hamric[5] believe this advanced level of judgment becomes particularly apparent when CNSs care for patients with complex physiologic and psychosocial problems. Because of the interaction and integration of graduate education in nursing practice and years of clinical experience, the CNS is able to exercise a level of discrimination that is unavailable to other experienced clinicians. These experienced CNSs can be described as having attained a form of maturity in a work role.

In Chapter 3 of this book, Klein describes several models of CNS role development and the characteristics of the mature CNS. The concept that role development occurs in sequential phases has been examined within nursing and within the CNS role.[6]

Oda et al.'s description[7] of role maturity is especially enlightening. The determinants of role maturity described by Oda et al. are proficiency, position, recognition, and reciprocity. *Proficiency* refers to competence in the CNS functional areas of clinical practice, education, consultation, and research. The hallmarks of proficiency in the CC-CNS are confidence in solving patient care issues either with the nursing staff or other disciplines, in-depth knowledge of pathophysiology of disease states (especially in the field of specialization), in-depth knowledge of information technology in the critical care environment, and implementation of theory-based and research-based nursing practice. *Position* refers to the movement of the CNS up the organizational ladder. Some CNSs have even reached the top of the organizational ladder. After time within the CNS role and interchange of experiences, a CNS is accorded *recognition* as an expert by peers and health care colleagues. Finally, this level of professional functioning is characterized by consistent *reciprocity,* that is, interpersonal exchanges of expertise with colleagues in patient care. What keeps CC-CNSs who have achieved this level of role maturity challenged and growing? What are other options for career advancement?

Career Opportunities for the Mature CC-CNS

The CC-CNS who has reached role maturity is a highly skilled and valuable individual with a number of highly marketable skills as well as in-depth knowledge of her or his specialty. Although these attributes seem obvious, CC-CNSs may not think of themselves as a commodity and therefore may fail to see the endless possibilities for advancement available within and outside their position.

Change away from the bedside is not necessary for continuous growth in the CC-CNS role. The CC-CNS can feel continuously challenged in the role and current position. Within the unit-based role, the mature CC-CNS has a number of role development options: (1) mentoring of graduate students and novice CNSs; (2) coordination of new projects within the unit or institution; (3) sabbatical from role responsibilities, for example, differentiated practice models; (4) focusing on a primary research role; (5) mentoring of a nurse fellow who could benefit from the guidance of the CC-CNS as well as work collaboratively with the CC-CNS on a research project of mutual interest; and (6) job sharing a full-time position with another CC-CNS.

For the CC-CNS who is ready for a change in position, the following possibilities exist: (1) movement into an administrator or nurse manager position; (2) a change to a joint faculty position in a school of nursing; (3) returning to school to pursue a doctorate degree or another nonnursing degree; or (4) a change to a position with a non–health care organization, such as a research specialist or educator for private industry.

RELATED RESEARCH AND LITERATURE

The unique aspect of a CNS position is its versatility and flexibility. Because of this, the advanced CC-CNS who has reached role maturity can easily take advantage of other career opportunities available. However, in changing jobs or areas of specialization, the experienced CC-CNS must allow time for adaptation to the new role. Time frames for developing expertise in the new role and experiencing some degree of success are individualized, but 1 or 2 years seem plausible.[7]

Anyone entering a new and complex role experiences a process of role development before being able to function with maximum effectiveness. It has been documented, however, that experienced CNSs who move to another position are able to advance in the role development phases more rapidly than those who are inexperienced.[8] According to experienced CNSs, their self-confidence and independence made movement through the phases of role development in their new role faster and more fluid. We believe that the mature CC-CNS's interpersonal and problem-solving skills support successful movement into any new role.

PRACTICE IMPLICATIONS

A sizeable percentage of CC-CNSs are reaching or have reached the top of their employment ladder.[7] Once role maturity is reached, strategies for role enhancement may prove beneficial for CC-CNS retention. According to Oda et al.,[7] examples of such strategies are providing creative challenges, sabbaticals for renewal, and monetary recognition of clinical excellence. The career opportunities mentioned above are elucidated in this section. The focus of this discussion is on the process of changing roles: How does one prepare for such a change? What questions need to be asked when making a change? Where does one find these positions? What are the advantages and disadvantages of different career options?

Mentoring Nursing Graduate Students and Novice CNSs

An opportunity for growth for experienced CC-CNSs is to serve as mentor both to novice CNSs or CNS graduate students (see also Chapters 3 and 10). Mentoring is an important concept that can be used in the evolutionary development of the effective CC-CNS. Mentoring involves the modeling of another CC-CNS in a specified environment through observation, orientation, and communication.[9]

Guidance and encouragement by the experienced and effective CC-CNS are valuable aids in the development of the graduate student CNS and the novice CNS. The university faculty member assigns a student to a selected, advanced-practice nurse in a specific clinical agency who serves as the preceptor or mentor. The preceptor guides the student through the necessary experiences that provide learning opportunities. Objectives and role expectations of both the mentor and student are identified before the beginning of the relationship. The CC-CNS should be aware of the exact amount of time being committed, including the number of days per week as well as the number of weeks the graduate student will be in the facility.

Mentoring the novice CC-CNS is unlike orienting or being a preceptor, because it is an active process that involves guidance, direction, sharing, and nurturing by one who is more experienced. Mentoring the novice CC-CNS may be seen as one way in which to ensure continuity and to pass on to the next generation of CC-CNSs a particular brand of leadership[10] or philosophy held by the mature CC-CNS.

There are several advantages to being a mentor. The mutuality of the mentoring experience enhances the self-concept and self-esteem of the mentor, which further supports the mentor's sense of competence and ability. The student or novice CNS may bring new knowledge and technologic advances as well as new and unbiased perceptions of the roles to further enhance the growth and development of the mentor. Through mutual sharing of wisdom and experience, there is growth of both mentor and student, thereby enhancing their self-worth, professional productivity, and value to the

organizational structure. Successful mentoring can be a highly productive, cost-effective way to increase performance levels, develop leadership skills, improve morale, and increase self-esteem and value of both the mentor and student or novice CNS.

CC-CNS as Director of Special Programs or Projects

Many changes in health care delivery systems today require an organized approach that will be least interruptive to organizational operations. The use of a program manager to implement a specific organizational change has several advantages. This approach obtains maximum input from everyone affected by the project while meeting project objectives in a timely manner. At the same time the organization is flattened and communication promoted through all levels of personnel. The program manager requires excellent interpersonal skills and an ability to work with people from all professional levels. The CC-CNS has been viewed as an ideal person to oversee such a program. Ryan-Merritt et al.[11] note that resourcefulness is a quality of most CNSs and that their extensive knowledge of the structure and content of the health care delivery systems contributes to their ability to promote organizational change. The most important characteristic that the CC-CNS brings to this role as a change agent is to help the project team and staff through the change process (see also Chapter 16).

The CC-CNS as director of program development is a recent addition to nursing. The director of special projects requires management skills in addition to CC-CNS skills. To assume this leadership role, the CC-CNS needs to consider developing skills in interactive leadership, resource allocation, marketing, negotiations, conflict resolution, and personnel management. This experience is advantageous for the CC-CNS who wishes to gain leadership experience before moving to a purely management position. Project director positions are available in most institutions and may present many options, including but not limited to coordinator of wound healing program, director of professional nursing services (including nursing research and quality assessment and improvement activities), trauma services coordinator, liver transplant program coordinator, and patient care delivery system coordinator. These positions allow the

CC-CNS to work in a specialized area with a very specific scope of responsibility.

The task, however, does not end once the change is implemented. The program manager needs to ensure the continuation of the project. It is during this period that the program manager assumes the majority of the responsibility in directing the program, since the team may no longer be necessary after the active part of the implementation process.

The CC-CNS contemplating taking the role of director of special projects should be prepared to ask these questions: What is the goal of the program in relation to patient care delivery? What kind of organizational support is available for the program? Who are the key people involved in the program? What kind of funding is available to carry out the program? And most importantly, what will happen to the CC-CNS position after the program is self-sufficient? The success of this career option can be evaluated by how well the CC-CNS in this position kept the program moving to full implementation and on target. How was conflict handled during program implementation? Ultimate success can be measured once the program is self-sufficient.

CC-CNS Sabbatical from Role Responsibilities

An innovative way for the mature CC-CNS to break from the routine of clinical practice is to take a paid sabbatical to work on a project that will benefit the institution and is of personal interest. Institutions that value their senior nursing staff are increasingly looking to this option as a way of rewarding an individual's long-standing contributions to the organization.

Sabbatical time can range from a few weeks to a few months, depending on how the CC-CNS wishes to use the time. Examples of projects that the CC-CNS may want to engage in include the following: professional writing, review and critique of the literature on an area of interest, a fellowship in another institution with a mentor, preparation of a research proposal, data collection for a research study, conduct of a national survey on a questioned practice in nursing, working in a clinic with a physician to improve physical assessment skills, working with a cardiologist to improve electrocardiogram (EKG) interpretation skills, and enrollment in educational programs. Few CC-CNSs would turn away an opportunity to pursue any one of these professional development options.

In considering this career option, the CC-CNS must come prepared with a specific proposal for how the time will be spent. Outcomes of the sabbatical are discussed in advance. The CC-CNS must also make plans for coverage of role responsibilities during the sabbatical. Who will make daily and weekly rounds? Who will take care of patients and families with special needs? Who will coordinate the new staff orientation? Who will cover teaching responsibilities?

One option is for the CC-CNS to prepare a senior staff nurse for coverage responsibilities. The CC-CNS could negotiate for the senior staff nurse to have 1 or 2 days per week to fulfill CNS responsibilities without a patient assignment. Although this may seem an almost impossible task in this era of cost containment, it is much less expensive to support a CC-CNS sabbatical than to hire and orient a new CC-CNS, particularly when it would probably be at least 2 years before the new person is able to make the kind of impact a mature CC-CNS can make.

CC-CNS in Research-Focused Role

CC-CNSs are expected to participate in research to use their education and clinical expertise to generate new knowledge ameliorating the profession. Nevertheless, for a variety of reasons the research component of the CC-CNS role has been slow to develop. The CC-CNS is in a position to encounter nursing problems that lend themselves to systematic study and therefore is the ideal person to study such problems. In addition, the recognition and reciprocity the CC-CNS has developed with physician and nonphysician colleagues are the ideal foundation for building a collaborative research program.

The characteristics and qualities needed in the nurse researcher role include the ability to critique the existing body of scientific literature and to synthesize information obtained from this critique. Additional qualities that the nurse researcher should possess are the ability to write research grants and knowledge of the different grant supports available. CC-CNSs without this knowledge can find a mentor from a school of nursing or a private agency who has a track record of obtaining grants. Another way to prepare for this role is to take courses in research design and grant writing.

Positions for pure nurse researchers are less

available and usually require doctoral preparation. However, this role is often found in large university-affiliated medical centers. In some cases the nurse researcher role may be integrated within a broad administrative title such as director of education or quality improvement.

The unit-based CC-CNS who is interested in expanding her or his current clinical role into a researcher role has two options: (1) gradual transition to a research-focused CNS role or (2) a formal change to a nurse researcher position with no responsibility for the other CNS role components. For the CC-CNS to take on a primary researcher role, other role responsibilities must be delegated to senior nursing staff. This delegation is one of transferring educational and other responsibilities to staff members who have demonstrated the ability to carry out some CNS responsibilities. The CC-CNS remains ultimately accountable for the quality of delegated responsibilities.

To move into a research-focused role, the CC-CNS must begin by developing a role change proposal. This proposal would outline the rationale for a role change, the new job responsibilities, and planning for how other role components (educator, practitioner, consultant, leader or manager) would be covered or how they would be incorporated into the new position focus. Important in this proposal would be a discussion on how the institution would benefit from this role change; for example, would the researcher bring grant money into the institution, what would be the cost benefits of this role, how would the CC-CNS's research activities improve patient care, would there be cost savings in patient care because of this role, and how would the nursing staff benefit?

In the early stages of proposal development, the CC-CNS should work closely with the nurse manager and unit director to ensure their support in the change. These individuals can help the CC-CNS evaluate the timing of such a change and can make recommendations for how to best present the proposal.

One of the reasons for the slow development of the research role component is that the accepted educational preparation for the CNS usually consists of only one or two research courses. Consequently, CNSs may not be academically prepared for the role of clinical researcher. Current debate focuses on the researcher role expectations, with some feeling that CNSs are only prepared to be consumers of research. Master's level statistics and research courses only provide a fundamental understanding of important conceptual and mathematic dynamics. How then does the CC-CNS obtain the knowledge and skill to assume a research-focused role?

One proposed solution is for the CC-CNS to collaborate with nurse scientists in research efforts. The advantages of such an approach for the CC-CNS are the following: (1) potential for access to resources not usually available to the CC-CNS, (2) opportunities for additional education regarding the research process, and (3) opportunities to network with other scientists who share a mutual area of interest. For the scientist who works with the CC-CNS, there are the advantages of having a clinical setting available, the CC-CNS's clinical expertise, which can be used when identifying variables that may impact results, and the opportunity to stay informed of new knowledge within the clinical setting. This model allows for a mutually beneficial marriage of practice and education. The CC-CNS has only to pursue this avenue to develop research knowledge.

The emphasis on research as a CC-CNS holds promise of great personal and professional satisfaction. The difficulty lies in the ability to secure support for this role given the current limitations on funding for new hospital positions.

Mentoring a Nursing Fellow in Critical Care

A career development option that has not been described in the literature is the CC-CNS's taking on another master's-prepared, novice CNS as a fellow in nursing. A fellow is a new CNS who has had little or no experience in the role and who works with the mature CC-CNS for 6 to 12 months to learn from the mature CC-CNS and obtain experience in the role. The fellowship is akin to nurse internships for new graduate nurses. On completion of the year, the fellow moves on to take a permanent position as a CC-CNS.

The benefits of this relationship for the mature CC-CNS are the following: (1) the mature CC-CNS has an opportunity to pass on personal philosophy and experience surrounding the role; (2) the fellow is able to take on many of the mentor's role responsibilities, freeing the mentor to develop professionally and pursue other interests; and (3) the fellow is able to assist the mentor with special projects that require assistance, such as clinical research data collection.

This model was tried by a mature cardiothoracic surgery CNS (CTS-CNS) at a university medical center. A proposal for the position was submitted to the director of nursing for the institution. The individual who was recommended for the fellowship was a cardiac surgery intensive care unit (ICU) nurse who had recently completed a master's program in nursing. This nurse was a senior nurse in the cardiovascular ICU who had demonstrated excellent clinical skills and good communication skills and was recognized as a leader in this unit. The CTS-CNS, who had been with the hospital for 8 years, needed assistance to implement some new programs for the staff in the cardiovascular ICU. In addition, she and the nurse manager had recently received a grant to conduct a research study with the cardiovascular ICU patients.

The CTS-CNS met with the director of nursing to discuss the fellowship position. In this meeting the CTS-CNS emphasized to the nursing director that this would be a way of rewarding the staff nurse for her loyalty to the institution as well as enable the mature CNS to complete some programs that would benefit the staff. The director of nursing was reluctant at first because of the cost (the salary for the fellow for the year). A research grant had been obtained by the CTS-CNS that could pay for part of the fellow's salary as a research assistant. The CC-CNS also obtained support from the unit medical director who could see the benefits of such a role. When the nurse manager and CTS-CNS figured the cost benefits of the program as a retention strategy and presented partial payment of the role by the grant, the position was approved. The fellow worked for 1 year with the CTS-CNS. A formal evaluation of the fellowship role using written questionnaires was conducted by the CTS-CNS. Survey results revealed that the fellow had made a positive impact on patient and staff nurse satisfaction. At the completion of a very successful year, the new CNS was hired by the department of surgery to work directly with the heart surgery patients.

Job Sharing the CC-CNS Role

Job sharing, a nontraditional work option supported in the business literature, is a viable alter-native for the CC-CNS who needs scheduling flexibility. Job sharing refers to a voluntary work arrangement in which two people are responsible for what was formerly one full-time position, dividing the hours, responsibilities, and benefits. Although successful job sharing has been well documented in other professions, it has received little attention within nursing. Job-sharing positions are rare and are usually created on an individual basis. Once a decision has been made to pursue this option, the job-sharing partner has to be approached and after a mutually acceptable proposition is reached, a proposal must be written and presented to an administrator. The proposal must include the suggested salary, number of hours worked, coverage for each other, benefits, committee participation, each CC-CNS's responsibilities, and the strengths and weaknesses of implementing job sharing. The importance of being thoroughly prepared to answer all arguments cannot be overemphasized when presenting a proposal.

Several advantages and disadvantages exist for both the employer and employee in a job-sharing situation. Increased scheduling flexibility is the most important aspect of job sharing for the employee and may result in a more effective use of employees' time to meet the needs of the position. Decreased turnover and increased productivity are among the other benefits observed among job sharers. The reduction in turnover may be due to the voluntary nature of the sharing. Productivity increases because of a desire to show appreciation for this unique opportunity and because morale is higher in a job that conforms to the employee's specific needs. Increased creativity and generation of ideas are other positive outcomes of job sharing. Last, reduced expenses are often cited as an advantage of job sharing in the areas of orientation and overtime, especially among nonsalaried employees.

The problems that job sharers frequently encounter are lack of continuity, supervision, and accountability. Communication or lack of it can make or break the job-sharing position. Because continuity and follow-up can be disrupted as a result of poor communication, personality conflicts and scheduling arrangements that hamper communication cannot be tolerated in this situation.

Several professional, personal, and situational factors affect the success of a job-sharing position.

Working with someone whose philosophy on patient care issues and professional nursing issues is similar to one's own is very important. Several factors need to be considered to ensure success of the job-sharing position. Compatibility begins during the selection of the job-sharing partner and continues as team building progresses, as evidenced by interactions when the job-sharing partners are together as well as alone on the job. It is important to walk through the steps of examining yourselves as a pair, identifying your strengths and weaknesses, and meshing these components with the job. Cooperation addresses the practicality of developing a work schedule that fits both partners. For continuity some job sharers arrange to have lunch together one day each week or work together one day each week, and essential meetings may be attended by both partners. Others have tried tape-recorded, daily reports to one another and have found these helpful. A communication book is another technique. It is also important to be able to fill in for each other when necessary so a loss of continuity will not be experienced by patients, staff, or administrators. This type of cooperation requires excellent communication skills and personal responsibility. A daily journal highlighting urgent items can be an integral component of the communication system. Daily telephone calls should be the norm, especially during the initial phase of job sharing.

Regardless of the problems that a job-sharing position has, the advantages still outweigh the disadvantages, especially for CC-CNSs who need a flexible work schedule such as those pursuing doctoral studies. In summary, compatible, flexible partners; awareness of the advantages and disadvantages of job sharing; and administrative support comprise integral components of successful job sharing. Job sharers should also have two evaluations: one addressing the individual's performance and the other evaluating the effectiveness of the team in meeting job responsibilities within the job description.

CC-CNS Who Becomes an Administrator/Nurse Manager

The abilities of the CC-CNS to function in a changing environment and to understand the dynamics of complex organizations are two important characteristics that can be used by CC-CNSs to sell themselves in applying for a management position. However, for the CC-CNS who is interested in entering the management track, the ideally suited beginning position is that of a nurse manager. First-line management positions come with certain regularity in every institution. This position builds on the experience and education of the CC-CNS, and as a nurse manager the CC-CNS will be responsible for the daily operations of a limited part of a larger organization. During this time the CC-CNS can also learn about fiscal responsibilities, legal matters, and political savvy. Other skills that a CC-CNS lacks to function efficiently in a management position are budgeting essentials, staffing and scheduling strategies, capital equipment management, and employer-employee relationships, especially in a collective bargaining environment. To prepare for this position the CC-CNS can attend leadership/management workshops within the institution and attend national meetings with sessions directed to managers (e.g., NTI, Leadership Forum). Books or references that may be helpful for the CC-CNS are those that discuss characteristics of a good leader or manager.[14]

The career opportunities present in nursing administration offer CC-CNSs the possibility to lead, direct, and impact the efforts of a clinical program or department. The role of the nurse manager is a dynamic one requiring a high degree of leadership skill and managerial competence intricately linked with clinical nursing knowledge and research.[14] The combination of a strong clinical base and sound educational preparation in leadership behaviors positions the CC-CNS in line for specific roles in formal nursing leadership. The CC-CNS who assumes a management position must integrate both practice and management components and must be comfortable and confident in doing so.

In an administrative position the CC-CNS will be able to execute other unspoken subroles.[8] We are well aware of the classic subroles of the CC-CNS—expert practitioner, educator, researcher, consultant, and leader—that exemplify how CC-CNSs practice on a day-to-day basis. Critical to the CC-CNS's success in actualizing these subroles are proficiency and sensitivity to the importance of being a role model, leader, change agent, and advocate for patients, families, and staff.

CC-CNS as Entrepreneur: Establishing a Business

There are several examples in the literature of CNSs who have moved out of a hospital-based role to establish a business that is built on CNS skills and expertise.[15] CNS-initiated businesses have offered such services as cardiopulmonary resuscitation (CPR) courses for large corporations, consultation for emergency room staff members on how to manage psychiatric emergencies, specialty-based educational programming for hospitals without CNSs, classes on trauma patient management for fire department personnel, and consultation on implementation of new patient care delivery systems.[13]

Becoming a nurse entrepreneur requires significant self-motivation, risk taking, and an ability to cope with an uncertain future. CC-CNSs who are considering this type of career change should perform a self-assessment, using one of the many instruments available.[13] These self-assessment tools will help an individual decide if being an entrepreneur is a viable career option. As these self-assessment tools demonstrate, not everyone has the personality to be an entrepreneur. Vogel and Doleysh[13] describe the characteristics of the entrepreneurial personality as follows: willingness to take moderate risks, self-confidence and an internal locus of control, determination and perseverance, interpersonal skills, low need for status, a need for achievement, a need to control and direct, and physical and mental resilience.

An entrepreneurial role offers several advantages: (1) work schedule independence, (2) total autonomy for how the work role is structured, (3) opportunities for improved income, (4) potential for enhanced self-confidence and self-esteem, and (5) new opportunities for application of problem-solving and leadership skills. Entrepreneurship, while not for every nurse, gives nurses a choice and creates new opportunities for autonomy, independence, and professional fulfillment.

CC-CNS as Faculty Member in a Joint Appointment Position

Another opportunity for growth for the experienced CNS is available in the academic setting. Functioning as a preceptor to undergraduate and graduate students and negotiating and balancing the demands of a joint or dual appointment are of interest to many CC-CNSs. The CC-CNS in this role is able to serve as a bridge between the clinical setting and academia. Over the years the camps of nursing education and nursing service have developed into very distant groups. Practitioners at the bedside think that nurses in academia live in an ivory tower and that students are taught ideal situations. Likewise, nurses in academia have limited communications with practitioners because of teaching responsibilities and research expectations. These situations result in limited access to the academic setting by practitioners and difficulty in conducting clinical research by academicians. The CC-CNS in a joint appointment position can bridge the gap between service and education.

A CC-CNS seeking a career opportunity as a faculty member needs answers to several questions. How will the joint or dual appointment role be accomplished? What are the expectations from both service and education for the person in this role? What percentage appointment will the CC-CNS commit to? How will the position be funded? What kind of organizational support will the person in this role have in carrying out the joint appointment position?

A joint appointment position can be salaried or nonsalaried (adjunct appointment) in the school of nursing. The nonsalaried faculty appointment or adjunct appointment is fully funded by the service institution and generally requires a minimum number of hours yearly that the CC-CNS contributes in the way of lectures, preceptorships, consultations, or thesis committee participation. An adjunct appointment permits the CC-CNS to incorporate the contributions of this role into daily patient-related activities, maximizing time utilization and role efficiency.

A salaried joint appointment may be the preferable alternative for personal or professional reasons. Although a salaried joint appointment may allow the CC-CNS to work toward seniority in the academic ranks, the main disadvantage of such an arrangement is that rarely does a part-time appointment remain part-time. The time spent in responding to patient needs competes with academic requirements, and the CC-CNS with salaried joint appointments will find that either two part-time positions have developed into two full-time needs or that a sense of dissatisfaction pervades because of doing neither job well.

In seeking the career opportunity as a faculty member, the CC-CNS must be very clear as to how the obligations attached to the CC-CNS role will be met and maintained in the light of the academic appointment. Clarifying the multiple responsibilities and activities involved in a joint appointment position must be a continuing effort since activities and time involvements may shift over the course of months. As educational commitments shift during an academic year, the CC-CNS may have more or less time for practice. Shoring up these expectations will enable the success of both roles.

Often joint appointment positions appear regularly within schools of nursing and are available in university-affiliated settings.[15] To take on this role the CC-CNS must be well versed in educational methodology, curriculum design and development, teaching strategies, test construction, and student evaluation methods. To prepare for this role the CC-CNS can attend workshops on the above mentioned subjects.

In the implementation of the joint appointment role the CC-CNS may need to post a weekly schedule (or monthly as appropriate) in both the clinical area and faculty office where clinical staff and faculty colleagues can see it. All regular meetings and activities should be reflected, including contact time with students (teaching, advising, office hours), class time, clinical practice, and lecture preparation time. This simple strategy may prevent others from thinking that the CC-CNS is not working when not in the clinical area or not visibly teaching. Another important factor in implementing the joint appointment role is to have a structured mechanism to facilitate student education and evaluation of the effectiveness of the education. CC-CNSs who stay in joint appointment roles have learned to make reasonable expectations of themselves and are able to identify sources of support. In addition, they have learned to deal with the ambiguity and frustration that occasionally come with the position. Last, CC-CNSs who have managed this dual responsibility recognize the unique pressures of time, feelings of split allegiances between nursing service and nursing education, and the challenges of dual responsibility.

CC-CNS as Doctoral Student

Nursing needs nurses with doctorates in nursing, education, and related disciplines, because it is only through doctoral education that a nurse can attain the breadth of background necessary to contribute to nursing science.[14] Making the decision to pursue doctoral studies is not an easy one for the practicing CC-CNS. Unfortunately 80% of the 5000 doctorally prepared nurses are in faculty positions.[16] However, a new breed of nurse scientists is emerging. CNSs are beginning to obtain doctoral degrees and return to the practice setting. This concept (role) of the doctorally prepared CNS is the major force that will bridge the gap between practice and research. The "single most important product of clinical research is the potential benefit it offers to clients."[17] Doctorally prepared CC-CNSs would bring much to the practice area. By maintaining a practice base, the CC-CNS would provide expert care to a select group of critically ill patients who would benefit from the additional knowledge the CC-CNS has gained through doctoral education.

The CC-CNS who plans to pursue doctoral education should evaluate programs for those that match the CC-CNS's interests and career goals. Downs[14] noted the importance of being clear about one's goals and aspirations in doctoral study.

Two doctoral programs existed in the United States in 1946.[15] Since then several programs have been initiated, and now there are nearly 50 programs in the United States.[18] Doctoral programs prepare nurses to be theoreticians, scholars, researchers, and teachers, but first and foremost, nurses with doctoral preparation are researchers. The three types of doctoral degrees offered in nursing are doctor of philosophy (PhD), doctor of nursing science (DNS), and doctor in education (EdD).

Finding a doctoral program that will foster one's professional development is the next step after deciding to pursue doctoral study. Information about available doctoral programs that can meet your goals comes from a variety of sources. Advisors and mentors are potential sources of information about doctoral programs. Networking at scientific meetings and well-attended conferences is also a potential source of information.

In choosing a program the CC-CNS must be aware of the following: time commitments, administrative support, financial support, acceptance or support by family members or social structure, quality of the program, personal goals, and to some extent geographic area. The CC-CNS must go through the following thought process to determine the timing of doctoral studies: What will happen with my current position while I return to school? Will I need to work part-time? Will the institution allow me to work part-time? What resources or opportunities exist to facilitate going back to school? Is financial support available?

Doctoral study generally requires some financial sacrifice. However, funding may be available through agencies such as the National Center for Nursing Research, National Institutes of Health, the Kellogg Foundation, and other specialty nursing organizations. Within the university information may be obtained regarding grants for career women and minority groups and individual National Research Service Awards (NRSAs). Individual NRSAs are usually available to registered nurses for research training leading to a doctoral degree.

In preparing for a doctoral program the CC-CNS must first identify her or his specific area of interest and goals for obtaining this advanced education. For example, the CC-CNS may decide she or he has a special interest in the healing process and wound management and has the professional goal of conducting clinical nursing research on wound healing. Once the area of study is identified, the CC-CNS then looks to different programs with faculty members who have a research background in the CNS's area of research. The CC-CNS may then investigate to see if there is a mentor with whom she could work.

Mentoring is the key ingredient in a successful doctoral study. The ideal mentorship starts with a conceptually sound, practicing researcher who is willing to share relevant issues and activities on a daily basis. The mentor must be an individual who the CC-CNS trusts and respects. This relationship will be the one that sees the CC-CNS through doctoral studies and one that will probably stay with the CC-CNS throughout her or his career. Although this creates an ideal match between the research interest of the CC-CNS and faculty, relocating oneself for doctoral studies may not be feasible because of costs, financial considerations, or family needs.

Despite the disadvantages, doctoral study has as its greatest advantage the development of productive researchers in nursing, which in turn is essential to the furthering of the goals of nursing science. A doctoral degree is a step toward achieving the high level of scientific productivity required to influence the future of nursing practice.

Career Change to Nonhospital Environment

A final career pathway the CC-CNS may consider is the movement into a nonhospital, corporate environment. Positions are available within the health care industry that require the skills of the CC-CNS. Examples of such positions are educational specialist for a product manufacturer, research specialist for a product manufacturer, consultant to health care management firms, consultant to insurance carriers and health maintenance organizations, and education and research specialist positions within nursing organizations (e.g., American Association of Critical Care Nurses). These positions offer a new perspective of the health care industry and provide an opportunity for the CC-CNS to broaden professional networks and experiences. The challenge for the CC-CNS who choses this type of position is to to keep abreast of changes in her or his area of specialization.

SUMMARY

A recurring theme within this book is the diversity within the CC-CNS role and the unique contributions of this individual. Institutions wishing to retain such a highly skilled and valuable person must be open to meeting the continued needs for mature CC-CNSs' career development. This chapter has provided several options for career enhancement within this role. In addition, this chapter outlines several career options for the mature CC-CNS who seeks an entirely new career but one that builds on CC-CNS skills. Limitless opportunities for career change are open to the CC-CNS.

References

1. Stevens BJ: Accountability of the clinical nurse specialist: the administrator's viewpoint, *J Nurs Admin* 6:30-32, 1976.
2. Reitner F: The nurse clinician, *Am J Nurs* 66:274-280, 1966.
3. Mayo A: Advanced courses in clinical nursing: a discussion of basic assumptions and guiding principles, *Am J Nurs* 44:579-585, 1944.
4. Benner P, Tanner C: Clinical judgment: how expert nurses use intuition, *Am J Nurs* 87:23-31, 1987.

5. Spross JA, Hamric AB: *The clinical nurse specialist in theory and practice,* ed 2, New York, 1989, Grune & Stratton.

6. Stetler CB, DiMaggio G: Research utilization among clinical nurse specialists, *Clin Nurse Specialist* 5:151-155, 1991.

7. Oda DS, Sparacino PA, Boyd P: Role advancement for the experienced clinical nurse specialist, *Clin Nurse Specialist* 2:167-171, 1988.

8. McCaffrey D: The unspoken subroles of the clinical nurse specialist, *Clin Nurse Specialist* 5:71-72, 1991.

9. Redland AR: Mentors and preceptors as models for professional development, *Clin Nurse Specialist* 3:70, 1989.

10. Caine RM: Mentoring the novice clinical nurse specialist, *Clin Nurse Specialist* 3:76-78, 1989.

11. Ryan-Merritt MV, Mitchell CA, Pagel I: Clinical nurse specialist role definition and operationalization, *Clin Nurse Specialist* 2:132-137, 1988.

12. Cardin S, Ward C: *Personnel management in critical care nursing,* Baltimore, 1989, Williams & Wilkins Co.

13. Vogel G, Doleysh N: *Entrepreneuring: a nurse's guide to starting a business,* New York, 1988, National League for Nursing.

14. Downs FS: Doctoral education: our claim to the future, *Nurs Outlook* 36:18-20, 1988.

15. American Association of Colleges of Nursing: *Essentials of college and university education for professional nursing,* Washington, DC, 1986, The Association.

16. U.S. Department of Health and Human Services: *Seventh report to the president and congress on the status of health personnel in the United States,* Rockville, Md, 1990, The Department.

17. Hickey M: The role of the clinical nurse specialist in the research utilization process, *Clin Nurse Specialist* 4(2):93-96, 1990.

18. Allen JC: *Consumer's guide to doctoral degree programs in nursing,* New York, 1990, National League for Nursing.

Chapter 21

Role Evaluation for the Critical Care Clinical Nurse Specialist

Marita G. Titler, RN, PhD
Karen M. Stenger, RN, MA, CCRN

Job performance evaluation is an essential component of critical care practice, particularly for the critical care clinical nurse specialist (CC-CNS). It is much more than the traditional subjective and ambiguous annual review that is periodically required by the organization; it is the critical analysis by self or others of how effective the CC-CNS is in meeting the expectations of the position. Evaluating job performance facilitates articulation and documentation of the value, purpose, and expectations of the role by the CC-CNS and nurse executive.[1,2] This chapter describes the theoretic perspective and practical components of CNS evaluation.

THEORETIC PERSPECTIVE

Evaluating one's role performance provides an opportunity to assess important aspects of the job, stimulate professional growth, document effectiveness, forecast practice and administrative trends, identify areas for improvement, and enhance collaboration with other members of the health care team. Through this process, the CC-CNS is able to point out how CC-CNS activities interface with the strategic plan of the department and help achieve the mission of the organization. Evaluating role performance also provides an opportunity to clarify priorities, negotiate role expectations, and determine potential salary adjustments or promotions.[1-3] Evaluation should begin when the CC-CNS interviews for the position and requests the job description and evaluation criteria. Clarifying job description and performance criteria before being hired into a position is essential to find the right fit between the organization and CC-CNS. Ongoing development and revision of job performance criteria are best done with the person to whom the CC-CNS is accountable, while negotiating for realistic measures and time frames for goal achievement.[2,4,5]

Theoretic Frameworks for CNS Evaluation

Several frameworks for CNS evaluation are described in the literature.[6-9] These frameworks have been used in varying degrees in critical care practice, but little empiric evidence is available to determine which are effective in evaluating job performance of CC-CNSs.

Functional Role Theory

The functional approach[8] is widely used and based on functionalist theory. According to the functionalist view, the CC-CNS role meets a socially conceived demand. The society in turn establishes norms or demands about the activities that should occur within the role. Roles evolve over time as the society or group determines the need for role development or change. In the functionalist perspective, certain expectations or competences are set by the employing organization or specialty.[10]

The American Association of Critical Care Nurses (AACN) competences reflect functional role theory with competence statements in each of the five functional role components: clinical, management, education, research, and consultation[11] (see Chapter 1). Evaluation criteria with measurable behaviors can be developed for each of these functional components using the competence statements as a guide. For example, evaluation of the clinical component includes actions that describe the CC-CNS as an advanced practitioner. Measurable process behaviors that a CC-CNS can use for this competence statement include (1) holding hemodynamic rounds weekly, (2) providing care for a patient with sepsis two times per month, (3) leading grand rounds on sepsis twice each year, (4) developing a multidisciplinary critical path for septic patients, and (5) leading a support group twice each week for families of critically ill patients. Measurable outcomes of these CNS activities would include (1) a 10% decrease in the variability of hemodynamic readings across shifts, (2) a 5% decrease in the mortality of septic patients, (3) a 24-hour decrease in length of intensive care unit (ICU) stay of septic patients, and (4) a 20% increase in patient and family satisfaction ratings regarding care.

Similar behaviors can be articulated for the other competences.[12] The types of behaviors selected will depend on the expertise of the CC-CNS, the values and goals of the organization, and the expectations of the employer. "The differences between CNSs functioning at different levels of role development are in the degree and sophistication with which these competences are met."[11] Table 21–1 outlines examples of first- and five-year competences.

Symbolic Interactionist Theory

The symbolic interactionist approach[10] to evaluation is based on the individual rather than society determining which activities have relevance for the role. In this case the CC-CNS has control in delineating activities and associated behaviors she or he views as important to the role. When using this framework, the CC-CNS is in tune to interpersonal interactions with others in the environment such as

TABLE 21–1 Examples of First-Year and Five-Year Competences for CC-CNS by Functional Component

Functional Components	First Year	Five Year
Clinical	Serves as role model for advanced nursing practice Demonstrates clinical expertise in problem-solving skills based on theoretical knowledge, expertise, and sound judgment	Serves as resource for nurses at all levels and for other health care providers for advanced clinical practice in area of expertise
Education	Facilitates acquisition and application of clinical knowledge, theoretic knowledge, and decision-making skills by nurses, nursing students, and other health care providers	Contributes to nursing knowledge through scholarly publications and presentations on clinical topics and issues in critical care nursing
Consultation	Provides consultation to staff on patient care and family problems	Provides consultation on research regarding clinical and administrative issues
Research	Identifies researchable topics related to clinical practice	Encourages and guides development and conduct of research process; facilitates research utilization activities
Management	Participates in development, implementation, and evaluation of annual budget in areas relating to clinical practice	Evaluates clinical outcomes of nursing practices, resources utilization, and environmental conditions Contributes to financial integrity of department through identification and implementation of cost-effective practices, direct generation of revenue, or both

Data from American Association of Critical Care Nurses.[11]

physicians, staff nurses, and administrators. The CC-CNS evaluates responses of others to the CC-CNS's behaviors and then decides to continue, modify, or abandon those activities. The CC-CNS is given the responsibility and freedom to shape the role and make decisions regarding role development within the complex social structure of the organization. Responses of people to CC-CNS activities are based on their perception of how these activities influence what they view as important. For example, staff nurses' reactions to CC-CNS performance may be based on how CNS activities empower them to make practice changes they perceive as important in affecting patient outcomes. In contrast, hospital administrators' reactions to CC-CNS performance are more likely to be based on how the CC-CNS activities contain costs while improving the quality of care.

Criteria used in evaluating the CC-CNS role with this approach include behaviors such as (1) actively listening to the overt and covert meaning that staff convey to the CC-CNS during interactions, (2) adjusting approaches used to allay the anxiety of family members based on their verbal and nonverbal cues, and (3) selecting appropriate negotiation strategies for conflict resolution based on the importance of what is to be achieved as perceived by each individual.

Hamric Approach

The approach described by Hamric[8] for evaluation of CC-CNS performance is based on the structure, process, and outcome theory of patient[13] and nursing care[14] evaluation. Table 21–2 gives examples of performance criteria for the CC-CNS using this approach.

The structure component focuses on the system in which the CNS practices.[8,15] Variables such as organizational placement of the CNS, administrative support, staff mix, and physical structure of the critical care unit are examples of systems components that the CNS may include in job performance evaluation. For example, one system criterion the CNS could use for evaluation is determining how effective she or he is in impacting the skill mix of staff in a particular ICU to improve efficiency and quality of care while decreasing costs. Planning, implementing, and evaluating the effects of a special unit for chronically critically ill patients are a second example of a systems com-

TABLE 21–2 Examples of Performance Criteria for CC-CNS Based on Hamric Approach

---

Performance dimension: consultation
- Structure: develops mechanism to document and charge for consultation services
- Process: consults with staff nurses, physicians, and respiratory therapists at least weekly regarding respiratory management of patients with complex cardiovascular problems
- Outcome: decreases average length of ventilator days for postoperative open heart surgery patients

---

ponent that could be incorporated into CC-CNS evaluation.[15,16]

The process component of CC-CNS evaluation focuses on the effectiveness of the CNS in performing activities such as facilitation, coordination, consultation, education, change, assessment, evaluation, and implementation.[8,17] Evaluation focuses on the CC-CNS as a process expert, and traditionally most CNS job performance evaluations have relied heavily on these types of criteria.[18]

The outcome component of CC-CNS job performance is becoming increasingly important in light of economic constraints in health care. CNS performance appraisals have traditionally not relied heavily on outcome criteria, perhaps because they are the most challenging to demonstrate. Examples of patient outcomes[3,19,20] the CC-CNS may incorporate into performance appraisals (1) a 10% reduction in symptom intensity such as pain, dyspnea, or fatigue; (2) a 10% improvement in functional health status as measured by the 12-minute walking distance test; (3) a 24- to 48-hour decrease in length of ICU stay; (4) a 25% reduction in the number of diagnostic related group (DRG) outliers for a specific patient population; (5) a 20% reduction of readmission of the ICU within 48 hours after ICU discharge; and (6) a 25% reduction in iatrogenic injuries or incidences such as urinary tract infections or spontaneous self-extubations.

Nursing Administration Approach

Nurse executives and nurse managers are responsible for creating an organizational climate that provides quality, cost-effective care to patients and families. The skills of the CC-CNS are valuable assets for the nurse executives to capitalize on in creating a professional practice environment.[21] CNS attributes that promote such an environment include expertise in the change process, ability to influence others through expert knowledge and skill, flexibility, ability to critically analyze and problem solve, and ability to develop and implement new innovations that can revolutionize critical care practice. CC-CNSs who use this type of evaluation approach focus on productivity with great consideration for what activities support and enhance the effectiveness of their nurse executives or nurse managers. Their performance criteria incorporate administrative concepts such as autonomy, job satisfaction, organizational climate, work redesign, staff nurse competency, and staff turnover.

Examples of performance criteria for CC-CNSs who use this approach are (1) a 10% improvement in job satisfaction of nurses as measured by the McCloskey/Mueller Satisfaction Scale,[22] (2) a 20% increase in nurse autonomy as measured by the Schutzenhofer Autonomy Index,[23] (3) a 10% increase in newly CCRN-certified staff members per year, (4) in addition of four nurses with competence in a certain specialty such as care of patients with a mechanical assist device, (5) a 20% decrease in staff turnover, and (6) a 40-hour decrease in the length of time for orientation of new staff.

RESEARCH AND LITERATURE REVIEW

The research and literature on methods of CC-CNS evaluation encompass (1) competencies and CC-CNS evaluation, (2) who evaluates the CC-CNS, (3) the tools used for evaluation, and (4) cost effectiveness of the CC-CNS role. Subsequent sections describe each of these aspects as it relates to CC-CNS evaluation.

Competences and CC-CNS Evaluation

Competences of the CNS role have been described through research. Most of the research, however, has focused on competence development for the CNS role in general rather than the CNS in a specific specialty.

Using a qualitative approach, Fenton[24] found that competences of the CNS were similar to the seven domains of skilled performance that Benner[25] describes as expert practice domains. As outlined in Table 21–3, another domain, the consulting

TABLE 21-3 Additional Competences in Selected Domains and in Consulting Role

Domain	Competence
Monitoring and ensuring quality of health care practices	Recognition of generic recurring event or problem that requires policy change
Organizational and work role	Building and maintaining therapeutic team to provide optimal therapy: • Providing emotional and situational support for nursing staff Competences developed to cope with staff and organizational resistance to change: • Showing acceptance of staff persons who resist system change • Using formal research findings to initiate and facilitate system change • Using concurrent or mandated charge to facilitate other system changes Making bureaucracy respond to patient's and family's needs (massaging the system)
Consulting role	Providing patient care consultation to nursing staff through direct patient care intervention and follow-up Interpreting role of nursing in specific clinical patient care situations for nursing and other professional staff Providing patient advocacy by sensitizing staff to dilemmas faced by patients and families seeking health care

Described by Fenton[24] and Steele and Fenton.[26]

role, emerged and several competences were added to Benner's expert practice domains.[24,26]

Another study found that perceptions between CNSs and nurse administrators regarding competences were congruent for all role components except research.[27] Nurse administrators consistently ranked research as more important to CNS functioning than CNSs. Specifically, rankings of nurse administrators were significantly higher than those of CNSs for the following research activities: (1) identifying relevant clinical questions for systematic study, (2) planning nursing studies according to accepted research standards, (3) conducting research relating to nursing practice, and (4) communicating results of research through presentation and publication. Wyers et al.[28] surveyed nurse administrators, graduate nurse educators, and CNSs to determine perceived essential competency behaviors in the role of the CNS, differences in perceptions of essential competences, and what subroles make up the CNS role. Developing an in-depth knowledge base, demonstrating clinical expertise in a selected area of clinical practice, and serving as a role model were the three competences considered most important by all three groups. Groups did not differ significantly regarding any of the behaviors. Based on factor analysis, investigators grouped the competence behaviors into the subroles of practitioner, educator, consultant, and researcher. Manager and change agent activities were mixed throughout the subroles.

Ryan-Merritt and colleagues,[29] using the nominal group process, defined six functional role components of the CNS (director of care, collaborator, teacher, consultant, researcher, and manager) and articulated competency statements for each. These were used for evaluation of students enrolled in a graduate program that prepared advanced-practice nurses in several specialty tracks.

Competence statements for the CC-CNS published by AACN[11] provide a useful beginning for writing CNS performance criteria. These competence statements are further clarified by example behaviors for implementing each role component.[11] A behavior anchored rating scale (BARS), as described in a subsequent section of this chapter, can be written for each role implementation behavior to evaluate CNS job performance. Table 21–4 gives an example of how BARS and AACN competence statements regarding education can be used to develop CNS evaluation criteria.

Who Evaluates?

One of the challenges in CNS evaluation is determining who will evaluate the CNS.[5] Because CNSs interact with several types and levels of staff, evaluation is often done by nurse executives (immediate supervisors), peers, the CNS (self-evaluation), and/or other staff (nurse managers, staff nurses, physicians).

Nurse Executive

CNSs perceive that evaluation by nurse executives is adversely influenced by the nurse executive's misunderstanding of the CNS role.[5] It is the CC-CNS's responsibility therefore to educate nurse executives about the CC-CNS role and to be clear about the contributions the CC-CNS makes to the organization. Methods CC-CNSs can use to do this are to ask nurse executives to shadow them as they work in the CC-CNS role, to provide nurse executives with weekly summaries of their CC-CNS activities, and to delineate in writing how CC-CNS activities have contributed to containing costs.

Periodic evaluation by the nurse executive provides an opportunity for the CC-CNS to clearly articulate how time is managed and what effect CC-CNS activities have on nursing staff and patient outcomes. This type of review promotes interfacing goals of the CNS with administrative and overall organizational goals. Points the CC-CNS can address with the nurse executive include the following:

- How the CC-CNS has contributed to maintaining the fiscal viability of the critical care division
- What the CC-CNS does to promote a professional practice environment for staff
- Positive feedback from patients, staff, and others as evidenced by letters, recognition, and so on

Peer Review

Peer review is a second important method of CNS evaluation. It is the process by which people of the same rank, profession, and setting critically appraise each other's work performance using established criteria.[30,31] The goals of peer review are to foster increased professionalism, responsibility, and accountability and to provide open communication among peers to achieve short- and long-term goals.[32–34]

Challenges in using peer review include costs accrued with respect to professional time, threats

TABLE 21-4 Example of AACN CNS Competence Statements, Implementation Behaviors, and BARS

Competence statement: education

"The CNS assesses learning needs and designs, implements, and evaluates comprehensive teaching programs for specific patient populations, health care providers, and community groups to improve patient outcomes."[11,p.6]

Implementation behavior for CC-CNS as educator

"Seeks to improve patient and family outcomes through the application of educational concept and skills."[11,p.9]

BARS

Excellent	5	Promotes attendance of staff at local, regional, and national educational meetings. Assists staff in preparing presentations. Leads discussions of how new knowledge can be applied in practice. Uses innovative teaching strategies such as educational rounds, computer-assisted instruction, and interactive sessions with patients and staff. Receives excellent evaluations from staff regarding teaching methods. Receives excellent feedback on patient/family satisfaction survey regarding patient or family instruction. Presents local, regional, and national continuing education unit programs.
Good	4	Uses variety of teaching strategies in orientation of new staff and education of current staff. Uses variety of teaching methods with patients and families. Regularly discusses with staff how newly acquired knowledge and skills can be used in practice. Receives positive evaluations from staff regarding teaching methods. Frequently receives positive feedback on patient and family satisfaction survey regarding patient and family instruction. Frequently presents at local and regional meetings. Occasionally presents at national meetings.
Average	3	Participates in planning and implementing educational activities for new staff. Uses didactic instruction as major teaching strategy for patients, families, and staff. Sporadically discusses with staff how newly acquired knowledge and skills can be applied in practice. Receives fair to positive evaluations from staff on educational programs. Regularly receives positive feedback on patient and family satisfaction survey regarding patient and family instruction. Occasionally presents at local and regional meetings. Seldom presents at national meetings.
Poor	2	Seldom participates in education of staff, patients, or families. Receives fair to poor evaluations from staff on in-service and CEU programs. Seldom presents at local and regional meetings. Never presents at national meetings. Discusses with staff infrequently how new knowledge and skills can be used to influence practice.
Unacceptable	1	Does not participate in education of staff, patients, or families. Refrains from presenting at local and regional meetings. Generates complaints from staff regarding inability to teach staff, patients, and families.

to objectivity, limited socialization and expertise of nurses in the evaluation process, and absence of reliable and valid performance appraisal criteria.[32,35] Advantages of using peer review are that the evaluator understands the role and can observe the process and outcome of the CC-CNS in the practice setting.[5] The reviewer and reviewee learn from one another, promote personal and professional growth, and have the potential for increasing their job satisfaction.

Several prerequisites are needed for success in peer review. These include administrative support, a cohesive and trustful group, understanding and appreciation of each other's role, commitment to the process, and at least 1 year of experience in the role.[33] Evaluation tools must be based on the job description, reflect the CC-CNS competences, and incorporate realistic and attainable performance criteria.

Questions that can be incorporated into the peer review process are as follows:

- What CC-CNS activities have a positive influence on outcomes of critically ill patients?
- What are two programs that the CC-CNS participates in that promote improvements in clinical decision making of new staff?
- How has the CC-CNS provided consultation to peers on clinical and organizational issues?

Peer review can be implemented in several ways. For example, Blanton and colleagues[33] describe a mechanism in which several CC-CNSs review the various components of the role. The peer review is separate from the nurse executive's evaluation in order to keep the review more realistic and free of threats associated with monetary rewards. The CC-CNS being evaluated decides whether or not to include the peer review information in a self-evaluation. Subsequent submission of the information to the nurse executive is optional.

A second method of implementation is for all CC-CNSs to meet and complete the evaluation collectively following an independent evaluation. Recommendations are then documented on one evaluation form. This cumulative evaluation is given to the CC-CNS being reviewed, who discusses it with the reviewers.[31]

Evaluation by Other Staff

To gain an accurate perception of CC-CNS effectiveness, eliciting evaluative feedback from other staff such as staff nurses, patients, and other disciplines is helpful.[20,36] Eliciting this type of feedback requires that a questionnaire or form is available for people to rate the CC-CNS on specific performance criteria. For example, a standardized instrument to elicit staff input for evaluation of the CC-CNS educational role component includes statements such as "The CNS promotes an environment in which new staff are encouraged to ask questions." and "The CNS uses a variety of teaching strategies to facilitate understanding of critical care content by new staff." Staff members are then asked to rate their agreement or disagreement with each of the statements about the CC-CNS on a 1

(strongly agree) to 5 (strongly disagree) Likert scale. Semistructured, open-ended questions regarding key role components of the CC-CNS can also be used to elicit feedback from staff. Table 21–5 illustrates the type of questions that might be asked of staff nurses regarding CC-CNS performance.

Issues in eliciting feedback from other staff members are similar to those addressed in peer evaluation. These include providing for anonymity of responses, determining where the information is sent (CC-CNS, nurse executives, or both), and deciding how the information is incorporated into the final evaluation form. Options for resolution of these issues are (1) having the information synthesized by the CC-CNS and incorporated as part of self-evaluation, (2) having the information summarized by a third party and forwarded to the CC-CNS and nurse executive for inclusion in their evaluations, or (3) having the feedback forms sent to both the nurse executive and CC-CNS simultaneously.

Self-evaluation

Self-evaluation, yet another method of CC-CNS evaluation,[5] provides an opportunity for the CC-CNS to articulate what she or he does well and areas in need of improvement. Self-evaluation should be done at least annually even if it is not required by the organization. It stimulates the CC-CNS to reflect on areas for career advancement and assists in developing an action plan to move forward in one's career. Key questions the CC-CNS will find helpful in doing a self-evaluation are as follows:

- What have been my major process- and outcome-focused accomplishments over the past year?
- How have I constributed to the fiscal viability of the organization, division, or unit?
- Have I achieved my goals that I set last year? If not, why not?
- Have I accomplished any major projects that were not included in the goals of the previous year? If so, why did I do the project or projects?
- What is my most rewarding accomplishment over the past year?
- What is the one thing, if any, that I am most

TABLE 21–5 Questions to Staff Nurses Regarding CC-CNS Performance

I am interested in receiving your feedback regarding how I perform as a clinical nurse specialist. I appreciate your comments; thanks for taking the time to answer these questions.

Date _____
Unit _____
Highest degree earned _____
Basic nursing education _____

1. In what ways have I as a CC-CNS been helpful to you in your staff nurse role?

2. What could I be doing as a CC-CNS that I am not doing now?

3. What activities of the CC-CNS have helped in the following categories?
   Patient care:

   Staff development:

   Education:

   Research:

   Management:

   Other:

4. What do you think are the major strengths of the CC-CNS you work with?

5. Other comments:

Return via campus mail to C512 GH by _____

disappointed about in terms of my CC-CNS role? How could I change or improve this?
- What do I want to be doing 1 year from now? Three years from now? Five years from now? Am I making progress toward these goals?

Self-evaluation is done in several ways. CC-CNSs can use the organization's CNS evaluation tool and rate themselves regarding each performance criterion. CC-CNSs can document what they perceive as their major contributions in each of the role components or delineate the degree to which they have achieved the goals they set the previous year. CC-CNSs can summarize the feedback received from their peers and comment on how congruent or incongruent their own perceptions are with those of their peers.

Self-evaluation, although commonly used, should not be the only form of CC-CNS evaluation. A multifocal approach to evaluation is beneficial to the CC-CNS, administrator, and other staff.[5]

Tools for CNS Evaluation

A variety of tools have been published to use in evaluating CNS performance.[1,2,4,18,32,33,37–41] Many of these tools have face or content validity but little documented reliability.[37,38] Additionally, few are for evaluation of the CC-CNS specifically, but many could be modified using the AACN CC-CNS role definition and competence statements.[11]

There is no one right instrument to use in evaluating the CC-CNS. The tools used for evaluation are influenced by the type of organization in which the CC-CNS practices and the manner in which the role is actualized.

Performance appraisal tools usually consist of two basic parts: the performance criteria and the rating scale. The performance criteria are developed from the job description and may include structure, process, and outcome criteria. The criteria should be objective, measurable, and based on the job description and competences of the CC-CNS rather than personality traits.[1,38,42] For example, an organization may have a generic CNS job description that addresses the five functional components with behavioral criteria for each. The CC-CNS distills from that job description a particular focus based on an area of specialization. The specific behavioral criteria are then negotiated with the nurse executive.[5]

Rating scales[1,2,32,38,42] to standardize job performance evaluations include the BARS and the task-oriented performance evaluation system (TOPES). As illustrated in Table 21-6, BARS uses job-related behavioral examples for each performance criterion to illustrate every point on a 1 (unacceptable) to 5 (excellent) scale. In contrast, TOPES uses behavioral descriptors of task accomplishments for each point on the scale, and these descriptors are the same for each performance criterion (Table 21-7).

When using BARS, the key job elements or criteria are first identified, and descriptive statements are formulated to reflect "excellent" and "weak" performance of that criterion. The BARS approach requires a considerable investment of time and money and is an extensive process involving those who will be evaluated and those who will do the evaluation to formulate each of the descriptive statements. CNS evaluation tools that use the BARS approach are available in the literature.[1,2,37,39]

TOPES concentrates directly on tasks required in a job rather than behaviors related to those tasks. It is less complex than BARS because a single basic evaluation scale is used for each job in the organization; only the task elements or criteria of the job are changed for each type of job performance evaluation tool. In addition, varying importance of different tasks can be incorporated by assigning weights to each task. Weights of the tasks are then multiplied by the numeric value received for that task, and a composite score is achieved for the evaluation.[38,42]

Cost Effectiveness of CC-CNS Role

In many ways, effectiveness of the CC-CNS is difficult to measure in dollars and cents. Because the nature of the role is supportive, it is hard to

TABLE 21-6 Example of BARS Performance Evaluation

Performance dimension: research
Performance criteria: impacts patient care through application of research findings in practice

	Rating	Behavioral Example
Excellent	5	Promotes research utilization by self and others. Always reviews current research to determine if critical care practice policies and procedures are current and appropriate. Completes at least one research utilization project per year. Applies for research utilization grants.
Good	4	Teaches staff about research utilization. Leads staff in critiquing critical care research. Uses research in his/her own practice. Participates in research utilization efforts led by others.
Average	3	Keeps current on critical care nursing research. Distributes pertinent critical care research articles to clinical areas. Uses research findings in own practice.
Poor	2	Seldom reads critical care research. Disseminates research articles to staff only on requests. Does not base own practice on research.
Unacceptable	1	Is antagonistic toward research utilization. Blocks efforts of others who are implementing research-based practices. Generates complaints from staff regarding assistance in finding pertinent research articles.

TABLE 21-7 Example of TOPES Performance Evaluation

Performance dimension: research
Performance criteria: does one research utilization project per year

	Rating	Behavioral Example
Excellent	5	Is superior with little room for improvement. Is eligible for maximum rewards available.
Good	4	Performance is better than average CNS, but there is still room for improvement. Is eligible for moderate individual rewards.
Average	3	Meets basic requirements of task, but there is substantial room for improvement. Is eligible for systems but not individual rewards.
Weak	2	Performance is barely adequate or marginal. Substantial improvement is needed in quality or efficiency in achieving task. Is not eligible for any rewards.
Unacceptable	1	Fails to meet minimum standards; does not accomplish specified task. Immediate improvement is warranted. Failure to improve will subject employee to disciplinary action and eventual dismissal.

extrapolate the empiric benefit of many CC-CNS activities such as reducing patient or family anxiety and increasing staff knowledge and skill in hemodynamic monitoring. Although activities such as these can be quantified, the cost benefit is difficult to capture. Additionally, CC-CNS effectiveness is shaped by organizational structure, clinical specialty and experience of the CC-CNS, and the manner in which the role components are implemented.[43-45]

The unique contribution of the CC-CNS is derived from application of an advanced body of knowledge that is versatile and practice based. The burden, however, is on the CC-CNS to demonstrate the value of the role in terms of both improved patient outcomes and institutional revenue.[46,47] CC-CNSs can show that they contribute to provision of cost-effective quality care via case management for DRG outliers, retention and recruitment of nurses, establishing consultation services, reducing product costs, and developing new revenue sources.[20,46,48-55] Decreasing turnover, for example, saves costs associated with orientation, estimated at $5000 to $10,000 per staff member.[54,55]

Demonstrating cost effectiveness requires (1) agreement among CC-CNSs and nurse executives regarding what forms CC-CNS practice will take in the institution, (2) quantifying the components of practice, (3) demonstrating that practice affects patient outcomes and nursing behaviors, and (4) linking these differences to hospital costs.[15] Table 21-8 lists variables useful in demonstrating CNS

effectiveness. As part of evaluation, CNSs should first determine what data are routinely collected in their organization and identify how these data may be used in quantifying CNS effectiveness.

Finding reliable and valid instruments to measure patient outcomes or changes in nurse behaviors is a challenge CC-CNSs encounter when documenting effectiveness of the role. Resources to locate useful measurement tools include (1) texts that review and publish research instruments,[56-63] such as *Measurement of Nursing Outcomes,* vol 1, *Measuring Client Outcomes*[61]; (2) national computerized data bases such as the Health Instruments File; (3) local instrument data bases[64]; and (4) researchers in your local area who may be investigating a particular patient outcome such as functional health status. Although justifying the CNS role has received national attention, few studies have quantified cost effectiveness of the role.[19,65-70] These studies, however, in combination with other empiric evidence clearly demonstrate that effective implementation of the CNS role saves money and has a positive impact on patient outcomes.[20,48,49,71-78]

For example, Brooten and colleagues[65,66] demonstrated that very low birth weight infants could be discharged early without adverse consequences when followed by master's-prepared CNSs, resulting in a net savings of $18,500 per infant. The incidence of mechanical- and skill-related complications was significantly reduced in an ICU staffed by a CC-CNS as compared to a similar ICU without

TABLE 21–8 Variables to Use in Quantifying CNS Effectiveness

Direct	Indirect
COST	
Length of stay	Employee turnover
Complication rates	Staff satisfaction and
Nosocomial infection rates	productivity
	Product evaluation
Patient compliance	Recruitment of experienced nurses
24-hour readmissions to ICU	Overtime pay
Charge reimbursements	Absenteeism and staff injuries
Number of DRG outliers	
QUALITY	
Anxiety	Knowledge and skills of staff
Pain	
Skin breakdown	Clinical decision making
Ventilator days	Variance in critical path
Patient or family satisfaction	Documentation
	Collaboration
Complication and infection rates	Communication
Unit-specific quality improvement monitors	

Data from Papenhausen and Beecroft.[3]

a CNS.[67] CNSs contributed to positive patient outcomes by identifying high-risk situations and potential complications that were then followed by timely interventions to prevent adverse outcomes.[79] A nurse-managed unit for chronically critically ill persons at University Hospitals, Cleveland, incorporated services provided by CNSs that resulted in decreased use of laboratory and diagnostic tests, more transfers out of the facility, and increased patient satisfaction with care.[15,16] Job satisfaction of nurses increased, and collegiality among nurses and between nurses and physicians was enhanced. A CNS practicing in a spinal cord injury center resulted in (1) noted improvements in documentation of physiologic and psychologic problems, (2) twice as many referrals for counseling, and (3) a decrease in length of time between patient admissions and initiation of expected interventions.[19] Surveys of nurse executives and other health care professionals have shown that the CNS role is perceived as an important component of providing cost-effective quality care and that elimination of the position would decrease quality of care.[80,81]

PRACTICE IMPLICATIONS

Strategies to maximize CC-CNS evaluation focus on (1) choosing an appropriate framework and method for evaluation, (2) setting realistic goals that flow directly from the job description and CC-CNS competences, and (3) using forms that facilitate documentation of CC-CNS activities and effectiveness, thus providing an empiric base for CC-CNS evaluation.

Choosing a Framework and Method

No one framework or method of evaluation is perfect. Factors to consider when choosing a framework and method are (1) the CC-CNS's level of role development; (2) the nature of the CNS evaluation tool used in the organization, if any tools are available; and (3) who participates in the evaluation process: nurse executives, nurse managers, staff nurses, other CNSs, physicians, the CC-CNS being evaluated, or some combination thereof. Factors such as these are important considerations during the interview process and throughout the CC-CNS's employment in the organization.

In selecting an evaluation framework it is essential to note the role development of the CC-CNS in conjunction with the presence and nature of the CNS evaluation tool used in the organization. For example, if the CNS evaluation tool is organized by the functional components of clinical, management, education, research, and consultation, then the functionalist approach rather than the symbolic interactionist approach should be used for evaluation. If the organization does not have a tool for CNS evaluation, the CC-CNS has more flexibility in selecting an evaluation framework and must consider the values of the organization in the selection process. For example, the symbolic interactionist approach is more likely to work in an organization that values collaboration and consensus building. In contrast, the Hamric approach and nursing administration approach are essential frameworks to consider if the organization focuses on fiscal viability and revenue generation. The advantage of using both frameworks is the inclusion of outcome components (Hamric approach) and productivity components (nursing administration approach), which clearly delineate CNS contributions to the organization. Additionally, a first-year CC-CNS is more likely to select a functionalist approach and focus on competences of advanced practice and education to establish credibility with staff and to carve out a content and process area of expertise. In contrast, a fifth-year CC-CNS is more likely to have already established clinical credibility and therefore would include more competences related to conduct and utilization of nursing research. Likewise, a CC-CNS with 5 or more years of experience in the role, hired as the first CNS in the organization, is more likely to use the symbolic interactionist approach, in which the role can be shaped within the complex structure of the organization. She or he is not confined by the way previous CNSs have practiced in the organization and can adjust behaviors based on interpersonal interactions.

Deciding who will participate in evaluation is an early step in carrying out the CC-CNS evaluation process. This decision may be set by organizational policy if there is a long-standing history of the CNS role in the organization, or it may be up to the CC-CNS to make this decision. Ideally, combining self-evaluation with evaluations from peers, other staff, and the nurse executive provides an opportunity for the CC-CNS to synthesize information from several levels of the organization and use it to enhance the effectiveness of the role. However, if evaluations from peers and other staff are not provided to the CC-CNS but are sent directly to the nurse executive with a subsequent impact on monetary rewards, then a CNS, particularly one new to the role, is likely to be threatened by this process and be less than enthusiastic about eliciting input from staff at several levels in the organization.

Factors to consider when deciding who should participate in CC-CNS evaluation include the following:

- Who the CC-CNS works with directly and indirectly (staff nurses, other CNSs, nurse managers, physicians, and other health care personnel such as physical therapists, social workers, and respiratory therapists)
- Whose professional behavior the CC-CNS is most likely to influence as part of the role
- Who the CC-CNS is most likely to collaborate with in impacting patient outcomes

- Availability and objectivity of the forms to elicit staff feedback
- Availability of staff members to respond
- Unbiased methods of eliciting staff input
- Necessity of maintaining anonymity of those providing feedback
- Where the elicited information is sent
- What can be gained in respect to professional development for all involved
- How the inclusion or exclusion of certain information impacts monetary rewards

For example, a division-based CC-CNS incorporates feedback from physicians with whom she or he collaborates (e.g., medical director of the units), nurse managers and staff nurses of units that she or he serves, other critical care and non–critical care CNSs, and selected respiratory therapists who work on committees with the CC-CNS. Staff nurses' feedback is elicited by selecting a 10% random sample of nurses from all units with which the CC-CNS works, making certain there is proportional representation from all shifts.

The personnel providing feedback are then sent an open-ended questionnaire (Table 21–9) or the standard CNS evaluation form and asked to complete and return it to the CC-CNS by a designated date. The feedback is elicited every 6 to 12 months, depending on the organization's standardized time frame for evaluation. The CC-CNS incorporates the feedback into the self-evaluation report and attaches a cumulative report of the feedback to the self-evaluation. These materials are submitted to the nurse executive, who reads them and considers the information when completing the CNS evaluation report. The CC-CNS and nurse executive then meet to discuss the evaluation, which is subsequently signed by both parties. Goals for the coming year are negotiated and attached to the evaluation.

Goal Setting

A critical strategy to maximize the benefits of CC-CNS evaluation is goal setting. Selected goals must be clearly linked with the CC-CNS job description, CC-CNS competence statements, and role definition behaviors.[11] Each goal is accompanied by action steps, a time frame for carrying out each action step, specifications of who carries out each action step, and methods of evaluating

TABLE 21-9 Questions to Elicit Feedback from Physicians Regarding CNS Performance

I am eliciting feedback from nursing and medical staff regarding my performance as a CNS. I would appreciate your insights into how I perform in the role. Please take the time to answer the following questions and return the questionnaire in a campus envelope to C512 GH. Thank you.

1. In your perception, what CC-CNS activities contribute to improving the quality of patient care in this unit?

2. Does the CC-CNS collaborate regularly with medical staff in providing patient care?

3. Do you make referrals to the CC-CNS on a regular basis? If so, what for?

4. In your mind, how might the CC-CNS be better utilized in this unit?

5. What do you perceive as the strengths of the CC-CNS?

6. Other comments:

---

goal achievement. The CC-CNS must also define how each goal interfaces with the strategic plan of the department and organization.

How goals are developed and written is influenced by the framework selected for evaluation and the proportion of time devoted to each role component. Goal setting must be done in collaboration with nurse executives, nurse managers, staff nurses, and other personnel with whom the CC-CNS collaborates. Incongruencies among CC-CNSs and nurse executives regarding CC-CNS goals can result in perceived poor performance by the nurse executive.

Concrete criteria CC-CNSs can use to determine the appropriateness of goal setting and evaluation are as follows:

1. Each goal has outcomes or evaluation criteria and identified methods for measuring them.
2. One or two goals in each of the CC-CNS

role components are realistic for the CC-CNS's level of role development.
3. The frequency of measuring the outcome is articulated.
4. The people involved in achieving the goal are identified.[4]

Table 21-10 illustrates an example of goal setting and evaluation.

Documentation

Documentation of CC-CNS practice is essential to provide information for performance criteria. Time documentation,[82] workload documentation,[83] and productivity flow sheets are three examples of how the CC-CNS can document practice. Keeping a daily log of CC-CNS activities, making notes in appointment calendars, and dictating accomplishments on a weekly or daily basis are three additional methods of documentation.

How CC-CNS practice is documented is influenced by the framework chosen for CC-CNS evaluation. For example, a CC-CNS using the functionalist theory documents practice using forms such as caseload cards, consultation reports, and continuous quality improvement reports to provide empiric evidence for goal attainment within each of the functional role components. In contrast, a CC-CNS using the symbolic interactionist approach might use letters from patients and families, recognition letters, thank-you cards from peers, and liaison reports from the community or national committees to illustrate goal achievement.

Other forms and reports the CC-CNS can use as empiric evidence for goal attainment include the following:

- Documentation tools for CC-CNS activities
- Letters and evaluations from staff, peers, physicians, and other colleagues
- End-of-year reports
- Updated curriculum vitae
- Patient and staff education materials
- Representative samples of standards, protocols, and procedures
- Publications
- Grants submitted
- Grants funded
- Research utilization reports
- Completed research

TABLE 21–10 Goal Setting and Evaluation

Goal	Outcome	Measurement	Frequency	Personnel Involved
CLINICAL PRACTICE				
Identify and implement nursing interventions to decrease risk of iatrogenic injuries	Decreased incident rate Decreased complication rate Decreased length of stay Decrease in threatened or actual lawsuits	Risk management data Continuous quality improvement Trends in type and frequency of lawsuits	Quarterly	Unit staff Nurse manager CC-CNS Legal counsel
Serve as case manager for patients on ventilator more than 7 days	Decreased cost of care Decreased length of stay Improved success rate in mechanical ventilatory weaning	Cost data to determine average supply and personnel costs per patient; multiply times number of patients seen per year	Quarterly	Financial manager CC-CNS
EDUCATION				
Develop computer-assisted instruction for critical care orientation of new employees	Revenue generation Decreased length of orientation Staff competency	Number of programs sold per year multiplied by cost of program Salary of employee multiplied by number of hours saved Competency checklist	Yearly	Orientees CC-CNS Unit staff
RESEARCH				
Implement research-based practice protocols (e.g., suctioning; hemodynamic monitoring; saline flushes for heparin locks)	Cost savings related to decreased complications, nursing time, supplies	Continuous quality improvement Track supply and personnel costs	Quarterly	CC-CNS Nurse manager Financial manager
Write grant proposals	Direct income National exposure for institution Enhanced use of research in practice	Dollars and equipment secured Use of research-based interventions in practice	Yearly	CC-CNS Nurse researcher
CONSULTATION				
Consult with area hospitals on research utilization	Visit three hospitals per year	Consultation fees generated	Yearly	CC-CNS

TABLE 21–10 Goal Setting and Evaluation *Continued*

Goal	Outcome	Measurement	Frequency	Personnel Involved
CONSULTATION—cont'd				
Consult with patients and families regarding DNR decisions	Increased satisfaction of staff, patients, and families Decision-making support provided for patients and families	Patient and family satisfaction survey Number of consultations provided per year Job satisfaction survey of nurses	Quarterly	Patients Families CC-CNS Unit staff
MANAGEMENT				
Provide divisional supervision as needed	Dispersion of appropriate staff for patient care	Number of days worked as supervisor	Quarterly	Nurse managers
Serve as resource in development of shared governance model for critical care	Implementation of shared governance	Number of in-service programs and retreats provided for staff Number and type of documents written Number of meetings attended for development and implementation	Yearly	CC-CNS Nurse managers Unit staff

Data from Sparacino et al.[45]

- Listing of educational classes completed for professional development
- Certifications achieved by the CC-CNS
- Certifications achieved by staff with assistance of CC-CNS

Collectively, these documentation strategies provide a way to quantify CC-CNS effectiveness.

CASE STUDY

SJ is a CC-CNS in a 600-bed community hospital with 30 adult critical care beds. She has been in this position for 4 years, and for the past 3 years her immediate supervisor has done her evaluation using the standard hospital CNS evaluation form that reflects her job description. SJ wants to broaden her evaluation process to get input from staff nurses, peers, nurse managers, and physicians. She consults with her immediate supervisor who is supportive of SJ's eliciting such feedback.

SJ uses the questions in Tables 21–5 and 21–9 to elicit feedback from staff nurses and physicians, respectively. She selects 10 names of staff nurses from each of the units she works with—medical, coronary, and surgical intensive care units. To attempt to elicit unbiased results, the names are selected from a hat with the understanding that there will be at least three nurses from each shift for each unit. Names of physicians who regularly admit patients to each of the units are also drawn from a hat for a total of four physicians per unit. In addition, SJ asks Dr. Smith to complete a questionnaire, because he has been working with her and other nursing staff members on a respiratory failure critical path for the past several months.

To elicit nurse managers' feedback, SJ asks them to respond in writing to the following questions:

1. What activities of the CC-CNS have helped you in your role as a nurse manager?
2. What does the CC-CNS do to improve the quality of care in your unit?
3. What are the strengths that the CC-CNS brings to your unit?
4. What would you like to see the CC-CNS do differently?

SJ receives all the questionnaires and provides another CNS in the hospital with copies. This CNS colleague summarizes the responses and meets with SJ to discuss them. This provides SJ with a peer who can help interpret the feedback and identify strategies for strengthening her role performance. SJ also provides her immediate supervisor with the summarized copy provided by her CNS colleague.

SUMMARY

Evaluation is a process of obtaining information for the purpose of self-growth and impact on clinical practice. This chapter discusses the theoretic bases for CC-CNS evaluation and provides practical tools for CC-CNSs. A case example was provided that demonstrates suggested steps CC-CNSs can use in the evaluation process.

References

1. Davis DS et al: Evaluating advance practice nurses, *Nurs Management* 15(3):44-47, 1984.
2. Houston S, Luquire R: Measuring success: CNS performance appraisal, *Clin Nurse Specialist* 5(4):204-209, 1991.
3. Papenhausen JL, Beecroft PC: Communicating clinical nurse specialist effectiveness, *Clin Nurse Specialist* 4(1):1-2, 1990.
4. Malone BL: Evaluation of the clinical nurse specialist, *Am J Nurs* 86(6):1375-1377, 1986.
5. Morath JM: The clinical nurse specialist: evaluation issues, *Nurse Management* 19(3):72-80, 1988.
6. Calkin JD: A model for advanced nursing practice, *J Nurs Admin* 14(1):24-30, 1984.
7. Dubrey RJ: The leadership role of the clinical nursing specialist: a quality of life nursing model, *Nurs Management* 19(5):71-80, 1987.
8. Hamric AB: A model for CNS evaluation. In Hamric AB et al, editors: *The clinical nurse specialist in theory and practice,* ed. 2, Philadelphia, 1989, WB Saunders Co.
9. Metcalf J, Werner M, Richmond TS: The clinical specialist in a clinical career ladder, *Nurs Admin Q,* pp 9-19, Fall 1984.
10. Clayton GM: The clinical nurse specialist as leader, *Topics Clin Nurs,* pp 17-27, April 1984.
11. American Association of Critical Care Nurses: *Competence statements for critical care clinical nurse specialists,* Laguna Niguel, Calif, 1989, The Association.
12. Noble MA: The critical care clinical nurse specialist: need for hospital and community, *Clin Nurse Specialist* 2(1):30-33, 1988.
13. Donabedian A: Evaluating the quality of medical care, *Milbank Mem Fund Q* 44(2):166-206, 1966.
14. Bloch D: Evaluation of nursing care in terms of process and outcomes: issues in research and quality assurance, *Nurse Res* 24(3):256-263, 1975.
15. Daly BJ et al: Development of a special care unit for chronically critically ill, *Heart Lung* 20:45-51, Jan 1991.
16. Rudy EB: Nurse-managed special care units. In French E et al, editors: *Nursing recruitment and retention,* Laguna Niguel, Calif. 1990, American Association of Critical Care Nurses.
17. Hamric AB: Clinical nurse specialist role evaluation, *Oncol Nurs Forum* 12(2):62-73, 1985
18. Harris J, Gallien E: Psychiatric mental health nursing specialist process evaluation criteria, *Nurs Management* 23(2):54-58, 1992.
19. Ingersoll GL: Evaluating the impact of a clinical nurse specialist, *Clin Nurse Specialist* 2(3):150-155, 1988.
20. Tierney MJ, Grant LM, Mazique SI: Cost accountability and clinical nurse specialist evaluation, *Nurse Management* 21(5):26-31, 1990.
21. Fralic MF: Nursing's precious resource: the clinical nurse specialist, *J Nurs Admin* 18(2):5-6, 1988.
22. McCloskey JC, Mueller C: *McCloskey/Mueller Satisfaction Scale,* 1990. (Available from J.C. McCloskey, University of Iowa, College of Nursing, Iowa City, Iowa, 52240.)
23. Schutzenhofer KK: Measuring professional autonomy in nurses. In Strickland OL et al, editors: *Measurement of nursing outcomes,* vol 2. New York, 1988, Springer Publishing Co.
24. Fenton MV: Identifying competences of clinical nurse specialists, *J Nurs Admin* 15(12):31-37, 1985.
25. Benner P: From novice to expert, Reading, Mass, 1984, Addison-Wesley Publishing Co.
26. Steele S, Fenton MV: Expert practice of clinical nurse specialists, *Clin Nurse Specialist* 2(1):45-51, 1988.
27. Tarsitano BJ, Brophy EB, Snyder DJ: A demystification of the clinical nurse specialist role: perceptions of clinical nurse specialists and nurse administrators, *J Nurs Educ* 25(1):4-9, 1986.
28. Wyers MEA, Grove SK, Pastorino C: Clinical nurse specialist: in search of the right role, *Nurs Health Care* 6(2):203-207, 1985.
29. Ryan-Merritt MV, Mitchell CA, Pagel I: Clinical nurse specialist role definition and operationalization, *Clin Nurse Specialist* 2(3):132-137, 1988.
30. Mullins AC, Colavecchio RE, Tescher BE: Peer review: a model for professional accountability, *J Nurs Admin* 9(12):25-30, 1979.

31. O'Loughlin EL, Kaulbach D: Peer review: a perspective for performance appraisal, *J Nurs Admin* 11(9):22-24, 1981.
32. Ackerman N: Effective peer review, *Nurs Management* 22(8):48A-48D, 1991.
33. Blanton NE et al: Putting peer review into practice, *Am J Nurs* 85(11):1284-1287, 1985.
34. Winch AE: Peer support and peer review. In Hamric AB et al, editors: *The clinical nurse specialist in theory and practice,* ed 2, Philadelphia, 1989, WB Saunders Co.
35. Hickey M: Peer review: a process of socialization, *J Nurs Educ* 25(2):69-71, 1986.
36. Hamric AB, Grescham ML, Eccard M: Staff evaluation of clinical leaders, J Nurs Admin 8(1):18-26, 1978.
37. Bond ML, Jackson E: Maternal-infant clinical nurse specialist performance assessment: development of an evaluation tool, *Clin Nurse Specialist* 4(4):180-185, 1990.
38. Brief AP: Developing a usable performance appraisal system, *J Nurs Admin* 9(10):7-10, 1979.
39. Cason CL et al: Maternal-infant clinical nurse specialist performance assessment: reliability and validity of an evaluation tool, *Clin Nurse Specialist* 4(4):187-193, 1990.
40. Girourard S, Spross J: Evaluation of the CNS: using an evaluation tool. In Hamric AB, Spross JA, editors: *The CNS in theory and practice,* New York, 1983, Grune & Stratton.
41. Hill KM, Ellsworth-Wolk J, DeBlase R: Capturing the multiple contributions of the CNS role: A criterion-based evaluation tool, *Clin Nurse Specialist* 7(5):267-273, 1993.
42. Bushardt SC, Fowler AR: Performance evaluation alternatives, *J Nurs Admin* 18(10):40-44, 1988.
43. Lucas MD: Organizational management style and clinical nurse specialist's job satisfaction, *Clin Nurse Specialist* 2(2):70-76, 1988.
44. Sample SA: Justifying and structuring the CNS role within a nursing organization. In Hamric AB et al, editors: *The clinical nurse specialist in theory and practice,* ed 2, Philadelphia, 1989, WB Saunders Co.
45. Sparacino PSA, Cooper DM, Minarik PA: *The clinical nurse specialist: implementation and impact,* Norwalk, Conn, 1990, Appleton & Lange.
46. American Association of Critical Care Nurses CNS-SIG: *New strategies to measure CNS effectiveness,* Laguna Niguel, Calif, 1989, The Association.
47. Lipetzky PW: Cost analysis and the clinical nurse specialist, *Nurs Management* 21(8):25-28, 1990.
48. Ahrens T, Padwojski A: Economic impact of advanced clinicians, *Nurs Management* 19(6):64A-64D-F, 1988.
49. Cronin CJ, Maklebust J: Case-managed care: capitalizing on the CNS, *Nurs Management,* 20(3):38-47, 1989.
50. Goode CJ et al: A meta-analysis of effects of heparin flush and saline flush: quality and cost implications, *Nurs Res* 40(6):324-330, 1991.
51. Hoffman SE, Fonteyn ME: Third party reimbursement for CNS consultation, *Nurs Econ* 6(5):245-274, 1988.
52. Howard JC et al: Cost-related variables: a pilot study, *Clin Nurse Specialist* 3(1):37-40, 1989.
53. Papenhausen JL: Case management: a model of advanced practice, *Clin Nurse Specialist* 4(4):169-170, 1990.
54. Hinshaw AS, Smeltzer CH, Atwood JR: Innovative reten-

tion strategies for nursing staff, *J Nurs Admin* 17(6):8-16, 1987.
55. Wise LC: Tracking turnover, *Nurs Econ* 8(1):45-51, 1990.
56. Cook JD et al: *The experience of work,* London, 1989, Academic Press.
57. Frank-Stromberg M: *Instruments for clinical nursing research,* Norwalk, Conn, 1988, Appleton & Lange.
58. Price JL, Mueller CW: *Handbook of organizational measurement,* Cambridge, Mass, 1986, Ballinger Publishing Co.
59. Strickland OL, Waltz CF: *Measurement of nursing outcomes,* vol 2. *Measuring nurse performance,* New York, 1988, Springer.
60. Strickland OL, Waltz CF: *Measurement of nursing outcomes,* vol 4. *Measuring client self-care and coping skills,* New York, 1988, Springer.
61. Waltz CF, Strickland OL: *Measurement of nursing outcomes,* vol 1. *Measuring client outcomes,* New York, 1988, Springer.
62. Waltz CF, Strickland OL: *Measurement of nursing outcomes,* vol 3. *Measuring clinical skills and professional development in education and practice,* New York, 1988, Springer.
63. Ward F: *Instruments for use in nursing education research,* Boulder, Col, 1979, WICH.
64. Clougherty J et al: Creating a resource database for nursing service administration, *Computers Nursing* 9(2):69-74, 1991.
65. Brooten D et al: Early discharge and specialist transitional care, *Image* 20(2):64-68, 1988.
66. Brooten D et al: A randomized clinical trial of early hospital discharge and home follow-up of very-low-birth-weight infants, *N Engl J Med* 15(15):934-939, 1986.
67. Goodnough SK, Bines A, Schneider W: The effect of clinical nursing expertise on patient outcome, *Crit Care Med* 14(4):358, 1986.
68. Litvak S et al: Early discharge of the postmastectomy patient: unbundling of the hospital service to improve patient profitability under DRGs, *Am J Surg* 229:577-579, 1987.
69. Naylor MD: Comprehensive discharge planning for hospitalized elderly: a pilot study, *Nurs Res* 39(3):156-161, 1990.
70. Neidlinger SH, Scroggins K, Kennedy LM: Cost evaluation of discharge planning for hospitalized elderly, *Nurs Econ* 5(5):225-230, 1987.
71. Fagin CM: The economic value of nursing research, *Am J Nurs* 82(12):1844-1849, 1982.
72. Fagin CM: Nursing's value proves itself, *Am J Nurs* 90(10):17-30, 1990.
73. Jacox A: The OTA report: a policy analysis, *Nurs Outlook* 35(6):262-267, 1987.
74. Kirkland SC, Tinsley D: CNS: special skill really contains costs, *Nurs Management* 21(9):97-98, 1990.
75. McGrath S: The cost-effectiveness of nurse practitioners, *Nurse Pract* 15(7):40-42, 1990.
76. National Commission on Nursing Implementation Project (NCNIP): *Features of high quality, cost-effective nursing care delivery systems of the future,* Milwaukee, 1988, The Commission.
77. Sweet JB: The cost-effectiveness of nurse practitioners, *Nurs Econ* 4(4):190-193, 1986.

78. Weinberg RM, Liljestrand JS, Moore S: Inpatient management by a nurse practitioner: effectiveness in a rehabilitation setting, *Arch Phys Med Rehabil* 64:588-590, 1983.

79. Gurka AM: Process and outcome components of clinical nurse specialist consultation, *Dimensions Crit Care Nurs* 10(3):169-175, 1991.

80. Sisson R: Co-worker's perceptions of the clinical nurse specialist role, *Clin Nurse Specialist* 1(1):13-17, 1987.

81. Walker ML: How nursing service administrators view clinical nurse specialists, *Nurs Management* 17(3):52-54, 1986.

82. Robichaud A, Hamric AB: Time documentation of clinical nurse specialist activities, *J Nurs Admin* 16(1):31-36, 1986.

83. Nevidjon B, Warren B: Documenting the activities of the oncology clinical nurse specialist, *Oncol Nurs Forum* 11(3):54-55, 1984.

Chapter 22

Issues and Future Trends for the Critical Care Clinical Nurse Specialist

Patricia S. A. Sparacino, RN, MS, FAAN

Since the first master's degree program was designed specifically for clinical nurse specialists (CNSs) by Peplau in 1954, development of the role has responded to the vast increase in clinical specialty knowledge, rapid development of patient care technology, and public need. Although the CNS role traditionally was used in acute care and tertiary care settings, more recently it is seen in a variety of practice settings and specialty areas. The role has grown from DeWitt's concept of the specialist nurse responding to the need for perfection within a limited domain[1] to the clearly defined and widely accepted role that it is today. The CNS role is multifaceted, with specialty boundaries defined by the knowledge and skill of the practitioner, organizational needs, and changing societal needs.[2,3]

The American Nurses' Association's (ANA's) support of and commitment to the development of the CNS role was clearly illustrated by creation of its Council of Clinical Nurse Specialists in 1982. Among its many functions, the council was a repository of documents and information about the role, and in 1986 the council published a CNS role statement.[3] The role statement describes four dimensions of the CNS role: clinician, educator, consultant, and researcher. It emphasizes the requirement for the CNS to have a patient-based practice and discusses factors influencing role implementation. One intended effect of the role statement was for specialty nursing organizations to use it as a framework on which to build specialty-specific statements. The American Association of Critical

Care Nurses (AACN) accomplished this with the role definition contained in *Competence Statements for Critical Care Clinical Nurse Specialists*.[4]

After the publication and acceptance of the ANA role statement, several other circumstances began to further clarify CNS role development. The issues confronting CNSs have been as follows:

- The identification of a core body of knowledge for CNS practice
- The use of the core body of knowledge as a basis for a standard graduate core curriculum
- Practice standards
- Credentialing at the advanced-practice level

In an effort to explore commonalities with other advanced nursing practice roles, discussions were held in the mid 1980s between groups of CNSs and nurse practitioners. These discussions focused on role similarities and differences[5] and addressed the concept of singular titling. In 1991 the ANA's Council of Clinical Nurse Specialists and Council of Primary Health Care Nurse Practitioners voted to merge, becoming the Council of Nurses in Advanced Practice. The benefit of the merger has been the power of combined effort: health care policy, legislative and reimbursement issues, and standards for education and practice are issues for all nurses in advanced practice.

The CNS role has never been, nor ever will be, static. The role is recognized as a magnet to recruit and retain highly committed professional nurses. Research on the role has begun to demonstrate a

293

positive impact on patient care outcomes while reducing the cost of health care delivery.[6-9] The CNS will continue to respond to changes in health care. Although the role is undergoing evolution, its core purposes must not change: (1) to provide advanced nursing practice to the population the CNS serves; (2) to apply new knowledge based on research, concepts, and theories to improve patient care; and (3) to integrate the areas of expert practice, education, consultation, research, and clinical leadership for the purpose of improved patient care. Now the responsibilities and activities of the CNS are shifting and broadening. The CNS is expected to be both a process expert (an expert in change, conflict management, nursing process application, and empowerment) and a content expert (an expert in the specialty area of practice, research-based practice, nursing diagnoses, and legal or ethical implications). The dilemma, then, for the CNS is to respond to these demands while struggling to remain within a patient-focused practice.

This chapter discusses the many historical and current factors that have influenced the CNS role, including role definition, educational preparation, practice standards, credentialing, and the merging of advanced nursing practice philosophies. Research related to the role will be reviewed, from its emphasis on role definition and implementation of the past to its present documentation of role impact. Practice implications will be addressed, especially as they relate to how CNSs must develop in order to keep pace with rapid changes in the health care environment. The challenge now for all CNSs is to maintain the integrity yet flexibility of the CNS role components while influencing organizational change. The chapter will discuss opportunities for the CNS's preferred future, especially in the areas of standards for an advanced core curriculum, advanced practice, advanced credentialing, health care policy development, and legislative reform. There is little in the literature on how these issues will affect the critical care CNS (CC-CNS). Therefore in this discussion, exemplars of how they may impact the CC-CNS are given.

THEORETIC FRAMEWORK

We must not hold nursing in today's standard; we must lift it and ourselves to tomorrow's possibilities . . . We must transcend the past; we must transcend ourselves.

Margretta M. Styles

Research on CNS Role Evaluation

From 1970 to 1978 most of the research related to the CNS role focused on the role itself,[10-14] its implementation,[15-17] and the effect of the role on practice characteristics of the generalist nurse.[18-22] No research at this time was specific to the CC-CNS role. Articles on the CC-CNS role were primarily case examples.[23,24]

Since 1978 advanced-practice nursing has been the subject of numerous studies. Benner et al.[25,26] have extensively analyzed nurse progression from beginner to expert, using the Dreyfus model of skill acquisition[27] as a framework. Benner et al. have described how the experienced nurse incorporates subtle knowledge into practice. Experience, however, is only one requirement for CNS expertise. The nurse who is an expert by experience has knowledge that is embedded in clinical practice and will operate on intuition but may not necessarily know how to justify a feeling or action. This does not mean that the expert nurse never uses an analytic approach to problem solving; however, what distinguish the CNS from the nurse who is an expert by experience are the depth and breadth of the theoretic foundation of knowledge, combined with advanced clinical judgment and clinical expertise.[28-31]

Other researchers have chosen to study this role by surveying the administrative view and co-workers' perceptions of CNS contributions. Walker[32] surveyed nursing service administrators to categorize perceptions of role effectiveness and factors related to utilization. Although the results of the questionnaire were limited by a geographically distinct population, the majority of nursing service administrators surveyed were using CNSs and were satisfied with the role, its impact on patient care quality, and the resulting cost effectiveness. Tarsitano et al.[33] found that perceptions between CNSs and nurse administrators regarding competencies were congruent for all role components except research. Nurse administrators placed a higher value on research than CNSs. Whereas the clinical practice and education role components were highly valued by both groups, the consultative component received the highest rating of all role functions.

Building on surveys of nurse administrators, Sisson[34] interviewed three groups of consumers at one university hospital: managers, staff nurses, and physicians. This assortment of health care workers perceived the two most discernable CNS role components were staff and patient educator and staff resource person. Whereas a majority of those interviewed felt that CNSs had a positive impact and were cost effective, the components that were identified as needing more attention were direct patient care and availability to staff members and patients. The ultimate balancing act is integrating and juggling the priorities of the five role components. A pilot study and follow-up study 2 years later by a group at Richland Memorial Hospital in Columbia, South Carolina,[35] tested the assumption that the roles of clinician, educator, and scholar could be successfully merged, as the literature on the CNS role had described. The investigators also wished to assess the merit and significance of the role. Their findings revealed that while the institution's prototype CNS spends a majority of time in clinical practice, the role components of clinician, consultant, educator, and researcher can be successfully implemented by one individual. The study concluded that there are implied cost savings in hiring CNSs, since so much is achieved by one individual.

Cason and Beck[36] surveyed CNSs, students, administrators, and faculty members regarding perceptions of the role and important role functions. Dimensions of the role found to be important by these groups were clinical knowledge and skills, problem-solving skills, ability to promote self-care, and ability to collaborate. CNSs and nurse administrators in this study were in greater agreement than CNSs and master's program faculty regarding role perceptions. Fenton[37] interviewed and observed 30 master's-prepared CNSs from all clinical areas who identified the following major role competencies: team building and maintenance, emotional support for the team, facilitation of organizational change, quality of care monitoring, consultation, and promotion of bureaucratic responsiveness to patient needs. Fenton concluded that CNSs function as advanced practitioners and that a part of their value is the ability to influence health care delivery by working through others.

From the research on perceptions of the CNS role, several observations can be made. In all studies the CNS was highly valued; however, different people value the role for different reasons. There are differing perceptions by individuals working with CNSs on what the role priorities should be. Some individuals found the consultative CNS role component the most important, whereas co-workers in another study valued direct patient care and responsiveness to staff needs. Others have identified specific behaviors desirable in the CNS such as collaboration and an ability to promote self-care. The challenges inherent in the CNS role are the multiple demands and expectations from patients, families, other health care providers, and the practice setting. The key element of success for the CNS role is flexibility.

Effects of CNS on Patient Care Outcomes

More essential to today's compelling needs in the health care environment has been the research on the effect of CNS interventions on patient care outcomes and cost of care. As early as 1967, Little and Carnevali[38] explored the variations in tuberculosis patients' responses to illness when patient-centered care was given by a psychiatric CNS. They measured specific variables' impact on improvement in radiologic and bacteriologic results, length of hospital stay, involvement in self-care, and deviant behaviors. The outcomes did not correlate with the patient-centered care, which may be explained by the fact that the CNS's area of expertise was psychiatric rather than pulmonary. In 1971 Pozen et al.[39] concluded that their experimental group, treated by a CNS, improved in most areas of recovery from myocardial infarction (MI). MI patients who received an educational and counseling intervention by the CNS returned to work sooner and at a higher frequency than control group patients. In addition, more of the experimental group either stopped or reduced smoking. In a more recent study, Burgess et al.[40] also studied the impact of CNS interventions on outcomes of MI patients. Psychosocial interventions by the CNS resulted in reduced psychologic distress at 3 months after discharge. The ability of the CNS to reduce psychologic distress may be a factor in MI patients' early return to work.

More recently, several significant studies have underscored the impact of the CNS on both patient care outcomes and the resultant cost savings. Brooten et al.[41] conducted a randomized, controlled clinical trial that used master's-prepared CNSs to provide continuity between the hospital and home to allow for earlier discharge of very low birth weight infants. The experimental group received instruction, counseling, home visits, and daily on-call availability of a hospital-based CNS for 18 months. The control group received routine care, instruction, and physician follow-up. The study demonstrated no difference between the early discharge experimental group and the control group in the number of rehospitalizations or acute care visits or in the measures of physical and mental growth. Thus the interventions by master's-prepared CNSs made an impact on the clinical outcomes of the very low birth weight infants, and the resulting net savings was $18,560 per infant for the early discharge group. A study by Neidlinger et al.[6] demonstrated that when a gerontologic CNS spent an average of 80 minutes per elder in comprehensive discharge planning with the experimental group, the length of stay was shorter and recidivism was reduced. Although limited by the single site of study and only 1 month of data collection, the study demonstrated a positive impact on patient care outcomes and cost savings of $35,000 generated by the experimental group in the 30-day study. Naylor's pilot study of comprehensive discharge planning for hospitalized elderly persons[9] built on the discharge planning protocol developed by Kennedy et al.,[42] and it refined Brooten's discharge planning strategies. Although the discharge planning process implemented by a gerontologic CNS did not significantly influence initial length of hospital stay or posthospital infections, there was a statistically significant difference in the fewer number of subjects rehospitalized. Russell[8] conducted a retrospective study comparing length of hospitalization and in-patient costs of patients undergoing a modified radical mastectomy. The patients who received intensive preoperative and postoperative counseling and instructions by a CNS working in collaboration with a surgical oncologist had a shorter hospital stay and lower hospital costs than the patients cared for by unit personnel under the guidance of an operating surgeon.

These studies have extended beyond historically more limited approaches, such as the effect of an intervention on hospital length of stay. By involving the CNS in preoperative and postoperative patient guidance and integrating discharge planning early in the hospital stay with data collected before

hospital discharge, such results as patient outcomes after discharge, the intervention effects on quality of care manifested in patient outcomes, and the cost of care have more value to both health care providers and policymakers.[7] The CNS has the ability to directly influence patient care delivery and the use and availability of health care resources. In this era of health care accountability, further research is needed to explain variations in patient outcomes attributable to the CNS. Although measuring outcomes in nursing is challenging,[43] a CC-CNS can examine a number of role-related outcomes: patient complications (such as dermal ulcers), patient length of stay in critical care, patient's or family's knowledge, staff assessment skills, staff competencies (e.g., response to an arrest situation), staff problem-solving skills (i.e., troubleshooting equipment failures), and resolution of nursing diagnoses. Through further outcome research, the CNS can demonstrate to health care professionals and the consumer how this role makes a difference in health care quality and cost.

Resource Allocation

The allocation of scarce health care resources is a dilemma of concern to all health care workers. For the CC-CNS the problems of effectiveness and cost containment within the critical care environment must be addressed. Critical care technology has advanced, yet there is only empiric evidence that the expanded capabilities of critical care units have actually improved patients' survival. Only a very small portion of hospitalized patients require critical care, but providing critical care consumes 15% of the hospital-directed health care dollar. Often severity of illness does not reflect the level of care required. The scope of case mix as well as the substantial differences in levels of intensive care, numbers of interventions used, and resources consumed confounds analysis of critical care outcomes.[44]

What is both clear and alarming is that the cost of critical care is neither logical nor predictable. Although a classification system (e.g., Acute Physiology and Chronic Health Evaluation [APACHE]) can reliably estimate the relationship between severity of illness and probability of death from diseases commonly treated in critical care units, the actual differences in the structure, process, and effectiveness of critical care are significantly influenced by the interaction and coordination of the unit physicians and nurses.[45] AACN endorses multidisciplinary health care teams, not as much from a proscriptive perspective but for the purpose of identifying criteria for decision making.[46] To achieve reforms that will provide available as well as affordable health care, certain changes will have to be made: better assessment of the medical efficacy and cost effectiveness of new technologies, agreement on the scope of standard medical practice through the development of practice guidelines and medical protocols, constraint on the amount of resources used, increased efficiency of resource delivery, and directives that will guide the matching of facility and health care provider supply to consumer need.[44,47]

Technology can mean medical equipment and devices, procedures, operative interventions, or drugs. The advantages of the technologic explosion have been nurses' increased autonomy as a result of objective criteria on which to make clinical judgments (e.g., titration of medications based on hemodynamic indices) and the autonomy to intervene (e.g., cardiac defibrillation).[48] With this new technology comes the responsibility for evaluation of its efficiency and impact. The CC-CNS is the ideal nurse to assess new technology. Technology assessment can encompass many dimensions: fiscal impact (purchase cost, efficacy, and the cost to educate staff in the use of new technology), environmental impact (allocation of space, storage, and noise impact), necessity (cost efficiency, usefulness of sophisticated technology), quality (expected performance, validity, and reliability of measures), patient response (benefits vs. undesired effects), and ease of use.

In an attempt to assist practicing clinicians to address these issues, the Society of Critical Care Medicine (SCCM) appointed a task force, The Technology Assessment Task Force, to develop a generic template that may be used to formulate practice policies for critical care technology.[49] This template, consisting of seven questions (Table 22–1), was recently applied to pulse oximetry. The task force reviewed research and manufacturers' literature on pulse oximetry and came up with the guidelines in Table 22–2. This type of assessment can be done by the CC-CNS to improve patient safety and reduce costs of care.

With the increasing responsibility for proficient

TABLE 22–1 Template for Technology Assessment

1. What is the basic science underlying the technology?
2. What are the indications for its use claimed by the manufacturers?
3. What are the common secondary indications claimed by frequent users?
4. Does the technology provide the basic function claimed by the manufacturer; by the frequent user? What are the efficacy data available to support its use?
5. Are there any appropriate impact data available? Data to consider include survival, morbidity, length of stay, benefits, and complications.
6. What are the costs of using the technology, including initial capital outlay, ongoing operating costs, labor impact, resource requirements, and indirect costs, such as special hospital space or program displacement? How is the total cost of patient care affected?
7. Should there be any special user requirements, such as knowledge base or experience, for safe and effective use of the technology?

From the Technology Assessment Task Force of the Society of Critical Care Medicine: A model for technology assessment applied to pulse oximetry, *Crit Care Med* 21(4):616, 1993. © Williams & Wilkins, 1993.

operation of technology, it becomes more challenging to provide humanistic patient care. The CC-CNS can serve as a role model for giving humanistic care by promoting open visiting for families, including families in the physical care of patients, teaching and using therapeutic touch, and giving patients more control over their care. The CC-CNS can also increase staff time available for patient care by decreasing the time spent on troubleshooting equipment by ensuring that staff members are thoroughly educated in its proper use.

Standards for CNS Role

Although the CNS role is well established within nursing, the premises of what comprises advanced practice are not. Health care is now in an era of accountability, and therefore it becomes important for nurses in all roles to articulate their value to the consumer. Four interrelated issues for advanced-practice nurses today are graduate preparation, standards for advanced practice, certification, and licensure.

TABLE 22-2 Guidelines for Use of Pulse Oximetry

1. All patients who require mechanical support of ventilation for an acute process or who have a critical airway (defined as an airway, artificial or natural, in a patient with physical and/or pharmacologic factors that might compromise its integrity) should be continuously monitored by pulse oximetry. This monitoring should be maintained during the transport of these patients.
2. During diagnostic procedures that may induce airway compromise or hypoxia, such as bronchoscopy, upper and lower gastrointestinal endoscopy, cardiac catheterization including bedside right heart catheterization, lumbar puncture or liver, and kidney biopsy.
3. Patients receiving supplemental oxygen should be monitored by intermittent measurement of oxygen saturation with the frequency of measurement based on the clinical status of the patient. Some of these patients would benefit from continuous monitoring of oxygen saturation.
4. Patients who require a tracheostomy and long-term mechanical support of ventilation for stable, chronic respiratory failure should be monitored by intermittent measurement of oxygen saturation with the frequency of measurement determined by the clinical status of the patient.
5. Pulse oximetry should not be used to monitor or diagnose in the following circumstances:
   Cardiopulmonary resuscitation
   Hyperoxia in newborns
   Hypovolemia
   The fine tuning of ventilatory (as opposed to oxygen) support

From The Technology Assessment Task Force of the Society of Critical Care Medicine: A model for technology assessment applied to pulse oximetry, *Crit Care Med* 21(4):623, 1993. © Williams & Wilkins, 1993.

Before standards for graduate preparation or advanced practice or criteria for credentialing can be appropriately developed, the nursing profession must identify a core body of knowledge for the nurse in advanced practice. An initial product of this effort is a working definition of advanced practice:

Nurses in advanced clinical nursing practice have a graduate degree in nursing. They conduct comprehensive health assessments, demonstrate a high level of autonomy and expert skill in the diagnosis and treatment of complex responses of individuals, families and communities to actual or potential health problems. They formulate clinical decisions to manage acute and chronic illness and promote wellness. Nurses in advanced practice integrate education, research, management, leadership, and consultation into their clinical role. They function in collegial relationships with nursing peers, physicians, professionals and others who influence the health environment.[50]

The significance of this working definition is that it clearly states that educational preparation requires a graduate degree in *nursing* and that the functional role components must be *integrated* into the clinical role.

Graduate Preparation

Periodic attempts have been made over the years to homogenize graduate preparation of nurses in general, with no concerted effort to standardize the graduate programs for CNS in particular. General as well as specific recommendations for curriculum content[51-53] have been extensive. The list of suggestions for general CNS and CC-CNS content includes the following:

1. Theories
   a. Organizational theories and strategies
   b. Nursing theory foundation
   c. Teaching-learning theory
   d. Change theory
   e. Role and role development theory
   f. Consultation theory
   g. Counseling theory
   h. Crisis intervention theory
   i. Stress and coping theory
2. Science
   a. Physiology and pathophysiology
   b. Pharmacology
   c. Biochemistry
   d. Immunology
   e. Genetics
   f. Physics
   g. Computer science
   h. Psychology
3. Skills
   a. Communication
   b. Group process
   c. Leadership and management
   d. Debate and negotiation
   e. Conflict resolution

f. Acquiring information through technology
g. Problem solving
4. Clinical practice
   a. Health assessment
   b. Clinical practicums for advanced skill development and refinement
   c. Residency for practicing change implementation, managing a patient caseload, and integrating clinical skills and judgment with consultation, education, and leadership skills
   d. Use of new technology
   e. Dealing with families in crisis
5. Research
   a. Analysis of research for application to practice
   b. Clinical investigations of nursing problems
   c. Collaborative practice-based research
6. Other
   a. Ethics
   b. Legislative issues
   c. Economic concepts
   d. Legal concepts

Although there has been agreement that content which represents the role components should be included in graduate preparation, there has been little agreement about the balance between teaching actual skills vs. a professionalization process that prepares the learner to continue to learn, nor has there been consistency among graduate curriculums in either program content or expected outcomes. In addition, some CNS programs do not have faculty members with practice experience as a CNS. It is unsettling that there appear to be as many ways of preparing a CNS as there are graduate nursing programs.

A core curriculum standard is needed to move advanced-practice nursing into the future. The process of developing such a standard would not be easy, because it would require consensus between CNSs who know what knowledge and skills are used in the practice setting, nursing administrators who have performance expectations for CNSs, and educators who must have the resources and teach the content within the customary 24-month time frame. However, the advantage of a core curriculum would be a base of knowledge common to all CNS graduates. Built on this core curriculum would be the area of subspecialization: the narrowing of focus on phenomena subsets, content and clinical practicums specific to a selected specialty (e.g., critical care), and content and a clinical residency specific to the specialty within a practice setting. A working model based on the cardiovascular CNS is given in Figure 22–1.

Once a core curriculum framework becomes uniform, there is a common basis for both a standard of advanced practice and a standard for certification, particularly at the advanced-practice level. This is an opportunity for a task force of experienced CC-CNSs to develop a graduate education standard that focuses on the unique knowledge needs of this group.

Advanced-Practice Standards

Advanced practice is the result not only of graduate education in nursing but also of the clinical expertise that is derived from learning by experience. Benner et al.[25] describe the learning process as the trajectory from the beginner who uses learned procedures and realizes success through completed tasks, to the competent nurse whose practice is guided by complex theoretic understandings and sophisticated goals, to the proficient nurse who can recognize the nuances and subtleties of a situation, to ultimately the expert who recognizes a clinical pattern, can manage a rapidly changing situation, and is responsible to and advocates for the patient and family. However, Benner's seven domains of skilled practice[26] need to be expanded to include competencies more reflective of the range of CNS responsibilities, as described in Chapter 3.

The standard of practice outlined by the professional nursing organization (the ANA) or a specialty nursing organization can be a template from which to develop a standard for each nursing or clinical specialty. Ideally the standard of practice would be developed collaboratively by both. The ANA has developed standards of practice for many specialty areas that focus on specialty knowledge rather than educational requirements but has not developed standards for advanced practice. The specialty organizations that to date have developed *advanced*-practice standards are the AACN, the Oncology Nursing Society, and the Emergency Nurses' Association. The CNS can use these prac-

A Core Curriculum for the Advanced Practice Nurse

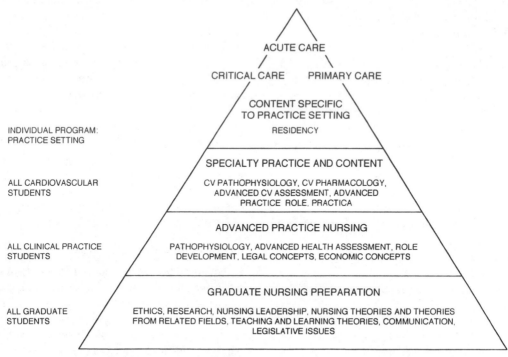

Figure 22-1 Core curriculum for the advanced-practice nurse.

tice standards to (1) develop the role, (2) guide daily practice, (3) standardize practice, (4) assist in professional development, and (5) develop a role evaluation process.

Certification

Certification is usually a voluntary process that demonstrates specialized knowledge and competence in an area of nursing practice. Its primary purpose is for consumer information, whether the consumer is the employer, the payer, or the patient. It is not a substitute for entry-level competence.[54] However, despite valiant efforts on the part of many persons, standards for certification continue to be inconsistent. This issue is of particular concern for the CNS, because certification may reflect only specialty content knowledge, rather than integrative process skills required of an advanced-practice nurse.

Many factors have challenged attempts to achieve professional conformity. Attempts to achieve uniformity confront the proliferation of specialties, a low correlation between graduate pro-

grams in nursing and certified practice specialties, the absence of uniform standards for specialties, the inability of nursing specialty organizations to agree to standards, and a lack of overall professional coordination.[55] As a result, more than 30 organizations offer certification,[56] but there are almost no standards for specific educational programs, degrees, or amount of practice experience required. Certification therefore provides limited guarantees to the consumer at this time.

In 1991 the American Nurses' Credentialing Center (ANCC) completed an administrative transition from an internal unit of the ANA to subsidiary status of the ANA. The ANCC offers certification for CNSs (adult psychiatric–mental health, child/adolescent psychiatric–mental health, gerontologic, medical-surgical, and community health) and nurse practitioners (gerontologic, pediatric, school, adult, and family). In 1992 the certification examination for CNSs and nurse practitioners was changed to reflect that both require graduate education and advanced practice. The credential earned is that of certified specialist; individuals previously certified as nurse practitioners are now identified as certified specialists.

In 1988 the Committee for the National Board of Nursing Specialties (NBNS), funded by the Macy Foundation, was formed to establish minimum standards for all certification programs.[57] In 1991 the American Board of Nursing Specialties (ABNS) evolved from the NBNS project. Eight charter organizations representing more than 120,000 certified nurses joined together in common purpose to ensure quality in specialty nursing and consistent standards of education and experience necessary to practice and to develop national standards for certification programs.

The ABNS addresses complex demands of the health care system by reviewing and approving nursing specialty certification boards. A certification board approved by the ABNS has met the highest standards established by a peer group. However, this body has not been supported by all nurse-certifying organizations; two of the reasons have been the disagreement over whether a baccalaureate in nursing is a criterion for certification and the argument that if credentialing were placed under the auspices of the ABNS, it would confuse the delineation between the distinct responsibilities of the professional specialty organizations and certifying organizations.[58]

The challenge that remains is to step beyond specialty certification for the expert nurse by experience and to address certification of advanced-practice nurses, specifically CNSs and nurse practitioners. CNSs need to remain informed and involved with these issues.

Licensure of Advanced-Practice Nurses

In an attempt to move individual states to achieve some consistency in regulatory language and activities pertaining to advanced nursing practice, the National Council of State Boards of Nursing (NCSBN) released in 1992 a position paper and a draft of model legislation recommending licensure of nurses in advanced practice. The position paper was the result of a 1991 survey that underscored the extensive variability of state requirements for advanced nursing practice, including education and certification requirements, competence requirements, physicians collaboration, and prescriptive authority.[59] This proposed second license is contrary to ANA's long-held position of supporting the least restrictive regulatory policy, based on the profession's responsibility to self-regulate through certification and professional peer review.

In response to the NCSBN proposal, the ANA Board of Directors convened an Ad Hoc Committee on Credentialing in Advanced Practice. After numerous hearings with representatives from state nurses' associations and specialty nursing organizations and the review of numerous reports and testimonies, the Ad Hoc Committee met in November 1992. In its report to the ANA Board of Directors, the committee recommended a definition for the nurse in advanced specialty practice, acknowledgment by statute of professional standards and certification, adoption of guidelines and recommendations for state nurses' associations and state licensing authorities for the development of state regulations, and support of the development and dissemination of model legislative language. Specifically related to the credentialing process, the Ad Hoc Committee recommended that state boards of nursing use the ABNS's *Reviewer Guidelines for Assessing Applications for ABNS Approval* to determine which professional certifications are accepted.[60]

PRACTICE IMPLICATIONS

Our system of health care delivery is changing rapidly. The CNS must focus on keeping pace with the rapid changes, strengthening the expert clinician component of the role, and improving the balance among and use of the role component responsibilities while influencing organizational change.

Current Issues

Current issues facing nursing can serve as a foundation for looking to the future[62]:

1. Practice patterns
   a. Patient acuity is increasing, with a rise in critical care unit mortality.
   b. The typical critical care unit patient is either premature or elderly.
   c. Physician demand for nursing expertise in general and for the CNS in particular is increasing.
   d. Nursing practice is becoming more research based.

e. Federal guidelines are influencing care and decision making.

f. There will be a refocus on the role of clinical practice to provide more effective service to patients and staff.

g. The geographic and specialty-specific nursing shortages require a rethinking of skill mix in the critical care unit.

h. Nursing care delivery is focusing on more cost-effective methods, but nurses are being challenged to maintain quality and ensure the professional practice model.

2. Ethical influence on direction of care
   a. The increase in patient acuity is resulting in an increase in ethical dilemmas.
   b. Traditional values are being challenged.
   c. Nurses are actively participating in ethical decisions.
   d. The patient's advance directive has stimulated discussion about the distinction between beneficence and autonomy.

3. Health care policy development
   a. Nurses are becoming more involved in health policy decisions, stimulated by a belief in individual rights and a respect for human dignity.

4. Influence of technology
   a. Advance-practice nurses are using humane principles to influence an appropriate balance in technology development.
   b. Use of advanced technology is expanding outside the critical care unit to home care.
   c. The power of medical technology is competing with the power of human values.

5. Health care resources
   a. We are witnessing the beginning of rationing of health care resources.
   b. Patients and families are beginning to take an active role in controlling the use of lifesaving technology.

Impact on CC-CNS Role: The Future

Current developments will influence the CC-CNS role of the future. How will these trends impact each role component? What prospects does the future hold?

Clinician

With the increasing emphasis on the CC-CNS becoming an organizational change agent, there is concern about what will happen to the traditional emphasis on patient care and patient-focused practice. What is the risk of the CC-CNS abdicating certain performance expectations? Who will assume responsibility for those relinquished responsibilities? When multiple requests compete with the CC-CNS's commitment to a patient-based practice, how will the CC-CNS maintain clinical expertise?

Case management, as discussed in Chapter 6, is one example of nursing's response to a health care dilemma of fragmented accountability for continuity of care and cost containment. Case management has focused on interdisciplinary collaboration as well as documentation of nursing's impact on patient care delivery and outcomes. The ideal patient population for case management is high-risk patients with complex and costly health care needs. Whereas case management has often developed where there was a shortage of nursing personnel and neither a CC-CNS nor a clinical ladder,[61] the CC-CNS has been recognized as the preferred case manager. The master's-prepared CC-CNS has the educational preparation and clinical expertise to effect system change and manage the goals of coordination of services and resources, involve the patient as an active participant, control costs, and improve quality of care.

Although the case management model does not recommend that nursing be responsible for monitoring physician practice and the business management of the hospital, it does provide an opportunity to quantify the specific responsibility and impact of nursing on patient outcomes. Although the CC-CNS is best suited for the case manager role, is this concept merely a new fad and another example of the profession's quest for what is quantifiable for nursing? Is case management a new delivery system that does not look at what service is actually being provided? Is case management really a new concept, or is it a contemporary term for the original intent of the CNS's patient care focus: to positively affect patient care and systems outcomes?[62]

Nurses in advanced practice may be encountering new spheres of impact and influence. In December 1992 the ANA and American Association of Nurse Anesthetists provided testimony before the Physician Payment Review Commission. The testimony was notable for one exception; namely, the draft paper "Financing Graduate Medical Education: Options for Reform" did not specifically mention CNSs as potential providers of hospital services. The testimony also made several recommendations for meeting hospital service needs if hospital residencies are reduced. Suggestions relevant to advanced-practice nurses included the following:

1. The use of advanced-practice nurses if residencies are to be decreased
2. The acknowledgment of advanced-practice nurses as either economic complements or economic substitutes for physicians in teaching hospitals
3. The use of "split care," in which the advanced-practice nurse manages patient care in consultation with physicians in hospitals, long-term care facilities, and primary care[63]

The use of advanced-practice nurses as physician substitutes is not a new idea; nurse practitioners have been doing it since 1968. The nurse in advanced practice is able to perform the necessary health assessments and interventions, make diagnoses, and prescribe, while retaining the nursing focus of providing health promotion guidelines, teaching about health status, and lending a completeness to the care process. The challenge for this role, however, will be to maintain a nursing focus without resorting to a medical model practice framework.

Consultant

With the rapidly changing configuration of health care delivery, the CC-CNS as a process expert will be an organizational systems consultant, called on to create change within the practice environment. This has advantages and disadvantages. To influence change the CC-CNS must be non-judgmental, be visible, and know how to collaborate. As shifts in power occur within the practice setting as well as the health care system, the CC-CNS will need political skills for negotiation and change.

As physician time becomes more limited (with higher patient volume to compensate for lower reimbursement), there will be a trend toward physician delegation of medical tasks to nurses. A current example is the trend for nurses to pull femoral sheaths after heart catheterization. Assuming that the nurse can pull the sheath with the same skill

and safety of a physician, one questions who will pay for the nurse's time to perform this new procedure. Is this time accounted for in the staffing patterns and unit budget (for which the hospital pays), is the nurse expected to work this procedure into an already hectic schedule without staffing compensation (for which the nurse pays), or should part of the reimbursement for the cardiac catheterization be appropriated to the hospital to cover the nurse's time and expertise (for which the patient pays)? The CC-CNS of the future will increasingly be involved in such decisions and will need to be particularly adept at negotiation and problem solving.

Increasingly, health care insurers are looking to quality indicators as they contract with hospitals for services. The savvy CC-CNS, in consultation with marketing personnel, can orchestrate cost-cutting programs and provide an informative package on quality and cost control measures to give the institution a competitive edge. Whereas past political strategy has used traditional paternalistic methods, newer models for political action will increase nurses' power and political involvement.[64]

Educator

With the need for expert and comprehensive knowledge stimulated by advanced technology and patient care, the CC-CNS will focus on further development of the proficient and expert nurse, delegating new employee orientation to senior staff members. Educational programs directed not only to the staff nurse as caregiver but also to the charge nurse as manager will increase staff independence and collaborative decision making to ensure quality patient care.[45] Increasingly the CC-CNS will be challenged on how to maintain staff competencies given the rapid increase in technology, the decrease in educational funding available, and the constantly changing staff. As CC-CNS time focuses more on system changes, there will be less time to allocate to more demands. CC-CNSs will begin to rely on other creative educational means, such as satellite video conferences, to keep staff informed.

Researcher

The research role of the CC-CNS is to assist nursing staff in answering clinical practice questions with research-based knowledge. With the increasing demand to document the impact of nursing and advanced nursing practice on patient care process and outcomes, the CC-CNS will continue to implement research utilization and will increase the level of involvement in practice-based research. Nursing interventions used by the CC-CNS are less likely to be embedded in practice convention and more likely to be the result of critical thinking applying theoretically based knowledge to diverse clinical situations. The researcher component of the role currently focuses on the advanced thinking demonstrated in clinical judgment, incorporating physiologic and psychologic variables into expert clinical practice, and the application of new knowledge to the improvement of nursing care. The next crucial step must be the CC-CNS's participation in the generation of clinically based knowledge, especially clinical outcomes research.

Research is an element of the CC-CNS role with significant cost impact. The ultimate foundation for the CC-CNS's commitment to and involvement in research must be an inner need to solve clinical problems. Research must be a commitment; the excitement for research will not thrive if it is a requirement. In spite of variations in extrinsic performance standards, administrative support, or a CC-CNS's academic preparation, strategies exist by which the CC-CNS can participate in research.

At the very least the CC-CNS can foster the spirit of inquiry by questioning the foundation of clinical procedures and nursing practice, as well as by incorporating findings into clinical practice. However, collaborative research and secondary data analysis make research feasible. Collaborative research bridges the real or perceived gap between clinical practice and academia to improve patient care delivery. Effective collaboration merges ideas from people with different perspectives. The reality is that the nurse researcher's expertise is theory and research methodology, whereas the CC-CNS's expertise is identification of clinical problems that need to be researched. The nurse researcher has access to resources, and the CC-CNS has access to patients. In successful collaborative research, each coinvestigator's viewpoints and concerns are incorporated into the collaborative project. The disadvantages of collaborative research are few: differences in ownership, authorship, accountability, commitment, and time allocation.

Another feasible approach to research is secondary data analysis, or the examination of data previously gathered for other research. The advantage of secondary data analysis is that it bypasses time-consuming data collection and permits reinspection and rethinking of data. The disadvantages are that the data must be on a computer file, the original researcher must be available, and the variables used must be those that the original investigator collected.[65]

Research-based advanced practice is an integral part of the AACN philosophy and goal. In 1991 the AACN convened 50 critical care nurse experts to determine research priorities. The identified topics were categorized into two areas: clinical practice and the context within which critical care nursing takes place. Of the topics identified within the context of the practice setting, two were resource allocation and ethical issues.

Clinical Leadership

With the external as well as internal demands being placed on the organizational structure of practice settings, the CC-CNS will increasingly provide the link between the provider and recipient of health care. The CC-CNS has the ability to facilitate concurrent change, maintaining the patient-focused practice as a primary target. Through the use of research findings, extensive literature reviews, and the ability to tolerate chaos and maintain hope, the CC-CNS initiates and provides concrete strategies for systems change and gives validity to the change.[66]

In this era of cost containment the CC-CNS can play a vital role. Instead of using a reactive cost-benefit approach to evaluate or justify a CC-CNS's position,[67] a proactive approach will be more effective. The CC-CNS must play an active role in reducing product costs, increasing hospital revenue, and examining other cost-related factors resulting from quality care.

National Issues

A variety of issues will also influence the future development of the CC-CNS role at both the institutional and national levels. Despite the fact that CC-CNSs and other categories of advanced-practice nurses have proven repeatedly to provide high-quality and cost-effective care with measurable outcomes, there are still legislative restrictions on scope of practice, perscriptive authority, and eligibility for reimbursement. Part of this problem is self-afflicted in that the multiplicity of roles and titles for advanced nurses ". . . resemble[s] the rubble of the Tower of Babel."[68] This confusion is especially problematic when attempting to achieve national uniformity and legislative recognition. Of particular concern to CC-CNSs is that the nurse practitioner title is more widely recognized; only in 1992 did the Health Care Financing Administration temporarily change their definition of CNS to better reflect practice characteristics and to make CNSs eligible for Medicare reimbursement.

The legal scope of practice is defined by health regulatory boards. However, a comparison of individual state regulatory language reveals restrictive and contradictory terminology. One problem is the lack of distinction between the advanced-practice nurse and the registered nurse. Those states with the fewest barriers to practice are regulated by a board of nursing. Those states with the most barriers to practice have either joint regulatory boards or a state legislature that gives limited statutory authority to the board of nursing.

Currently 43 states give nurse practitioners prescriptive authority, but there is wide disparity in the degree of autonomy. Of the 43 states, 22 give nurse practitioners independent authority. Those states are notable for (1) a board of nursing as the final authorization for administering the prescriptive authority, (2) prescriptive authority without a physician's signature, and (3) prescribing being considered within the nurse's scope of practice.[69] Since most of the current health care policy debate focuses on access to care, discussion has focused on nurse practitioners who provide primary care rather than on the broader range of advanced practice nurses. Nonetheless, the Drug Enforcement Agency's proposed rule to permit registration of mid-level practitioners, including advanced-practice nurses, would allow a new group to prescribe controlled substances, consistent with state-granted authority.[70]

The struggle to achieve direct reimbursement for advanced nursing practice is an important one for the CNS, because it will give the provider recognition and visibility, recognize advanced-practice nurses as independent health care practitioners, place a value on the service provided, improve data on the service and research of costs and outcomes, and increase the advanced-practice nurse's autonomy and authority.[71] Currently advanced-practice nurses are eligible, in varying degrees, for some federal, state, and private payer reimbursement. Federal reimbursement depends on the type of advanced-practice nurse, the health care setting, and the payment level. To date, nursing home care and rural care are the only direct reimbursement provisions. Forty-two states have enabling rules and regulations for Medicaid reimbursement to specified advanced-practice nurses, most often nurse practitioners. States provide variable percentages of reimbursement, from 100% to 60%. Private payer reimbursement differs from state to state, with the approach and compliance varying and often depending on the state's regulatory language.[69] The CC-CNS must continue to keep abreast of state and national legislation and actively participate in lobbying and voting on issues affecting CC-CNS reimbursement.

CONCLUSION

Challenges confront the CC-CNS. The challenges are also opportunities to shape the CC-CNS's preferred future.

We face internal challenges. The CC-CNS role is sometimes no better understood by CC-CNSs than by those with whom we collaborate: physicians, consumers, educators, administrators, and legislators. The definition of advanced practice is used by some to describe both the nurse who is an expert by experience and the CC-CNS. We have not helped this confusion by our multiplicity of titles. The internal changes needed are a standard for a core curriculum, to provide a common basis for advanced practice; a standard for advanced practice, to delineate CC-CNS competencies; and a standard for advanced certification, without which advanced-practice credentials will not be recognized or reimbursed. We also need clarification of the intent and purpose of the role so that the scope of advanced practice and its influence can be expanded.

In addition, we face external challenges. Interstate inconsistency exists in regulation of advanced nursing practice, including definition, titling, standards, recognition of certification, prescriptive authority, and compliance with federal reimbursement mandates. Safriet[68] concludes that the three most significant barriers to effective advanced nursing practice are (1) restrictive and contradictory definitions of scope of practice that prevent services, (2) restrictions on prescriptive authority that must accompany the expanded scope of practice, and (3) few avenues for reimbursement for the services provided by an expanded scope of practice. The barriers are in statutes and regulations; the barriers can be removed by legislative reform. Current federal legislative activity gives CC-CNSs a prime opportunity to influence reform. To facilitate this process, however, there must be a single statutory designation, a single title. This would provide symmetry to states' statutes and to federal policymakers.[67]

What does the future hold for every CNS, regardless of specialty or practice setting? It holds challenges and exciting opportunities. We must concur on the issues and goals, and, although we may be uncertain of the outcomes, together we must pursue those goals relentlessly.

Acknowledgment

I would like to thank Pamela Minarik, RN, MS, FAAN, who provided invaluable expertise in editing the manuscript.

References

1. DeWitt K: Specialties in nursing, *Am J Nurs* 1:14-17, 1900.
2. American Nurses' Association: *Nursing: a social policy statement,* Kansas City, Mo, 1980, The Association.
3. American Nurses' Association: *The role of the clinical nurse specialist,* Kansas City, Mo, 1986, The Association.
4. American Association of Critical Care Nurses: *AACN competence statements for the critical care clinical nurse specialist,* Newport Beach, Calif, 1989, The Association.
5. Sparacino PSA, Durand BA: Specialization in advanced nursing practice, *Momentum* 4(2):2-3, 1986 (editorial).
6. Neidlinger S, Kennedy L, Scroggins K: Effective and cost efficient discharge planning for hospitalized elders, *Nurs Economics* 5:225-230, 1987.
7. Brooten D et al: Early discharge and specialist transitional care, *Image* 20:64-68, 1988.
8. Russell LC: Cost containment of modified radical mastectomy: the impact of the clinical nurse specialist, *Ethicon* 26(3):18-19, 1989.
9. Naylor MD: Comprehensive discharge planning for hospitalized elderly: a pilot study, *Nurs Res* 39:156-161, 1990.
10. Baker C, Kramer M: To define or not to define: the role of the clinical specialist, *Nurs Forum* 9(1):41-55, 1970.
11. Barrett J: Administrative factors in development of new nursing practice roles, *J Nurs Admin* 1(4):25-29, 1971.
12. Aradine C, Deynes MJ: Activities and pressures of clinical nurse specialists, *Nurs Res* 21:411-418, 1972.
13. Shaefer J: The satisfied clinical: administrative support makes the difference, *J Nurs Admin* 3(4):17-20, 1983.
14. Davidson KR et al: A descriptive study of the attitudes of psychiatrists toward the new role of the nurse therapist, *J Psychiatr Nurs Mental Health Services* 16(11):24-28, 1978.
15. Boucher R: *Similarities and differences in the perception of the role of the clinical specialist,* vol 1, Kansas City, Mo, 1972, American Nurses' Association.
16. Bruce S: *Valuation of functions of the role of the clinical nursing specialist,* vol 2, Kansas City, Mo, 1972, American Nurses' Association.
17. Smith M: Perceptions of head nurses, clinical nurse specialists, nursing educators, and nursing office personnel regarding performance of selected nursing activities, *Nurs Res* 23:505-511, 1974.
18. Georgopoulos B, Christman L: The clinical nurse specialist: a role model, *Am J Nurs* 70:1030-1039, 1970.
19. Georgopoulos G, Jackson M: Nursing kardex behavior in an experimental study of patient units with and without clinical nurse specialists, *Nurs Res* 19:196-218, 1970.
20. Georgopoulos G, Sana J: Clinical nursing specialization and intershift report behaviour, *Am J Nurs* 71:538-545, 1971.
21. Ayers R et al: *The clinical nurse specialist: an experiment in role effectiveness and role development,* Duarte, Calif, 1971, City of Hope National Medical Center.
22. Girouard S: The role of the clinical nurse specialist as change agent: an experiment in preoperative teaching, *Intern J Nurs Studies* 15(2):57-65, 1978.
23. Yokes JA: The clinical nurse specialist in cardiovascular nursing, *Am J Nurs* 66:2667-2670, 1966.
24. Zschoche D, Brown LE: Intensive care nursing: specialism, junior doctoring or just nursing? *Am J Nurs* 69:2370-2374, 1969.
25. Benner P, Tanner C, Chesla C: From beginner to expert: gaining a differentiated clinical world in critical care nursing, *Adv Nurs Sci* 14(3):13-28, 1992.
26. Benner P: *From novice to expert,* Menlo Park, Calif, 1984, Addison-Wesley.
27. Dreyfus SE, Dreyfus HL: *A five-stage model of the mental activities involved in directed skill acquisition.* Unpublished report supported by the Air Force Office of Scientific Research (AFSC), USAF (Contract F49620-79-C-0063), University of California, Berkeley, Feb 1980.
28. Kitzman HJ: The CNS and the nurse practitioner. In Hamric AB, Spross JA, editors: *The clinical nurse specialist in theory and practice,* Philadelphia, 1989, WB Saunders Co.
29. Spross JA, Baggerly J: Models of advanced nursing practice. In Hamric AB, Spross JA, editors: *The clinical nurse specialist in theory and practice,* Philadelphia, 1989, WB Saunders Co.
30. Murphy SA, Hoeffer B: Role of the specialties in nursing science, *Adv Nurs Sci* 5(4):31-39, 1983.
31. Pridham KF: Why clinical field study? *Nurs Outlook* 38(1):26-30, 1990.
32. Walker ML: How nursing service administrators view clinical nurse specialists, *Nurs Management* 17(3):52-54, 1986.
33. Tarsitano BJ, Brophy EB, Snyder DJ: A demystification of the CNS role: perceptions of CNSs and nurse administrators, *J Nurs Educ* 25(4):4-9, 1986.

34. Sisson R: Co-workers' perceptions of the clinical nurse specialist role, *Clin Nurs Specialist* 1:13-17, 1987.
35. Boyd NJ et al: The merit and significance of clinical nurse specialists, *J Nurs Admin* 21(9):35-43, 1991.
36. Cason CL, Beck CM: CNS role development, *Nurs Health Care* 3(1):35-38, 1982.
37. Fenton MV: Identifying competencies of clinical nurse specialists, *J Nurs Admin* 15(12):31-37, 1985.
38. Little D, Carnevali D: Nurse specialist effect on tuberculosis, *Nurs Res* 16(4):321-326, 1967.
39. Pozen MW et al: A nurse rehabilitator's impact on patients with myocardial infarction, *Med Care* 15:830-837, 1977.
40. Burgess AW et al: A randomized controlled trial of cardiac rehabilitation, *Soc Sci Med* 24(4):359-370, 1987.
41. Brooten D et al: A randomized clinical trial of early hospital discharge and home follow-up of very-low-birth-weight infants, *N Engl J Med* 315(15):934-939, 1986.
42. Kennedy L, Neidlinger S, Scroggins K: Effective comprehensive discharge planning for hospitalized elderly, *Gerontologist* 27:577-580, 1987.
43. U.S. Department of Health and Human Services: *Proceedings of a conference sponsored by the National Center for Nursing Research. Patient outcomes research: examining the effectiveness of nursing practice.* NIH Pub. No. 93-3411, Washington, DC, 1992, The Department.
44. Birnbaum ML: Cost-containment in critical care, *Crit Care Med* 14:1068-1077, 1986.
45. Knaus WA et al: An evaluation of outcome from intensive care in major medical centers, *Ann Int Med* 104:410-418, 1986.
46. Reigle J: Resource allocation decisions in critical care nursing, *Nurs Clin North Am* 24:1009-1015, 1989.
47. Schramm CJ: Health care financing for all Americans, *JAMA* 265:3296-3299, 1991.
48. Marsden C: Technology assessment in critical care, *Heart Lung* 20:93-94, 1991.
49. The Technology Assessment Task Force of the Society of Critical Care Medicine: A model for technology assessment applied to pulse oximetry, *Crit Care Med* 21(4):615-624, 1993.
50. McLoughlin S: Congress of Nursing Practice meets, *Am Nurse* 18:23, March 1992.
51. Lewis ER: The purposes and characteristics of master's education. In National League for Nursing: *Developing the functional role in master's education in nursing (NLN #15-1840),* New York, 1980, The League.
52. McCormick K: Preparing nurses for the technological future, *Nurs Health Care* 4:379-382, 1983.
53. Sparacino PSA: A historical perspective on the development of the clinical nurse specialist role. In Sparacino PSA, Cooper DM, Minarik PA, editors: *The clinical nurse specialist: implementation and impact,* Norwalk, Conn, 1990. Appleton & Lange.
54. Kennerly SM: Imperatives for the future of critical care nursing, *Focus Crit Care* 17:123-127, 1990.
55. Styles MM: Bridging the gap between competence and excellence, *ANNA J* 18:353-360, 366, 1991.
56. Hartshorn JC: A national board for nursing certification, *Nurs Outlook* 39:226-229, 1991.
57. Parker J: Envisioning a national board of nursing specialties: an interview with Jeanette Hartshorn, *ANNA J* 17:217-223, 1990.
58. American Association of Critical Care Nurses: Certification corporation unable to support proposed national certification board. *CCRN News,* Spring 1991.
59. National Council of State Boards of Nursing: *Postion paper on the licensure of advanced practice nursing,* Chicago, May 18, 1992, NCSBN Subcommittee to Study the Regulation of Advanced Nursing Practice.
60. American Board of Nursing Specialties: *Reviewer guidelines for assessing applications for ABNS approval.*
61. Zander K: Nursing case management: resolving the DRG paradox, *Nurs Clin North Am* 23:503-520, 1988.
62. Sparacino PSA: The CNS-case manager relationship, *Clin Nurs Specialist* 5:180-181, 1991.
63. Keane A: *Testimony of the American Nurses Association, American Association of Nurse Anesthetists before the Physician Payment Review Commission,* Washington, DC, Dec 9, 1992.
64. Mason DJ, Backer BA, Georges CA: Toward a feminist model for the political empowerment of nurses, *Image,* 23:72-77, 1991.
65. Herron DG: Secondary analysis: research method for the clinical nurse specialist, *Clin Nurse Specialist* 3:66-69, 1989.
66. Fenton MV: Education for the advanced practice of clinical nurse specialists, *Oncol Nurs Forum* 19(suppl):16-20, 1992.
67. Lipetzky PW: Cost analysis and the clinical nurse specialist, *Nurs Management* 21(8):25, 28, 1990.
68. Safriet BJ: Health care dollars and regulatory sense: the role of advanced practice nursing, *Yale J Regulation* 9:417-488, 1992.
69. Pearson LJ: 1992-93 update: how each state stands on legislative issues affecting advanced nursing practice, *Nurse Practitioner* 18:23-28, 1993.
70. Minarik PA: Federal action on prescriptive authority, *Clin Nurse Specialist* 7:46, 1993.
71. Mittelstadt PC: Federal reimbursement of advanced practice nurses' services empowers the profession, *Nurse Practitioner* 18:43, 47-48, 1993.

Index

Note: Page numbers in *italics* refer to illustrations; page numbers followed by t refer to tables.